MYOCARDIAL INFARCTION

electrocardiographic differential diagnosis

MYOCARDIAL INFARCTION

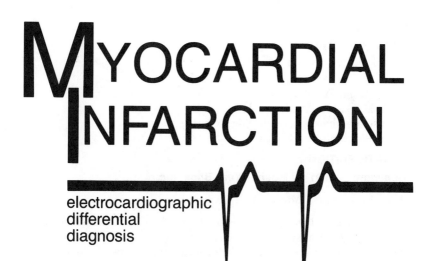

electrocardiographic
differential
diagnosis

ARY L. GOLDBERGER, M.D.
Associate Professor of Medicine,
Harvard Medical School;
Director of Electrocardiography Laboratory,
Beth Israel Hospital,
Boston, Massachusetts

FOURTH EDITION

with 210 *illustrations*

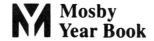
Mosby
Year Book

St. Louis   Baltimore   Boston   Chicago   London   Philadelphia   Sydney   Toronto

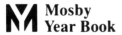 **Mosby**
Year Book

Dedicated to Publishing Excellence

Editor: Nancy Megley
Editorial assistant: Anthony Alves
Manuscript editor: George B. Stericker, Jr.
Production: Kathleen L. Teal

FOURTH EDITION

Mosby–Year Book, Inc.
11830 Westline Industrial Drive, St. Louis, Missouri 63146

Library of Congress Cataloging in Publication Data

Goldberger, Ary Louis, 1949-
    Myocardial infarction: electrocardiographic differential
diagnosis/Ary Goldberger,—4th ed.
        p.   cm.
    Includes bibliographical references.
    Includes index.
    ISBN 0-8016-6080-7
    1. Heart—Infarction—Diagnosis.   2. Electrocardiography.
3. Diagnosis, Differential.   I. Title.
    [DNLM: 1. Diagnosis, Differential.   2. Electrocardiography.
3. Myocardial Infarction—diagnosis.   WG 300 G618m]
RC685.I6G64   1991
616.1'23707547—dc20
DNLM/DLC
for Library of Congress   91-10561
CL/MY 9 8 7 6 5 4 3 2 1   CIP

For
ELLEN and ZACH
and LEXY

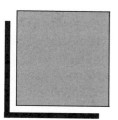

Foreword

The diagnosis of myocardial infarction cannot always be readily made, as the electrocardiogram may not be diagnostic even in the presence of an established infarction. Similarly, the electrocardiogram may be misleading in that it may suggest the presence of an infarction when in fact one has not occurred in either the remote or the recent past. Knowledge of the pitfalls in the electrocardiographic interpretation of infarction will inevitably help physicians to provide better care for their patients. The emotional and economic savings to a patient whose condition is not misdiagnosed as a myocardial infarction are at the least satisfying and at the most capable of changing the course of his life.

Dr. Goldberger has written a comprehensive, authoritative, and scholarly text that will be the definitive work in this field for decades to come. He provides examples and explanations of virtually all the simulators of myocardial infarction. The book is written in a clear style and is richly illustrated with examples of each aberration described. I predict that it will be a classic in its own time. It was my privilege to be able to be associated with him during the preparation of this book.

Lawrence S. Cohen, M.D.

The Ebenezer K. Hunt
Professor of Medicine,
Yale University School of Medicine

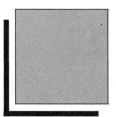

Preface

The art of clinical medicine is in large measure the art of differential diagnosis. Each facet of clinical evaluation—patient history, physical examination, and laboratory testing—entails its own, unfortunately often large, list of differential possibilities.

Perhaps nowhere are these problems so well illustrated as in the diagnosis of myocardial infarction. The so-called pathognomonic electrocardiographic changes of Q waves, ST segment deviations, T wave inversions, and tall positive T waves are often as elusive and misleading as the crushing chest pains that prove to be acute cholecystitis or costochondritis.

The main purpose of this book is to help refine the electrocardiographic diagnosis of myocardial infarction. The clinician who misinterprets the Q waves of the Wolff-Parkinson-White pattern or hypertrophic cardiomyopathy and assigns the diagnosis of coronary artery disease commits one error. However, his regrets are certainly no less than those of a colleague who overlooks the subtle "hyperacute" T wave changes of an incipient myocardial infarction and sends the patient home with antacids. The now routine use of thrombolytic therapy for suspected acute myocardial infarction has made the electrocardiographic differential diagnosis of this condition even more important.

The fourth edition of this book includes new material on numerous pseudo-infarct patterns, cardiomyopathies, "silent" ischemia, and exercise testing, as well as revised discussions of the pathophysiology of the QRS and ST-T changes of myocardial infarction. New material also has been added on numerous other topics, including thrombolysis, pulmonary embolism, right ventricular infarction, congenital heart disease, and myocarditis, and on the diagnosis of infarction with pacemakers and bundle branch block.

In writing this book, I assumed a familiarity with basic electrocardiography on the part of the reader and attempted to continue where most textbook discussions end. As the clinician involved in the daily evaluation of patients soon discovers, it is the exceptions to the rule and the variations on classic themes that make up a large, and by far the most interesting, part of clinical practice.

I would like to thank my colleagues who contributed illustrative ECGs. Most of all, I would like to thank my wife, Ellen, for again abiding my absence and presence during the preparation of this new edition.

Ary L. Goldberger

Contents

Introductory concepts

Over the past two decades major new diagnostic technologies have been introduced into clinical cardiology, particularly in the areas of biochemistry, electrophysiology, and cardiac imaging. The next decade promises further advances. Given these rapid changes, the future role of the conventional electrocardiogram might be questioned. Undoubtedly, new technologies will permit greater resolution in diagnosing metabolic and structural cardiac abnormalities. However, in the daily assessment of patients and the emergency evaluation of the critically ill, the ECG will retain its prominent and unique role as a noninvasive, immediately available, inexpensive, and highly versatile test.[16] Furthermore, in recent years, there have been important refinements in ECG diagnosis. Analysis of electrocardiographic changes has contributed new insights into the pathophysiology of ischemia and infarction. In addition, the advent of the *thrombolytic era*[3,5,25] has refocused clinical attention on the ECG signs and simulators of acute infarction. Familiarity with the uses and limitations of this important test therefore continues to be essential to all clinicians.

ECG PATTERNS OF MYOCARDIAL ISCHEMIA AND INFARCTION

One of the pivotal aspects of electrocardiography centers on the recognition and differential diagnosis of myocardial ischemia and infarction. Unfortunately for clinicians, there is no single ECG pattern associated with myocardial ischemia. Rather, as depicted in Fig. 1-1, the ECG may show a variety of depolarization (QRS) and repolarization (ST-T) changes, including Q waves, ST segment elevations, ST segment depressions, tall (positive) T waves, and deeply inverted (negative) T waves.

Three major factors account for this variability: the extent of ischemic injury ("transmural" vs. "subendocardial"), the locus of ischemia (anterior vs. inferoposterior part of the left and sometimes the right ventricle), and the duration of ischemia (hyperacute or acute vs. evolving or chronic).

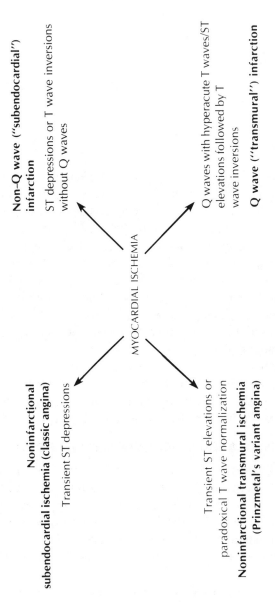

FIG. 1-1. Variability of electrocardiographic patterns associated with myocardial ischemia. As discussed in the text, the ECG may be normal or nonspecifically abnormal. Furthermore, these categorizations are not mutually exclusive. In other words, a non–Q wave infarct may evolve into a Q wave infarct (p. 177), a non–Q wave infarct (p. 25), ST elevations may be followed by a non–Q wave infarct (p. 25), or ST depressions and T wave inversions may be followed by a Q wave infarct (p. 25).

Extent of Ischemic Injury: "Transmural" Versus "Subendocardial"

Traditionally, myocardial infarctions have been divided on the basis of ECG-pathologic correlations into two groups: *transmural* (Q wave) infarcts, associated with a full or nearly full thickness of subepicardial and subendocardial necrosis, and *nontransmural,* or *subendocardial,* infarcts (without Q waves), in which the zone of necrosis is limited to the inner layer of the ventricle. However, as critics have appropriately pointed out,[40,41,47] this pathologic stratification based on ECG criteria is oversimplified and often misleading. Q waves may appear with subendocardial infarcts, whereas not all transmural infarcts are associated with Q waves. Therefore in this book the terms *Q wave infarct* and *non-Q wave infarct*[41] have been adopted in preference to the usual "transmural" and "nontransmural" appellations. A detailed review of this somewhat controversial subject is provided in Chapter 2.

A related question is whether ST segment elevation is a reliable indicator of transmural ischemia and whether ST segment depression is a reliable indicator of subendocardial ischemia. This classic distinction, based on the polarity of the ST segment, has also been challenged; the debate over the pathogenesis of ischemic repolarization changes is reviewed in Chapters 8 and 11. The weight of evidence seems to support the association of ST segment elevation with transmural ischemia and ST segment depression with subendocardial ischemia, although the precise mechanism of these changes is still unresolved. ST segment depression associated with predominant *subendocardial* ischemia may occur with typical anginal attacks, as shown in Fig. 1-1, or during exercise stress testing (Chapters 11 and 13). In addition, ST depression noted during exercise testing or ambulatory ECG monitoring may be a marker of "silent ischemia" (Chapters 12 and 13). By contrast, *transmural* ischemia without infarction may be associated with transient ST segment elevation (Prinzmetal's variant angina, Chapter 8) or with paradoxical normalization of T waves (Chapter 18).

Locus of Ischemia

Q wave infarcts tend to be localized to a region of the anterior or inferoposterior wall of the left ventricle. This topographic localization, discussed in detail in Chapter 2, reflects the regional distribution of the coronary arteries. Right ventricular infarction is discussed separately (Chapters 2 and 21).

Duration of Ischemic Injury

The timing of the ECG in relation to the onset of myocardial infarction is of major importance. For example, the evolution of a classic Q wave infarct is generally also marked by a progression of distinctive changes in the ST segment and T wave (Figs. 1-2 and 1-3). These changes can be temporally divided into *acute* and *evolving* (subacute, chronic) patterns. The hallmark of the acute phase is primary elevation of the ST segment ("current of injury") in one or

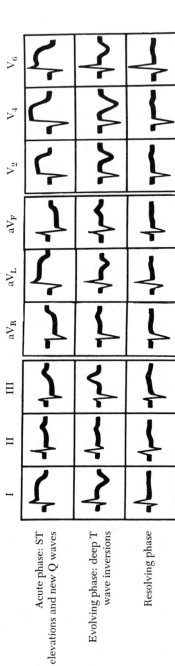

FIG. 1-2. Sequential QRS and ST-T changes seen with anterior wall Q wave infarction. Note the reciprocal ST-T changes in II, III, and aV$_F$. (From Goldberger AL, Goldberger E: Clinical electrocardiography, ed 4, St Louis, 1990, The CV Mosby Co.)

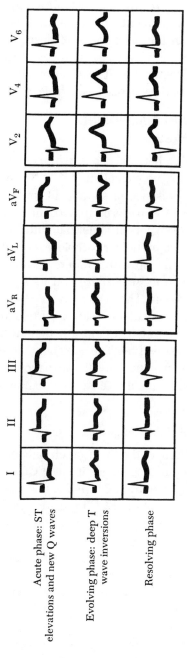

FIG. 1-3. Sequential QRS and ST-T changes with inferior wall Q wave infarction. Note the reciprocal ST-T changes in the anterior leads. (From Goldberger AL, Goldberger E: Clinical electrocardiography, ed 4, St Louis, 1990, The CV Mosby Co.)

more leads, sometimes with *reciprocal* ST depressions in other leads (p. 231). Occasionally this ST segment elevation is preceded or accompanied by tall positive T waves, the so-called *hyperacute* T waves of infarction. These hyperacute T wave changes and acute ST segment alterations are then typically followed by inversion of the T wave, with the appearance of deep "coved plane" or "coronary" T waves in leads reflecting the area of infarction during the evolving (subacute or chronic) phase (Chapter 14). The electrophysiologic basis for these evolutionary repolarization changes is discussed in Part Two.

LIMITATIONS OF THE ECG IN DIAGNOSING CORONARY ARTERY DISEASE

Most clinical tests produce both false-positive and false-negative results.[22] The ECG, despite its utility, is no exception.[14,18,45] Normal ECGs (*false-negatives*) may be found in the presence of significant underlying cardiac disease (Chapter 20). *False-positive* ECG patterns may occur either when an entirely normal ECG variant is mistaken for an abnormal pattern or when a definitely abnormal pattern caused by one particular pathologic condition is mistaken for a similar pattern found in conjunction with a different abnormality.

The ECG is limited in both its *sensitivity* and its *specificity* in diagnosing myocardial ischemia or infarction. The sensitivity of a test is a measure of the percentage of abnormal tests in patients with a particular disease. The more false-negative results (e.g., a normal ECG in a patient with underlying infarction), the less sensitive the test will be. The specificity of any test is a measure of the percentage of normal (negative) results in patients without a particular disease: the more false-positive results (e.g., pseudoinfarct patterns), the less specific the test.[16,22]

Sensitivity: The Problem of False-Negatives

Limitations in sensitivity reflect the fact that chronic or even acute ischemia does not always produce diagnostic changes in the ECG.

Assessment of the sensitivity of the ECG in diagnosing myocardial infarction is also complicated by the timing of the ECG in relation to the onset of ischemia. For example, in the very earliest phase of an infarct the ECG may be normal or show only nondiagnostic changes, resulting in a falsely negative test. Within hours or days the classic changes of infarction generally evolve. However, as described in Chapter 2, in the weeks and months following the myocardial infarction these diagnostic ECG changes (Q waves and ST-T deviations) may remit or resolve completely, leading again to a falsely negative test. Therefore the sensitivity of the ECG in diagnosing infarction must be considered in a temporal context. These and other limitations in the diagnostic sensitivity of the ECG are discussed throughout this text and summarized in Chapter 20.

Specificity: The Problem of False-Positives (Pseudoinfarction)

The specificity of the ECG in diagnosing ischemic heart disease is limited, because other conditions can be associated with patterns similar or even identical to the classic changes of infarction. The present study focuses primarily on the specificity of the ECG in ischemic heart disease, examining in detail those patterns that may simulate actual infarction, the so-called pseudoinfarct patterns, or coronary false-positive patterns.

Part One of the text deals with *depolarization patterns* that simulate myocardial infarction. These include both normal variant patterns and noninfarctional abnormal patterns associated with prominent Q waves.

Part Two deals with *repolarization patterns* that simulate myocardial infarction. These include both normal variant and noninfarctional abnormal patterns that may be associated with ST segment elevation, ST segment depression, deep T wave inversions, or tall positive T waves.

There is some unavoidable overlap between these two subsections. For example, certain Q wave patterns, as may occur for instance with left bundle branch block, are frequently associated with ST-T changes simulating ischemia; in such cases both the depolarization and the repolarization pseudoinfarct patterns are described together.

Part Three is devoted to special topics related to the ECG differential diagnosis of ischemia and infarction, including the sensitivity of the ECG in detecting ischemic heart disease (Chapter 20) and the ECG findings associated with the major mechanical complications of acute myocardial infarction (Chapter 21). Finally, Chapter 22 reviews the complementary roles of electrocardiography, enzyme analysis, nuclear cardiology, and echocardiography in the differential diagnosis of infarction.

NONSPECIFIC ST AND T WAVE CHANGES

In addition to the classic ST-T changes noted above, myocardial ischemia (with or without infarction) is also one of the major causes of so-called nonspecific ST-T changes,[10,18,26,34] which include minor deviations of the ST segment, T wave flattening, and slight T wave inversions (Fig. 1-4). No attempt is made in this discussion of pseudoinfarct patterns to describe in detail the literally dozens of other factors that can produce such nonspecific repolarization changes. A partial list of these factors appears in the box on pp. 8 and 9.

In clinical practice there is a tendency to overlook the multiplicity of normal and pathologic factors affecting repolarization and to automatically ascribe such nonspecific ST and T wave alterations to ischemia. As a consequence the term *coronary disease* is inappropriately applied to many persons with such nonspecific repolarization changes. At the same time, other causes of nonspecific ST-T changes, such as drug effects or mitral valve prolapse, important in their own

PARTIAL LIST OF FACTORS CAUSING NONSPECIFIC ST-T CHANGES*

A. Normal and functional variants
1. Juvenile T wave inversions†
2. Pectus excavatum†
3. Postural (orthostatic) changes
4. Postprandial T wave flattening
5. Benign early repolarization variants†
6. Ingestion of ice water
7. Cold pack on chest wall
8. Tachycardia
9. Anxiety or sudden fright
10. Hyperventilation†
11. Sauna bath[48]
12. Upper gastrointestinal endoscopy[27]

B. Pharmacologic agents
1. Digitalis
2. Quinidine, procainamide, and other antiarrhythmic agents
3. Psychotropic drugs (e.g., phenothiazines, lithium, tricyclic antidepressants)
4. Norepinephrine and other sympathomimetic agents
5. Emetine
6. Antimony
7. Amyl nitrite
8. Doxorubicin hydrochloride (Adriamycin)†

C. Primary ischemia or hypoxemia
1. Myocardial infarction†
2. Transient reversible ischemia associated with hypotension,† tachyarrhythmias,† angina,† etc.
3. Anomalous origin of the left coronary artery†
4. Anemia
5. Carbon monoxide poisoning‡

D. Direct myocardial injury
1. Penetrating myocardial wounds†
2. Myocardial contusion†
3. Lightning stroke†

E. Ventricular hypertrophy and dilation
1. Left ventricular hypertrophy and "strain"†
2. Right ventricular hypertrophy and "strain"†
3. Hypertrophic cardiomyopathy†
4. Acute and chronic cor pulmonale†

F. Electrolyte and acid-base disturbances
1. Hyperkalemia†/hypokalemia†
2. Hypercalcemia/hypocalcemia
3. Hypermagnesemia/hypomagnesemia
4. Acidosis/alkalosis

G. Endocrine and other metabolic disorders
1. Addison's disease
2. Hypopituitarism
3. Acromegaly
4. Hypothyroidism/hyperthyroidism
5. Hypothermia†/hyperthermia
6. Pheochromocytoma†

H. Infiltrative myocardial diseases
1. Primary or metastatic cardiac tumors†
2. Amyloidosis†
3. Hemochromatosis

*Nonspecific ST-T changes are defined here as either slight deviations of the ST segment (elevation or depression) or T wave alterations (flattening or slight inversion of the T wave).

†Indicates factors that are also reported to be associated with actual infarction patterns (characteristic ST-T changes or prominent Q waves), discussed in detail in the text.

‡Myocardial hypoxia resulting from carbon monoxide poisoning may be associated with nonspecific ST-T changes or with more prominent repolarization abnormalities.[1a,44] Rarely the pattern of acute myocardial infarction has been reported.[5] Arrhythmias and conduction disturbances may also occur.[1a]

PARTIAL LIST OF FACTORS CAUSING NONSPECIFIC ST-T CHANGES—cont'd

I. **Myocarditis: infectious or noninfectious**
 1. Viral†
 2. Bacterial†
 3. Parasitic (e.g., Chagas' disease,† echinococcosis†)
 4. Acute syphilitic myocarditis†
 5. Rickettsial
 6. Tuberculous
 7 Sarcoid†
 8. Idiopathic†
J. **Toxic myocardial agents**
 1. Phosphorus†
 2. Scorpion sting venom†
K. **Pericarditis**
 1. Acute pericarditis†
 2. Chronic constrictive pericarditis†
L. **Conduction defects with secondary ST-T changes**
 1. Left bundle branch block†
 2. Right bundle branch block†
 3. Wolff-Parkinson-White syndrome†
 4. Pacemaker patterns†
 5. Left anterior hemiblock†
M. **Central nervous system disorders**
 1. Acute cerebrovascular accident†
 2. Head injury, neurosurgery, tumors†
N. **Neuromuscular diseases with associated cardiomyopathy**
 1. Myotonia atrophica†
 2. Friedreich's ataxia†
 3. Muscular dystrophy†

O. **Other cardiomyopathies**
 1. Endocardial fibroelastosis†
 2. Alcoholic cardiomyopathy†
 3. Idiopathic dilated cardiomyopathy†
 4. Glycogen storage disease of the heart
 5. Arrhythmogenic right ventricular dysplasia†
P. **Allergic reactions**
 1. Drug reactions†
 2. Serum sickness
Q. **Collagen vascular and other autoimmune conditions**
 1. Scleroderma†
 2. Dermatomyositis
 3. Polyarteritis nodosa
 4. Rheumatic fever
 5. Systemic lupus erythematosus§
R. **Miscellaneous**
 1. Stokes-Adams T wave pattern†
 2. Truncal vagotomy†
 3. Radical neck dissection†
 4. Postpacemaker T wave pattern†
 5. Posttachycardia T wave pattern†
 6. Postextrasystolic ST-T changes
 7. QT prolongation–syncope syndromes†
 8. Mitral valve prolapse†
 9. Acute pancreatitis (see Chapter 6)
 10. Biliary tract disease‖
 11. Acquired immunodeficiency syndrome (AIDS)¶

§Nonspecific ST-T changes are common in systemic lupus erythematosus (SLE) secondary to the associated pericarditis or myocarditis. Actual infarct patterns (with Q waves and characteristic ST-T changes) have also been reported in association with SLE and were ascribable either to lupus arteritis or to concomitant coronary atherosclerosis leading to true infarction.[4,24,49] There is no evidence to suggest that lupus myocarditis alone causes pseudoinfarct patterns.

‖Although sometimes cited as a cause of false coronary patterns, biliary tract disease per se is probably associated with at most only nonspecific ST-T alterations. Q waves or marked ST-T changes should *not* be ascribed to biliary tract disease alone.[11]

¶The ECG changes in AIDS can represent a variety of cardiac abnormalities, including myocarditis or pericarditis due to idiopathic causes or opportunistic infection, dilated cardiomyopathy, and metastatic Kaposi's sarcoma.[1]

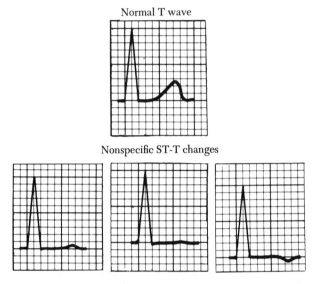

FIG. 1-4. Nonspecific ST-T changes include slight T wave flattening or inversion and may be caused by a multiplicity of factors (pp. 8 and 9). (From Goldberger AL, Goldberger E: Clinical electrocardiography, ed 4, St Louis, 1990, The CV Mosby Co.)

right, may be overlooked. Discussion of repolarization changes has been deliberately limited to a consideration of more marked alterations in the ST-T complex. For example, the section on T wave inversions focuses primarily on conditions that may be associated with *deeply* negative T waves, which for the purposes of this text are arbitrarily defined as greater than 5 mm (0.5 mV) deep.

VALIDATION OF PSEUDOINFARCT PATTERNS

A recurrent problem in any discussion of pseudoinfarct patterns is establishing the validity of a particular pattern. Before a new pseudoinfarct pattern can be accepted, there must be adequate demonstration of two key points: (1) that myocardial ischemia was not present at the time the ECG was recorded, and (2) that no other condition known to be associated with a pseudoinfarct pattern was present. However, strict application of these criteria makes "canonization" of pseudoinfarct patterns problematic if not at times impossible.

For example, definite exclusion of myocardial ischemia may prove difficult. The absence of chest pain, presence of normal cardiac enzymes, even a normal coronary arteriogram or postmortem examination, may be strong evidence against ischemia, but they do not definitely exclude it. Patients may have "silent" infarcts with atypical symptoms or no symptoms at all. Transient noninfarctional ischemia may lead to marked ST-T changes and even Q waves without serum enzyme elevations or pathologic changes at postmortem examination (Chapter 6). Finally, myocardial infarction with "normal" coronary arteries is a well-recognized syndrome (due, for example, to vasospasm [Chapter 8]).

The second criterion for establishment of a pseudoinfarct variant requires that other conditions known to simulate ischemic ECG patterns be excluded. For example, several types of cardiomyopathies have been reported to cause Q waves and ST-T changes suggesting infarction (p. 159). However, such patterns are also well described in association with the left or right ventricular enlargement that frequently accompanies the myopathy. For these reasons isolated case reports of "new" pseudoinfarct patterns should be evaluated with proper caution.

Despite these problems, many well-documented pseudoinfarct patterns are described in the following chapters. Some of the more controversial questions, such as the significance of ECG changes with acute pancreatitis, are also reviewed.

SIGNIFICANCE OF PSEUDOINFARCT PATTERNS

The clinician frequently is faced with the problem of deciding whether a tracing represents a true infarct pattern or a false-positive result. In 1947 Wilson et al.[51] cautioned, "Electrocardiographic abnormalities are not diseases." Mistaking a normal variant for a sign of coronary disease may condemn a patient to a life of cardiac invalidism[20] because of what Marriott[31] has called an *electrocardiographogenic disease.* On the other hand, by incorrectly ascribing an abnormal pattern to infarction one may be overlooking another pathologic condition, such as hypertrophic cardiomyopathy or pulmonary embolism, with similar ECG manifestations but different clinical and therapeutic implications.

Aside from their obvious clinical significance, pseudoinfarct patterns are also important from a theoretical standpoint. The electrophysiologic basis of coronary Q waves and ischemic ST-T changes is still incompletely understood. Examination of the cause of certain pseudoinfarct patterns can sometimes provide a better understanding of the pathogenesis of true infarct patterns. For example, the concept of *early repolarization* has been cited to explain both the pattern of benign ST elevations and the ST elevations seen during acute infarction. However, in other cases it appears that identical ECG patterns can be produced by disparate conditions (e.g., myocardial infarction and hypertrophic cardiomyopathy) through different pathophysiologic mechanisms (necrosis vs. hypertrophy).

Pseudoinfarct patterns are also important in their own right. For example, the discovery that acute cerebrovascular accidents can induce marked repolarization abnormalities mimicking myocardial infarction has stimulated new research into the relationships between the central nervous system and cardiac function (Chapter 16).

Because of these clinical and basic science applications, pseudoinfarct patterns have been of interest for many years. The subject was first reviewed in 1950 by Myers[35-38] in a series of four articles, and over the ensuing years there have been a number of shorter reviews.* Many ECG textbooks† devote some at-

---

*References 6-8, 9, 13-15, 17, 29-33, 39, 42, 50.
†References 2, 12, 19, 21, 33, 43, 46.

tention to the differential diagnosis of infarction. In addition, scores of individual articles, referenced in the appropriate sections in this book, deal with specific pseudoinfarct patterns.

Despite this considerable bibliography, no single previous publication has systematically categorized the pseudoinfarct patterns, described their differential diagnosis, and compared their underlying electrophysiology. This book attempts to consider comprehensively both the clinical and the theoretical aspects of the ECG differential diagnosis of myocardial infarction.

REFERENCES

1. Anderson DW, et al: Prevalent myocarditis at necropsy in the acquired immunodeficiency syndrome, J Am Coll Cardiol 11:792, 1988.

1a. Anderson RD, et al: Myocardial toxicity from carbon monoxide poisoning, Ann Intern Med 67:1172, 1967.

2. Arbeit SR, et al: Differential diagnosis of the electrocardiogram, Philadelphia, 1960, FA Davis Co.

3. Blankenship JC, Almquist AK: Cardiovascular complications of thrombolytic therapy in patients with a mistaken diagnosis of acute myocardial infarction, J Am Coll Cardiol 14:1579, 1989.

4. Bor I: Cardiac infarction in Libman-Sacks endocarditis [Letter to the editor], N Engl J Med 279, 164, 1968.

5. Braunwald EB (editor): Symposium on modern thrombolytic therapy, J Am Coll Cardiol 10(suppl B):1, 1987.

6. Chou TC: Pseudo-infarction (noninfarction Q waves). In Fisch C (editor): Complex electrocardiography, Philadelphia, 1973, FA Davis Co., vol 1.

7. Chung EK, Duca PR: ECG recognition of true vs pseudo myocardial infarction. In Brest AN (editor): Cardiovascular clinics: innovations in the diagnosis and management of acute myocardial infarction, Philadelphia, 1975, FA Davis Co.

8. Epstein M, Wasserburger RH: Electrocardiograms simulating myocardial infarction in the presence of normal coronary arteries, Vasc Dis 4:215, 1967.

9. Fisch C: Electrocardiographic diagnosis of myocardial infarction: pitfalls of a graphic technique. In Likoff W, et al (editors): Atherosclerosis and coronary artery disease, New York, 1972, Grune & Stratton Inc.

10. Friedberg CK, Zager A: "Nonspecific" ST and T-wave changes, Circulation 23:655, 1961.

11. Friedman GD: The relationship between coronary heart disease and gallbladder disease: a critical review, Ann Intern Med 68:222, 1968.

12. Friedman HH: Diagnostic electrocardiography and vectorcardiography, ed 2, New York, 1977, McGraw-Hill Book Co.

13. Goldberger AL: Recognition of ECG pseudoinfarct patterns, Mod Conc Cardiovasc Dis 49:13, 1980.

14. Goldberger AL: ECG simulators of myocardial infarction. I. Pathophysiology and differential diagnosis of pseudo-infarct Q waves, PACE 5:106, 1982.

15. Goldberger AL: ECG simulators of myocardial infarction. II. Pathophysiology and differential diagnosis of pseudo-infarction ST and T patterns, PACE 5:414, 1982.

16. Goldberger AL: Utility of the routine electrocardiogram before surgery and on general hospital admission. Critical review and new guidelines, Ann Intern Med 105:552, 1986.

17. Goldberger AL: Normal and noninfarct Q waves, Cardiol Clin 5:357, 1987.

18. Goldberger AL, Goldberger E: Clinical electrocardiography, ed 4, St Louis, 1990, The CV Mosby Co.

19. Goldberger E: Unipolar lead electrocardiography and vectorcardiography, ed 3, Philadelphia 1953, Lea & Febiger.

20. Goldman MJ: Normal variants in the electrocardiogram leading to cardiac invalidism, Am Heart J 59:71, 1960.

21. Goldman MJ: Principles of clinical electrocardiography, ed 12, Los Altos Calif, 1986, Lange Medical Publications.

22. Griner PF, et al: Selection and interpretation of diagnostic tests and procedures:

principles and applications, Ann Intern Med 94:559, 1981.

23. Hayes JM, Hall GV: The myocardial toxicity of carbon monoxide, Med J Aust 1:865, 1964.

24. Hejtmancik MR, et al: The cardiovascular manifestations of systemic lupus erythematosus, Am Heart J 68:119, 1964.

25. Lee TH, et al: Candidates for thrombolysis among emergency room patients with acute chest pain. Potential true- and false-positive rates, Ann Intern Med 110:957, 1989.

26. Levine HD: Non-specificity of the electrogram associated with coronary artery disease, Am J Med 15:344, 1953.

27. Levy N, Abinader E: Continuous electrocardiographic monitoring with Holter electrocardiocorder throughout all stages of gastroscopy, Am J Dig Dis 22:1091, 1977.

28. Lipman BS, et al: Clinical scalar electrocardiography, ed 7, Chicago, 1984, Year Book Medical Publishers Inc.

29. Marriott HJL: Coronary mimicry: normal variants and physiologic, pharmacologic, and pathologic influences that simulate coronary patterns in the electrocardiogram, Ann Intern Med 52:411, 1960.

30. Marriott HJL: Normal electrocardiographic variants simulating ischemic heart disease, JAMA 199:325, 1967.

31. Marriott HJL: Practical electrocardiography, ed 8, Baltimore, 1988, The Williams & Wilkins Co.

32. Marriott HJL, Nizet PM: Physiologic stimuli simulating ischemic heart disease, JAMA 200:715, 1967.

33. Marriott HJL, Slonim R: False patterns of myocardial infarction, Heart Bull 16:71, 1967.

34. Mirvis DM, et al: Clinical and pathophysiologic correlates of ST-T wave abnormalities in coronary artery disease, Am J Cardiol 66:699, 1990.

35. Myers GB: QRS-T patterns in multiple precordial leads that may be mistaken for myocardial infarction. I. Left ventricular hypertrophy and dilatation, Circulation 1:844, 1950.

36. Myers GB: QRS-T patterns in multiple precordial leads that may be mistaken for myocardial infarction. II. Right ventricular hypertrophy and dilatation, Circulation 1:860, 1950.

37. Myers GB: QRS-T patterns in multiple pre-cordial leads that may be mistaken for myocardial infarction. III. Bundle branch block, Circulation 2:60, 1950.

38. Myers GB: Other QRS-T patterns that may be mistaken for myocardial infarction. IV. Alterations in blood potassium; myocardial ischemia; subepicardial myocarditis, distortion associated with arrhythmias, Circulation 2:75, 1950.

39. Pec L, Enderle J: Ondes Q pathologiques en l'absence d'infarctus du myocarde: classification et considerations électrophysiologiques, Acta Cardiol 24:242, 1969.

40. Phibbs B: "Transmural" versus "subendocardial" myocardial infarction: an electrocardiographic myth, J Am Coll Cardiol 1:561, 1983.

41. Pipberger HV, Lopez EA: "Silent" subendocardial infarcts: fact or fiction? Am Heart J 100:597, 1980.

42. Proudfit WL, et al: Electrocardiographic evidence suggestive of myocardial infarction without significant organic heart disease, Am Heart J 110:448, 1985.

43. Schamroth L: The electrocardiology of coronary artery disease, Oxford, 1975, Blackwell Scientific Publications.

44. Shafer N, et al: Primary myocardial disease in man resulting from acute carbon monoxide poisoning, Am J Med 38:316, 1965.

45. Silverman ME, Silverman BD: The diagnostic capabilities and limitations of the electrocardiogram. In Hurst JW (editor): The heart: update I, New York, 1979, McGraw-Hill Book Co.

46. Sodi-Pallares D: New bases of electrocardiography, St Louis, 1956, The CV Mosby Co.

47. Spodick DH: Q-wave infarction versus S-T infarction: nonspecificity of electrocardiographic criteria for differentiating transmural and nontransmural lesions, Am J Cardiol 51:913, 1983.

48. Taggart P, et al: Cardiac responses to thermal, physical, and emotional stress, Br Med J 3:71, 1972.

49. Taubenhaus M, et al: Cardiovascular manifestations of collagen diseases, Circulation 12:903, 1955.

50. Timio M, et al: Alterazioni elettrocardiografiche pseudo-infartuali, Cuore Circulaz 53:313, 1969.

51. Wilson FN, et al: Interpretation of the ventricular complex of the electrocardiogram, Adv Intern Med 2:1, 1947.

Depolarization (Q Wave) Patterns Simulating Myocardial Infarction

The abnormal Q wave is the most characteristic ECG manifestation of myocardial infarction. This section examines the current theoretical understanding of coronary Q waves and then presents a detailed discussion of other patterns (normal and abnormal) that may simulate the Q waves of infarction.

A Q wave is, by definition, an initial negative deflection of the ventricular depolarization complex (QRS). The lowercase letter *q* is used to indicate an initial negative deflection of relatively short duration, small amplitude, or both. If the entire complex is negative, it is termed a QS. This Q wave nomenclature is illustrated below.

A Q or QS pattern per se is not necessarily abnormal, nor do all abnormal Q waves invariably represent myocardial infarction. The normality of any Q wave depends on a number of factors: the particular lead in which it is recorded, its amplitude, its duration, and also its configuration. The criteria for assessing Q wave normality are discussed further in the following chapters.

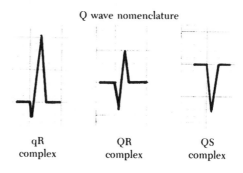

Q wave nomenclature

qR
complex

QR
complex

QS
complex

Q waves of myocardial infarction

The purpose of this chapter is to consider the depolarization changes associated with myocardial infarction, focusing in particular on theoretical and clinical aspects of pathologic Q waves.

THEORY OF INFARCTIONAL Q WAVES

There have been two general theoretical approaches to understanding the Q waves of myocardial infarction: Wilson's classic cavity potential theory, with its subsequent modifications, and the vectorial theory of Q waves.

Wilson's Cavity Potential Theory of Coronary Q Waves

Wilson's classic Q wave theory was based on experimental coronary ligation in dogs with records of intracavity and intramural potentials.[90,91] Wilson and his colleagues proposed that during *transmural* infarction the potentials of the subjacent ventricular cavity are transmitted through the electrically inert infarcted myocardium to an electrode overlying the infarct. Since the potentials of the left ventricular cavity are normally entirely negative, an electrode overlying an area of transmural left ventricular infarction should also record an entirely negative (QS) complex. In this way, according to the cavity potential theory, the necrotic myocardium acts as a figurative "window" or "hole" in the heart, transmitting negative cavity potentials to epicardial and surface electrodes.

Subsequent experimental observations by Durrer, van Lier, and Büller,[24] Maxwell, Kennamer, and Prinzmetal,[57] and Prinzmetal et al.[66] supported Wilson's theory of transmural Q waves. Prinzmetal's group produced through-and-through transmural infarcts in dogs so the affected myocardium was functionally akinetic, electrically incapable of generating a current of injury, and histologically necrotic. In such cases of definite transmural damage, the electrical potentials recorded in the ventricular cavity were identical in timing and configuration to the potentials recorded at all levels within the infarcted wall and also on the epicardial surface. These experimental findings were interpreted as supporting Wilson's basic theory—that cavity potentials appear to be transmitted unaltered to epicardial and surface leads in cases of transmural infarction.

Wilson et al.[91] also described cases in which the cavity potentials were not transmitted in pure form to the surface. For example, electrically viable muscle surviving in the infarcted area might generate enough potentials to modify the basic QS complex of the cavity and produce an actual R wave (as part of a QR complex); or it might give rise only to an embryonic r wave or produce notching of the basic cavity QS complex.

Prinzmetal et al.[66] and Maxwell, Kennamer, and Prinzmetal[57] found that in cases of experimental infarction in dogs, QS waves recorded over regions containing live muscle differed from the cavity QS wave. They called these modified QS complexes *mural QS waves,* to differentiate them from the pure *cavity* QS waves recorded over areas of complete transmural infarction. They suggested that mural QS waves represented a combination of the purely negative cavity potentials modified by the positive potentials of muscle still alive in the infarcted region. Prinzmetal's observations on transmural myocardial infarction and his distinction between mural and cavity QS complexes are entirely consistent with the cavity potential theory of Q waves proposed by Wilson.

Wilson et al.[91] also observed that *transient* QS waves could occur clinically during a typical ischemic attack. They attributed these Q waves to a temporary loss of myocardial excitability secondary to reversible ischemia. The subject of transient Q wave patterns is described in more detail in Chapter 6.

Finally, Wilson et al.[91] reported that in cases of subendocardial infarction a QR type of complex could appear.

In summary, the salient points of Wilson's Q wave theory were as follows:

1. The coronary QS wave represents actual transmission of negative left ventricular cavity potentials through an area of transmural myocardial injury.
2. The basic cavity QS complex in nontransmural infarction can be modified by residual positive potentials of still viable muscle in the infarcted area to produce QR, Qr, or notched QS waves.

Vectorial Theory of Q Waves

Q waves can also be conceptualized in vectorial theory in terms of a balance of myocardial electrical forces (vectors).[36] The deflections seen on the scalar electrocardiogram represent a complex spatial and temporal summation of potentials from a myriad of myocardial fibers. A Q wave in any given lead indicates that the net vectorial sum of initial ventricular depolarization forces is negative (i.e., oriented at greater than right angles to the positive pole of that particular lead).

In vectorial terms the Q wave of infarction results from a primary loss of myocardial forces caused by ischemic injury. Furthermore, loss of forces in one direction must result in a reciprocal gain in potentials oriented in the opposite direction, according to vectorial theory. For example, infarction of the anterior wall results in a loss of initial forces directed toward the precordial leads. Consequently, abnormal Q waves appear in these leads. However, leads placed around the back or in the esophagus would necessarily record a reciprocal increase in positive forces (taller R waves). The opposite pattern obtains when the posterior portion of the heart is infarcted. When posterior wall infarction occurs, tall wide R waves characteristically appear anteriorly in the right precordial leads. These do *not* represent a primary increase in right ventricular forces, as seen with right ventricular hypertrophy. Instead, they signify a net loss of posteriorly directed forces, which leaves the anterior forces in the horizontal plane relatively less opposed.

In general, abnormal Q waves caused by a loss of electrical potentials can occur with any process that results in significant myocardial injury. This injury may be ischemic or nonischemic, reversible or irreversible. The noncoronary causes of myocardial injury constitute an important category of pseudoinfarct Q waves and are discussed in Chapters 6 and 7.

Wilson's Cavity Potential Theory Versus the Vectorial Theory

The vectorial explanation of pathologic Q waves is a general mathematical formulation that conceptualizes all ECG patterns in terms of a balance of positive and negative forces (vectors). Wilson's cavity theory, on the other hand, is a very concrete model that equates the abnormal negative potentials seen with infarction to the negative potentials that actually are recorded in the left ventricular cavity.

Although Wilson's cavity theory has never been disproved and is in fact supported by a number of experimental observations, the vectorial model is more generally advocated today for a number of reasons. Proponents of the vectorial approach have criticized the cavity potential theory of infarction for its apparent failure to explain the ECG pattern in such cases as posterior wall infarction, which is generally recognized by an increase in precordial R wave voltage rather than the presence of pathologic Q waves.[87] Posterior wall infarction, however, *does* produce Q waves, although these will be recorded only by posterior leads (e.g., esophageal leads) not generally used in routine clinical practice. The example of posterior wall infarction therefore does not disprove or negate the cavity potential theory. Nevertheless, it does illustrate one of the main weaknesses of Wilson's theory: the failure to explain adequately the reciprocal *increase* in voltage in leads facing away from the infarct (in addition to the primary loss of forces seen over the infarct).[87]

The vectorial model has an added advantage in that it can be used to conceptualize noninfarctional Q waves. For example, Q waves may result not only from a net decrease in positive forces (as seen with infarction and other types of myocardial injury) but also from a net increase in negative forces (as in some cases of hypertrophy). The vectorial model is also useful in explaining the Q waves caused by altered conduction (e.g., bundle branch block), in which there is no net augmentation or decrement in myocardial forces but only an abberation in the sequence of myocardial activation.* Finally, the vectorial theory is helpful in accounting for the *transient* Q waves that may occur with noninfarctional myocardial injury (ischemic or nonischemic)[6] (Chapter 6).

Subendocardial Versus Transmural Infarctions

A topic of considerable confusion and controversy relating to the presence or absence of pathologic Q waves centers on the diagnosis of transmural versus subendocardial infarcts. This confusion stems from contradictory data reported from previous experimental and clinical studies. The major question is this: do subendocardial infarcts result in pathologic Q waves or is the subendocardium "electrically silent" in terms of its contribution to the QRS complex recorded on the body surface?

Conflicting claims have been made concerning the process of subendocardial activation and its contribution to surface R waves. According to traditional theory, the ventricular myocardium depolarizes in an orderly fashion from endocardium to epicardium. Consequently, points at varying distances inside the myocardium should all be expected to record an R wave as a reflection of this outward spread of positive potentials—that is, points just inside the subendocardium, where a small r wave is predicted, as well as points at the epicardial surface, where a tall R wave should be registered (reflecting depolarization of the entire width of the myocardium).[56]

However, when actual intramural recordings were made by Prinzmetal et al.[66] and by Sodi-Pallares et al.,[77] a QS complex and not the predicted rS was found in the subendocardial layers of normal canine hearts. This region of subendocardial negativity extended in some places more than halfway through the myocardium.[77] The expected R wave progression was seen only in the more peripheral subepicardial areas.

Furthermore, it was observed that the depolarization of the subendocardium, where the QS complexes were recorded, occurred almost instantaneously, in marked contrast to the relatively slower pace of depolarization in the subepicardial layers. Massumi et al.[56] suggested that the subendocardial area might actually depolarize too rapidly to be recorded with the conventional electrodes. They theorized that the extensive ramifications of Purkinje fibers in the subendocardium could account for the rapid spread of depolarization in that area.

Based on similar observations, Sodi-Pallares et al.[77] conceptualized the left ventricular myocardium in terms of an inner electrical subendocardium and an outer electrical subepicardium. The electrical subepicardium appeared to depolarize according to the classic model of a simple outward-spreading wave of ex-

---

*Delayed epicardial activation may also play an important role in the pathogenesis of Q waves in some cases of nontransmural infarction (pp. 21 and 22).

citation. The electrical subendocardium, however, appeared to depolarize very rapidly and irregularly,[65] so that an electrode placed in this region recorded mainly the spread of the slower epicardial forces away from the endocardium.

The term *electrical subendocardium* therefore was used to define an electrophysiologic entity rather than a discrete anatomic area. The basic characteristic of the electrical subendocardium is its electrical negativity, which is similar to that of the ventricular cavity. In dogs this region was reported to extend for a variable distance into the myocardium. According to Pipberger et al.,[65] the subendocardial QS zone comprised from 27% to 39% of the whole thickness of the ventricular wall. In humans it was estimated to constitute the inner 50% of the anatomic myocardium.[77]

Support for this concept of subendocardial "silence" also came from a number of experimental and clinical observations suggesting that pure subendocardial infarctions do not cause pathologic Q waves. For example, Maxwell, Kennamer, and Prinzmetal[57] in experiments with dogs did not observe Q waves when subendocardial infarction was produced either by coronary artery ligation or by direct thermal injury. In contrast, these investigators did observe QS waves when only the subepicardium of canine hearts was damaged (by heat, chemicals, or excision) and the subendocardium was left intact. These findings were consistent with the claim that the subendocardium does not contribute significantly to surface R wave positivity.

A number of early studies correlating pathologic and electrocardiographic data also supported this concept.[*] In some of the reported cases, subendocardial infarction was associated with a diminution in R wave amplitude. However, the general absence of Q waves with infarction limited to the inner half of the left ventricular wall was noteworthy[67] even when the infarcts were otherwise extensive enough to cause cardiogenic shock.[32] Cook, Edwards, and Pruitt[17] did observe Q waves with nontransmural infarcts that extended more than halfway into the myocardium, consistent with the boundary of the "electrical subendocardium" defined by others[56,77] in the canine ventricle.

This notion of an electrically silent subendocardium, however, has been vigorously challenged[63,64,79] based on apparently countervailing data. As noted on p. 18, Wilson et al.[91] initially suggested that nontransmural (subendocardial) infarcts could be associated with QR-type complexes. However, detailed pathologic correlations were not provided. Subsequently, Durrer, van Lier, and Büller[24] in canine experiments were unable to define a zone of subendocardial negativity and reported QR complexes in the surface leads in some cases of small subendocardial infarcts. Similarly, Abildskov et al.[1] reported pathologic Q waves with nontransmural injury in dogs and also in clinicopathologic studies of subendocardial infarction.[88] Mirvis et al.[60] confirmed the appearance of Q waves in

---

[*]References 17, 18, 47, 67, 92.

nontransmural infarction in dogs. In this and other experimental studies,[19,24] Q wave pathogenesis with nontransmural infarction correlated with delayed activation of the surviving subepicardial tissue overlying the necrotic zone. A number of more recent clinical studies have also corroborated the association of Q waves with nontransmural infarction.[29,68,74,80]

From a clinical viewpoint it is clear that the traditional equation of Q waves with transmural infarction and the absence of Q waves with subendocardial infarction is inaccurate. Subendocardial infarcts, particularly when they involve more than one third to one half the thickness of the ventricular wall, may be associated with prominent Q waves. On the other hand, not all transmural infarcts result in pathologic Q waves. From the electrocardiographer's vantage point, the terms Q *wave* and *non–Q wave* infarction are clearly preferable to the standard categorization of infarcts as "transmural" or "subendocardial" based solely on the ECG.[3,79]

The effects of subendocardial ischemia and infarction on the repolarization (ST-T) complex are discussed separately in Chapters 11 and 14.

CLINICAL ASPECTS OF INFARCTIONAL Q WAVES

When coronary occlusion is produced experimentally, Q waves may appear within minutes of the onset of ischemia. Clinically, Q waves generally appear within 24 hours of the onset of infarction. Occasionally there is longer lag between the advent of ischemic chest pain and the appearance of Q waves (see also p. 25). In persons without symptoms and without definite history of prior infarction, it is not uncommon to find Q waves as the remnants of prior unrecognized and sometimes completely "silent" infarcts.[42]

Angiographic studies of patients with ischemic heart disease have shown a strong correlation between the presence of Q waves and ventricular wall motion abnormalities (asynergy).[13,14,35] Bodenheimer et al.[14] found asynergic zones in 60 of 64 patients (95%) with abnormal Q waves. The absence of Q waves in patients with ischemic heart disease, however, did not exclude the possibility of ventricular asynergy or even ventricular aneurysm. Thus Q waves are a specific although insensitive marker of an underlying wall motion disorder.

Localization of Infarction

Infarcts can be localized geographically as either *anterior* or *inferoposterior (diaphragmatic)* on the basis of whether the abnormal Q waves are found in one or more of the anterior leads (I, aV_L, V_1 to V_6) or in the inferior limb leads. Furthermore, standard textbooks traditionally consider anterior infarcts as anteroseptal (Q waves in V_1 to V_3) or anterolateral (Q waves in V_4 to V_6). In addition, some authors label infarcts that produce Q waves in V_3 to V_5 as anteroapical, since these leads are thought to reflect the left ventricular apex. Finally, inferoposterior infarcts are generally separated into strictly inferior (Q waves in II, III, and aV_F) and strictly posterior (tall R waves in the right precordial leads).

Meticulous correlative studies[70,74,80] have confirmed the general accuracy of distinguishing anterior versus inferoposterior infarcts based on the ECG. However, these same studies have indicated important limitations in the criteria that are clinically used to categorize anterior wall infarctions as "anteroseptal" or "anterolateral" or to predict whether necrosis will involve the inferior or true posterior wall of the left ventricle. Pathologic studies[70] reveal that infarction is rarely limited to the left ventricular lateral wall or interventricular septum. Similarly, the ECG does not reliably differentiate between strictly posterior and strictly inferior infarcts based on standard criteria: Q waves in II, III, and aV_F may occur with true posterior infarction whereas tall right precordial R waves may be found with inferior (or lateral) wall involvement.[70]

Anterior wall infarcts (diagnosed by ST elevation and/or Q waves in V_1 to V_4) generally correlate with high-grade obstruction in the left anterior descending coronary system. Similarly, T wave inversions in V_1 to V_4 with anginal syndromes suggest high-grade left anterior descending obstruction (p. 276). However, the electrocardiographic patterns of inferior wall infarction (changes in II, III, and aV_F) may occur with occlusion of either the right coronary artery or the left circumflex coronary artery.[11,31] (See also p. 52.)

Right Ventricular Infarction

The subject of right ventricular infarction has received increasing attention in recent years. Electrocardiographic evidence of acute right ventricular infarction may be obtained by examining the right precordial leads for ST segment elevation (see Fig. 21-1). The diagnosis of right ventricular infarction is discussed in detail in Chapter 21.

Atrial Infarction

Infarction of the atria may also occur in association with ventricular infarction. Atrial infarction may be electrocardiographically silent or may be associated with nonspecific findings, including alterations in P wave morphology, PR segment deviation, and atrial arrhythmias.[46] The differential diagnosis of PR segment changes associated with atrial infarction is briefly described on p. 213.

Q Wave Versus Non–Q Wave Infarcts: Clinical Differences

Although the presence or absence of Q waves is of limited value in predicting whether infarction is transmural or subendocardial, there are important clinical differences between "Q wave" and "non–Q wave" infarcts* (Table 2-1). Gibson[33] has provided a useful summary of data from the "prethrombolytic" era in an exhaustive review of this subject. As a group, patients with non–Q wave infarcts have a smaller amount of myocardial necrosis than those with Q wave

---

*References 3, 22, 30, 33, 40, 48, 54, 55, 69, 79.

TABLE 2-1. Non−Q wave versus Q-wave infarction

Creatine kinase release	Lower
Short-term mortality	Lower
Postinfarction angina	Higher
Reinfarction rate	Higher
Multivessel disease	Comparable
Prevalence of patent infarct-related artery	Higher
Long-term mortality	Comparable

infarcts and a better short-term prognosis (i.e., days to weeks). However, the subsequent course of patients with non−Q wave infarcts appears to be more malignant, with a high rate of reinfarction. As a result, late mortality for these patients is comparable to, and in some studies worse than, that of patients with Q wave infarcts.[33]

The instability of non−Q wave infarcts is consistent with current concepts of their underlying pathophysiology.[3,33] DeWood et al.[22] reported that total occlusion of the infarct-related vessel is infrequently observed in the early hours of non−Q wave infarction. Furthermore, even when total occlusion is present, perfusion of the distal vessel is usually maintained by collateral vessels. These anatomic findings support the suggestion that non−Q wave infarction often indicates an *incomplete* ischemic event, with additional territory at risk. This postulate is supported by the observation that subsequent infarcts in these patients tend to occur in the same location as the initial one.[3]

It has been appreciated for many years that non−Q wave infarction is not a monolithic syndrome.[29,51] From an electrocardiographic viewpoint, patients with this diagnosis can be further divided into those who present with T wave inversion and those who present with ST deviations.[61] This simple classification may be of some clinical relevance. A number of studies[51,75,83] suggest that non−Q wave infarctions associated with ST depression carry a greater risk than such infarctions associated with T wave inversion. Furthermore, Schechtman et al.[75] found that persistent ST depression (present on admission and discharge) was a particularly strong indicator of subsequent mortality at 1-year follow-up. The authors speculated that persistent ST depression following infarction might be a marker of "silent" ischemia (p. 247) emanating from a zone of chronically hypoperfused ("hibernating") myocardium. Such a jeopardized zone, in turn, might be the site of reinfarction or ventricular tachyarrhythmias. Non−Q wave infarcts may also be preceded by ST segment elevation.[12,39,89] This topic is discussed at greater length on p. 177.

Finally, it should be recognized that patients who initially present with non−Q wave infarction may evolve pathologic Q waves during their hospitalization. Kleiger et al.[45] observed this transition from non-Q to Q wave infarction in 76 of 544 patients (14%) in the Diltiazem Reinfarction Study database. Of interest, the majority of patients who evolved Q waves did not have enzymatic evidence of infarct extension. The authors referred to the late development of Q waves following an acute and initially non–Q wave infarction as an electrocardiographic "lag" phenomenon; its precise mechanism remains uncertain.

Overestimation, Underestimation, and Mislocalization of Infarcts

As noted, the ECG is generally accurate in localizing infarcts to the anterior versus inferoposterior wall of the left ventricle. However, in cases of anteroapical infarction the ECG may show abnormal Q waves in both inferior and anterior leads, possibly leading to an "overestimation" of the extent of infarction.[14]

In other cases the ECG may underestimate the degree of myocardial necrosis. For example, Bodenheimer et al.[14] studied the correlation between pathologic Q waves on the standard 12-lead ECG and the epicardial ECG obtained at the time of cardiac surgery. In a number of cases pathologic Q waves were detected only by the epicardial electrogram and were "lost" on the standard surface ECG. Similarly, in a correlative study of healed myocardial infarction, Sullivan et al.[80] found that the ECG frequently underestimated the extent of necrosis.

A variety of quantitative ECG indices have been proposed to estimate infarct size and left ventricular ejection fraction after Q wave infarctions. These scoring systems are discussed briefly on p. 357, and interested readers are referred to the literature.[85]

Finally, in some instances the presence of Q waves may not exactly represent the area of infarction.[38] For example, right ventricular infarcts are generally associated with the pattern of inferior wall infarction.* Confusion over the localization of infarction also occurs with left bundle branch block. The diagnosis of infarction with left bundle branch block is fraught with difficulty. Left bundle branch block commonly produces pseudoinfarctional QS complexes in the anterior or inferior leads. However, the appearance of a QR pattern in the lateral chest leads (V_5 and V_6) with a left bundle branch block pattern generally reflects infarction of the interventricular septum, *not* the lateral wall. The cause of these paradoxical patterns with left bundle branch block is described in detail in Chapter 5.

Regression of Q Waves After Infarction

In the months following an acute infarction, the pathologic Q waves in the anterior or inferior leads may persist unchanged or they may regress in size, in

---

*As described on p. 358, diagnostic confusion with acute right ventricular infarctions may also arise because the ST elevations rarely extend as far left as V_5, simulating anterior infarction.

some cases disappearing entirely.* For example, in one serial study of postinfarction ECGs[43] the abnormal Q waves disappeared or regressed to normal limits in 15% of the cases reviewed after a mean period of about 18 months. Furthermore, in 6% of the cases there was complete normalization of the ECG 42 months after the acute transmural infarction. *Therefore the absence of abnormal Q waves or even the presence of an entirely normal ECG does not rule out previous "transmural" infarction.* Even patients with severe heart failure caused by multiple previous infarctions (ischemic cardiomyopathy) may not have Q waves. Coll et al.[16] studied 313 patients for a mean of 63 months after Q wave infarction and reported a loss of pathologic Q waves in 34 cases (11%). In this study, patients with Q wave regression had smaller-sized infarcts than those with persistent Q waves. In a similar study of patients who sustained a first acute Q wave infarction,[41] Q waves disappeared in 12 of 53 cases (23%). Not surprisingly, wall motion abnormalities were more severe in patients with persistent Q waves as compared to those with Q wave disappearance. Limitations of the ECG in the diagnosis of chronic as well as acute infarction are described in detail in Chapter 20.

There are five potential explanations for the regression of ischemic Q waves:

1. Q waves appearing during the course of myocardial ischemia do not necessarily indicate irreversible myocardial necrosis but may denote transient reversible "electrical shutdown" (stunning) of myocardial cells. If there is sufficient recovery of electrical function, R waves will "regenerate" over all or part of the ischemic tissue. (See "Effects of Reperfusion on Q Wave Evolution" below and Chapter 6.)

2. Q waves may regress following actual infarction if there is sufficient "scarring down" of the infarcted myocardium that the fibrotic zone has a smaller size than the original precinct of myocardial damage.

3. Q wave regression may occur paradoxically if a second new infarction develops involving the contralateral wall of the myocardium and produces what Evans[26] has called a *contrecoup effect.*† In such cases the new infarct will cause a loss of myocardial potentials in the opposing direction

---

*References 16, 41, 43, 62, 86, 93.

†Bassan et al.[7] cited the contrecoup principle to explain the apparently paradoxical appearance of new Q waves following aortocoronary bypass surgery in patients without evidence of new infarcts. The authors studied 11 patients in whom new Q waves developed postoperatively. In 7 there was definite evidence of new infarction to account for the Q waves; however, in 4, who had angiographic evidence of inferior wall dysfunction without Q waves before surgery, new inferior wall Q waves developed after surgery without evidence of reinfarction. The authors suggested that in these four cases the ECG pattern of inferior wall infarction was canceled by concomitant anterior wall injury. Postoperative improvement in anterior wall function may have allowed these latent inferior wall Q waves to become manifest. In this way the contrecoup principle has been cited to explain both the regression of Q waves seen in some cases of multiple infarctions and the unmasking of latent Q waves seen sometimes after successful myocardial revascularization. It should be emphasized, however, that the appearance of new Q waves following coronary artery bypass grafting generally indicates perioperative infarction.

(i.e., toward the first infarct). This realignment of depolarization vectors produced by the new infarct helps explain the diminution in negative forces (Q waves) over the area of the first infarct.

4. The Q waves of myocardial infarction may be masked by the appearance of a ventricular conduction disturbance. Left bundle branch block and the Wolff-Parkinson-White pattern both may mask anterior or inferior infarcts. Left anterior hemiblock occasionally masks an inferior wall infarct. (The effects of conduction disturbances on the ECG patterns of infarction are described in Chapter 5.)

5. Q wave regression may occur if there is hypertrophy of myocardial fibers near the infarcted zone. In such cases local augmentation in cardiac potentials may partially counterbalance the original loss of QRS forces.

Effects of Reperfusion on Q Wave Evolution

Reperfusion following acute total occlusion of a coronary artery may occur spontaneously (due to resolution of vasospasm or clot autolysis) or result from interventions (e.g., thrombolytic therapy, coronary angioplasty, coronary bypass graft surgery). Under any of these circumstances, the effects of reperfusion on Q wave evolution are likely to be quite variable and related to a number of factors, including the duration of coronary occlusion, the extent and location of necrosis, and the presence or absence of collateral blood flow. For example, very early reperfusion may entirely abrogate the appearance of Q waves. This scenario is perhaps best illustrated by the patient who presents with evidence of acute transmural ischemia (ST elevations) and in whom only a small non–Q wave infarct subsequently evolves associated with spontaneous reperfusion, prompt thrombolytic therapy (Fig. 2-1),* or coronary angioplasty.[37,39]

In most patients with acute infarction and ST segment elevations who receive thrombolytic therapy (intracoronary or intravenous), Q waves do evolve (Fig. 2-2). Indeed, both animal[6] and human[2] studies suggest that reperfusion may paradoxically *accelerate* R wave regression or Q wave appearance within the first minutes or hours of therapy. Beller et al.[8] correlated the rapid evolution of Q waves in dogs with a reperfusion-related injury characterized by subendocardial hemorrhage and transmural edema. In the days immediately following thrombolytic therapy, regeneration of R waves seems more likely to occur,[2,10,84] perhaps due to salvage of the myocardium and resolution of the reperfusion injury. However, for the reasons noted above, there is considerable variability in the electrocardiographic response to thrombolytic therapy and thus specific predictions in individual patients are not possible.[2,10,82,84] The effect of reperfusion on ischemic ST changes is discussed elsewhere (p. 175).

---

*note: Unless otherwise indicated, ECGs in this book are standardized so that 1 mV = 10 mm. In some cases original ECGs have been retouched for clarity.

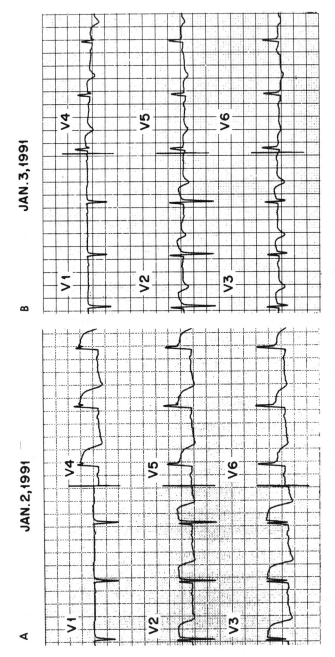

FIG. 2-1. A, Pronounced ST elevations (monophasic-type current of injury pattern). Intravenous thrombolytic therapy was given. **B,** The follow-up ECG shows evolving ischemic T wave inversions but no new Q waves. Creatine kinase peaked at 950 IU, with 6% MB fraction, on 1-2-91.

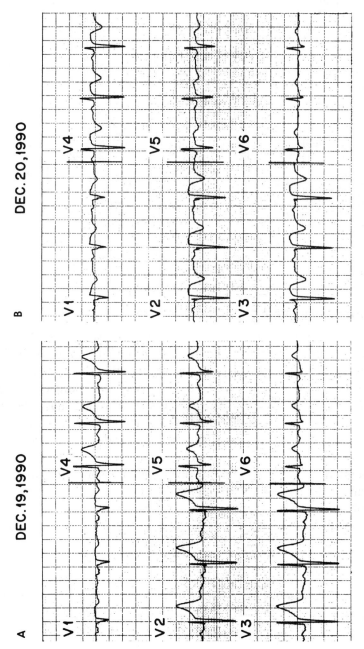

FIG. 2-2. A, ST elevations, most apparent in V_2 to V_4, on a tracing obtained from a 65-year-old man with chest pain. Note the minuscule Q wave in V_2. Left atrial abnormality is also present. The patient was given intravenous thrombolytic therapy. **B,** One day later, notice the classic evolution of an anterior wall Q wave infarction pattern with ST-T changes. Creatine kinase peaked at 1348 IU, with 16% MB fraction, on 12-20-90.

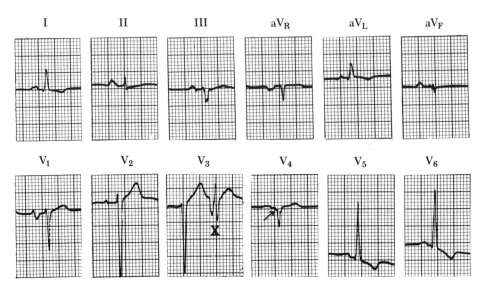

FIG. 2-3. Anterior wall infarction. The ECG of this 47-year-old woman with a history of previous infarction shows poor R wave progression in the precordial leads, with a QS complex in V_4. There is slight notching *(arrow)* on the descending arm of the QS. In V_3 the wide Q (as part of a QRS wave) in the ventricular premature beat *(X)* also is suggestive of underlying infarction.

Diagnosis of Myocardial Infarction from Premature Beats

Premature ventricular beats arising in either ventricle lead to asynchronous ventricular depolarization. In some cases this asynchrony may unmask the loss of electrical potentials caused by prior myocardial infarction that may not have been seen in normally conducted beats.* Fig. 2-3 shows an example of an infarct diagnosed from an extrasystole. The diagnosis of infarction should be suspected whenever the premature beat shows a QR or QRS morphology with a Q wave of at least 0.04 second duration in one or more leads (except aV_R). The specificity of this sign, based on a small number of patients,[20] appears to be relatively high. Premature ventricular contractions frequently show a QS morphology in the absence of infarction. Therefore only a QR or equivalent pattern is of diagnostic significance.[78] Finally, pathologic Q waves may sometimes be unmasked by aberrantly conducted supraventricular (atrial or AV junctional) beats.

Tall R Waves with Acute Myocardial Infarction

Q waves are a hallmark of infarction. In some cases, however, the earliest depolarization (QRS) change seen with acute coronary occlusion may be a paradoxical *increase* in R wave amplitude (and a decrease in S wave amplitude) in leads showing ST segment elevation.[25,52] The ECG in such cases resembles a

---

*References 9, 20, 23, 44, 49, 73, 76, 78, 81.

monophasic curve. This augmentation of R wave voltage has been described both during the earliest phase of acute myocardial infarction (Fig. 2-1) and with severe noninfarctional transmural ischemia (Fig. 8-9). The pattern is always transient and often followed by the appearance of Q waves.

The mechanism of such a paradoxical increase in R wave amplitude is not clear. Ekmekci et al.[25] were able to produce similar changes in dogs with intra-coronary infusions of hyperkalemic, hyponatremic, or 5% dextrose solutions. They speculated that the increase in R wave height might relate to an augmentation of the action potential, a local change in conductivity, or an aberration in ventricular depolarization. Subsequent observations in animals[4,21,37] and humans[4,5] have supported the role of decreased intramyocardial conduction velocity, possibly related to leakage of intracellular potassium from actively ischemic cells.[37] Clinically the appearance of tall R waves with prominent ST elevations during acute ischemia may indicate enhanced electrical instability associated with an increased susceptibility to ventricular fibrillation.[54]

Effect of Myocardial Infarction on Middle and Late QRS Forces

Clinical interest has focused primarily on the effect of infarction on the earliest phase of ventricular activation, which results in the appearance of pathologic Q waves. For many years there has also been recognition of the effects of infarction on the middle and late phases of ventricular depolarization. In some cases these changes can be recognized by the appearance of abnormal but nonspecific notching or slurring of the QRS following infarction. Subsequently investigators have used body surface maps[28,59] based on multiple leads to further study depolarization changes during the middle and late phases of ventricular activation. The potential clinical relevance of such techniques remains to be established, however.

In the past there has been particular interest in the possible effects of myocardial infarction on the terminal QRS forces, specifically on the relationship of such changes to ventricular conduction abnormalities. Discussion of these problems has generated considerable semantic confusion in the literature, centering on the relative merits of such concepts as *periinfarction block, parietal (focal) block, hemiblock,* etc. This topic has been surveyed in detail by Rosenbaum et al.[71] and is only briefly outlined here.

The possible effects of *chronic* myocardial infarction on terminal QRS forces were initially investigated by First, Bayley, and Bedford.[27] They described an ECG pattern following infarction characterized by a wide QRS, with QR waves in either the inferior or the anterior leads depending on the location of the infarct. These changes were ascribed to a local periinfarction block that could disrupt the normal subendocardial to epicardial spread of activation. As a consequence the injured zone might be depolarized in a delayed fashion by way of alternate pathways, with widening of the QRS and discordance of the initial (Q) and terminal (R) depolarization vectors. Grant and Murray[36] subsequently proposed that some cases of apparent periinfarction block might result from more proximal conduction delays in one of the fascicular subdivisions of the left bundle system. This concept of fascicular blocks and hemiblocks (p. 109) was expanded by Rosenbaum, Elizari, and Lazzari[71] and cited as an explanation for the terminal conduction changes seen with infarction as well as in many other settings. Subsequent analyses favored the importance of proximal versus more distal (parietal) left ventricular conduction blocks in explaining terminal QRS changes with myocardial infarction. However, there has been renewed interest more recently[29] in local periinfarction blocks and their relation to *late potentials* and ventricular arrhythmogenesis.

The effects of *acute* ischemia on the middle and later phases of ventricular activation have been described in connection with the pathogenesis of paradoxically tall R waves during the hyperacute phase of infarction or with variant angina (noninfarctional transmural ischemia) (p. 30).

Q WAVE GENESIS AND PATHOGENESIS: REVIEW AND PREVIEW

From a theoretical point of view, all Q waves may be placed in one or more of the following categories (see box):

1. *Physiologic or positional variants.* Depending on either the anatomic or the "electrical" position of the heart, Q waves may appear in certain leads in the absence of infarction or other pathologic findings; physiologic pseudoinfarct patterns are described in Chapter 3.
2. *Primary increase in negative cardiac potentials.* When cardiac hypertrophy occurs, leads facing the hypertrophied myocardium record an increase in positive voltage; leads facing away record a reciprocal increase in negative potentials, which may produce Q waves in some cases (see Chapter 4).
3. *Altered conduction.* Any significant change in the pathway of ventricular activation will affect the ECG pattern, and Q waves may appear in certain leads because of a change in the orientation of initial depolarization forces (see Chapter 5).
4. *Primary loss of positive myocardial potentials.* Any type of myocardial injury, ischemic or nonischemic, acute or chronic, that produces a sufficient deficit of positive depolarization forces can result in abnormal Q waves; pseudoinfarct patterns resulting from noninfarctional myocardial injury are described in Chapters 6 and 7.

In some cases a Q wave can be ascribed to a combination of factors. For example, the noninfarctional Q waves seen with right ventricular volume or pressure overload may be caused both by underlying right ventricular hypertrophy and by an alteration in cardiac position resulting from right-sided dilation.

EXAMPLES OF FACTORS ASSOCIATED WITH PSEUDOINFARCT Q WAVES*

1. **Physiologic or positional variants**
   Septal Q waves
   Left pneumothorax
2. **Ventricular enlargement**
   Right or left ventricular enlargement
   Hypertrophic cardiomyopathy
3. **Altered ventricular activation**
   Left bundle branch block
   Wolff-Parkinson-White patterns
4. **Myocardial damage or replacement**
   Dilated cardiomyopathies
   Amyloid heart disease

---

*See pp. 170 and 171 for a detailed summary of the differential diagnosis of Q waves.

REFERENCES

1. Abildskov JA, et al: An experimental study of the electrocardiographic effects of localized myocardial lesions, Am J Cardiol 8:485, 1961.
2. Anderson JL, et al: A randomized trial of streptokinase in the treatment of acute myocardial infarction, N Engl J Med 308, 1312, 1983.
3. Andre-Fouet X, et al: "Non–Q wave," alias "nontransmural," myocardial infarction: a specific entity, Am Heart J 117:892, 1989.
4. Barnhill JE, et al: The QRS complex during transient myocardial ischemia: studies in patients with variant angina pectoris and in a canine preparation, Circulation 71:901, 1985.
5. Barnhill JE et al: Depolarization changes early in the course of myocardial infarction: significance of changes in the terminal portion of the QRS complex, J Am Coll Cardiol 14:1413, 1989.
6. Barold SS, et al: Significance of transient electrocardiographic Q waves in coronary artery disease, Cardiol Clin 5:367, 1987.
7. Bassan MM, et al: New Q waves after aortocoronary bypass surgery: unmasking of an old infarction, N Engl J Med 290:349, 1974.
8. Beller GA, et al: Effects of ischaemia and coronary reperfusion on regional myocardial blood flow and on the epicardial electrogram, Cardiovasc Res 11:489, 1977.
9. Bisteni A, et al: Ventricular premature beats in the diagnosis of myocardial infarction, Br Heart J 23:521, 1961.
10. Blanke H, et al: Electrocardiographic changes after streptokinase-induced recanalization in patients with acute left anterior descending obstruction, Circulation 68:406, 1983.
11. Blanke H, et al: Electrocardiographic and coronary arteriographic correlations during acute myocardial infarction, Am J Cardiol 54:249, 1984.
12. Boden WE, et al: ST segment shifts are poor predictors of subsequent Q wave evolution in acute myocardial infarction. A natural history study of early non–Q wave infarction, Circulation 79:537, 1989.
13. Bodenheimer MM, et al: Q waves and ventricular asynergy: predictive value and hemodynamic significance of anatomic localization, Am J Cardiol 36:615, 1975.
14. Bodenheimer MM, et al: Correlation of pathologic Q waves on the standard electrocardiogram and the epicardial electrogram of the human heart, Circulation 54:213, 1976.
15. Bren GB, et al: The electrocardiogram in patients undergoing thrombolysis for myocardial infarction, Circulation 76(suppl II):18, 1987.
16. Coll S, et al: Significance of Q-wave regression after transmural acute myocardial infarction, Am J Cardiol 61:739, 1988.
17. Cook RW, et al: Electrocardiographic changes in acute subendocardial infarction. I. Large subendocardial and large nontransmural infarcts, Circulation 18:603, 1958.

18. Cook RW, et al: Electrocardiographic changes in acute subendocardial infarction. II. Small subendocardial infarcts, Circulation 18:613, 1958.
19. Daniels TM, et al: Comparison of human ventricular activation with a canine model in chronic myocardial infarction, Circulation 44:74, 1971.
20. Dash H, Ciotola TJ: Morphology of ventricular premature beats as an aid in the electrocardiographic diagnosis of myocardial infarction, Am J Cardiol 52:458, 1983.
21. David D, et al: Intramyocardial conduction: a major determinant of R-wave amplitude during myocardial ischemia, Circulation 65:161, 1982.
22. DeWood MA, et al: Coronary arteriographic findings soon after non–Q-wave myocardial infarction, N Engl J Med 315:417, 1986.
23. Dressler W: A case of myocardial infarction masked by bundle branch block but revealed by occasional premature ventricular beats, Am J Med Sci 206:361, 1943.
24. Durrer D, et al: Epicardial and intramural excitation in chronic myocardial infarction, Am Heart J 68:765, 1964.
25. Ekmekci A, et al: Angina pectoris. V. Giant R and receding S wave in myocardial ischemia and certain non-ischemic conditions, Am J Cardiol 7:521, 1961.
26. Evans W: Cardiographic contrecoup in the course of cardiac infarction, Br Heart J 25:713, 1963.
27. First SR, et al: Peri-infarction block: electrocardiographic abnormality occasionally resembling bundle branch block and local ventricular blocks of other types, Circulation 2:31, 1950.
28. Flowers NC, et al: New evidence for inferoposterior myocardial infarction on surface potential maps, Am J Cardiol 38:576, 1976.
29. Flowers NC, et al: Relation of peri-infarction block to ventricular late potentials in patients with inferior wall myocardial infarction, Am J Cardiol 66:568, 1990.
30. Freifeld AG, et al: Nontransmural versus subendocardial infarction. A morphologic study, Am J Med 75:423, 1983.
31. Fuchs RM, et al: Electrocardiographic localization of coronary artery narrowing: studies during myocardial ischemia and infarction in patients with one-vessel disease, Circulation 66:1168, 1982.
32. Georas CS, et al: Subendocardial infarction, Arch Intern Med 111:448, 1963.
33. Gibson RS: Non–Q-wave myocardial infarction: diagnosis, prognosis, and management, Curr Probl Cardiol 13:9, 1988.
34. Goldberger AL: Normal and noninfarct Q waves, Cardiol Clin 5:357, 1987.
35. Gottlieb RS, et al: Correlation of abnormal Q waves, coronary pathology, and ventricular contractility, Am Heart J 90:451, 1975.
36. Grant RP, Murray RH: The QRS complex deformity of myocardial infarction in the human subject, Am J Med 17:587, 1954.
37. Holland RP, Brooks H: The QRS complex during myocardial ischemia: an experimental analysis in the porcine heart, J Clin Invest 57:541, 1976.
38. Horan LG, et al: Significance of the diagnostic Q wave of myocardial infarction, Circulation 43:428, 1971.
39. Huey BL, et al: Acute non–Q wave myocardial infarction associated with early ST segment elevation: evidence for spontaneous coronary reperfusion and implications for thrombolytic trials, J Am Coll Cardiol 9:18, 1987.
40. Hutter AM Jr, et al: Nontransmural myocardial infarction: a comparison of hospital and late clinical course of patients with that of matched patients with transmural anterior and transmural inferior myocardial infarction, Am J Cardiol 48:595, 1981.
41. Jaarsma W, et al: Left ventricular wall motion with and without Q-wave disappearance after acute myocardial infarction, Am J Cardiol 59:516, 1987.
42. Kannel WB, Abbott RD: Incidence and prognosis of unrecognized myocardial infarction: an update on the Framingham study, N Engl J Med 311:1144, 1984.
43. Kaplan BM, Berkson DM: Serial electrocardiograms after myocardial infarction, Ann Intern Med 60:430, 1964.
44. Katz KH, et al: Acute myocardial infarction revealed by an isolated premature ventricular beat, Circulation 18:897, 1958.
45. Kleiger RE, et al: Frequency and significance of late evolution of Q waves in patients with initial non–Q wave acute myocardial infarction, Am J Cardiol 65:23, 1990.
46. Lazar EJ, et al: Atrial infarction. Diagnosis and management, Am Heart J 116:1058, 1988.
47. Levine HD, Ford RV: Subendocardial infarction: report of six cases and critical survey of literature, Circulation 1:246, 1950.

48. Levy W, et al: The nontransmural myocardial infarction in perspective, Cardiovasc Rev Rep 2:1285, 1981.
49. Lichtenberg SB, et al: Value of premature ventricular contraction morphology in the detection of myocardial infarction, J Electrocardiol 13:167, 1980.
50. Liu CK, et al: Atrial infarction of the heart, Circulation 23:331, 1961.
51. Lown B, et al: Unresolved problems in coronary care, Am J Cardiol 20:494, 1967.
52. Madias JE: The earliest electrocardiographic sign of acute transmural myocardial infarction, J Electrocardiol 10:193, 1977.
53. Madias JE, Krikelis EN: Transient giant R waves in the early phase of acute myocardial infarction: association with ventricular fibrillation, Clin Cardiol 4:339, 1981.
54. Madias JE, et al: A comparison of transmural and nontransmural acute myocardial infarction Circulation 49:498, 1974.
55. Madigan NP, et al: The clinical course, early prognosis, and coronary anatomy of subendocardial infarction, Am J Med 60:634, 1976.
56. Massumi RA, et al: Studies on the mechanism of ventricular activity. XVI. Activation of the human ventricle, Am J Med 19:832, 1955.
57. Maxwell M, et al: Studies on the mechanism of ventricular activity. VIII. The genesis of the coronary QS wave in through-and-through infarction, Am J Med 17:610, 1954.
58. Maxwell M, et al: Studies on the mechanism of ventricular activity. IX. The "mural-type" coronary QS wave, Am J Med 17:614, 1954.
59. Mirvis DM: Current status of body surface electrocardiographic mapping, Circulation 75:684, 1987.
60. Mirvis DM, et al: Electrocardiographic effects of experimental nontransmural myocardial infarction, Circulation 71:1206, 1985.
61. Ogawa H, et al: Classification of non-Q wave MI according to electrocardiographic changes, Br Heart J 54:473, 1985.
62. Pappas MP: Disappearance of pathological Q waves after infarction, Br Heart J 20:123, 1958.
63. Phibbs B: "Transmural" vs "subendocardial" myocardial infarction: an electrocardiographic myth, J Am Coll Cardiol 1:561, 1983.
64. Pipberger HV, Lopez EA: "Silent" subendocardial infarcts: fact or fiction, Am Heart J 100:597, 1980.
65. Pipberger HV, et al: Studies on the mechanism of ventricular activity. XXI. The origin of the depolarization complex with clinical applications, Am Heart J 54:511, 1957.
66. Prinzmetal M, et al: Intramural depolarization potentials in myocardial infarction: a preliminary report, Circulation 7:1, 1953.
67. Pruitt RD, et al: Certain clinical states associated with deeply inverted T waves in the precordial electrocardiogram, Circulation 11:517, 1955.
68. Raunio H, et al: Changes in the QRS complex and ST segment in transmural and subendocardial myocardial infarctions: a clinicopathologic study, Am Heart J 98:176, 1979.
69. Roberts R: Recognition, pathogenesis, and management of non-Q-wave infarction, Mod Conc Cardiovasc Dis 56:17, 1987.
70. Roberts WC, Gardin JM: Location of myocardial infarcts: a confusion of terms and definitions, Am J Cardiol 42:868, 1978.
71. Rosenbaum M, et al: The hemiblocks, Oldsmar Fla, 1970, Tampa Tracings.
72. Ross AM, et al: Electrocardiographic and angiographic correlations in myocardial infarction patients treated with thrombolytic agents. A report from the NHLBI Thrombolysis in Myocardial Infarction (TIMI) trial, J Am Coll Cardiol 2:495, 1985.
73. Salomon S, Silverman JJ: Myocardial infarction pattern disclosed by ventricular extrasystoles, Am J Cardiol 4:695, 1959.
74. Savage RM, et al: Correlation of postmortem anatomic findings with electrocardiographic changes in patients with myocardial infarction, Circulation 55:279, 1977.
75. Schechtman KB: Risk stratification of patients with non-Q wave myocardial infarction. The critical role of ST segment depression, Circulation 80:1148, 1989.
76. Simonson E, et al: Coronary insufficiency revealed by ectopic nodal and ventricular beats in the presence of left bundle branch block, Am J Med Sci 209:349, 1945.
77. Sodi-Pallares D, et al: Unipolar QS morphology and Purkinje potential of the free left ventricular wall: the concept of electrical endocardium, Circulation 23:836, 1961.
78. Sodi-Pallares D, et al: Electrocardiographic diagnosis of myocardial infarction in the presence of bundle branch block (right and left), ventricular premature beats, and

Wolff-Parkinson-White syndrome, Prog Cardiovasc Dis 6:107, 1963.

79. Spodick DH: Q-wave infarction versus S-T infarction: nonspecificity of electrocardiographic criteria for differentiating transmural and nontransmural lesions, Am J Cardiol 51:913, 1983.

80. Sullivan W, et al: Correlation of electrocardiographic and pathologic findings in healed myocardial infarction, Am J Cardiol 42:724, 1978.

81. Szilagyi N, Ginsburg M: Acute myocardial infarction revealed in the presence of right bundle branch block and ventricular extrasystoles, Am J Cardiol 9:632, 1962.

82. Timmis GC: Electrocardiographic effects of reperfusion, Cardiol Clin 5:427, 1987.

83. Varat MA: Non-transmural infarction: clinical distinction between patients with ST depression and those with T wave inversion, J Electrocardiol 18:15, 1985.

84. Von Essen R, et al: Myocardial infarction and thrombolysis: electrocardiographic short term and long term results using precordial mapping, Br Heart J 54:6, 1985.

85. Wagner GS: Clinical usefulness of quantitative ECG methods for evaluating ischemic and infarcted myocardium, Cardiol Clin 5:447, 1987.

86. Wasserman AG, et al: Prognostic implications of diagnostic Q waves after myocardial infarction, Circulation 65:1451, 1982.

87. Whipple GH: Current concepts in electrocardiography: a critique of the unipolar approach to interpretation, Med Clin North Am 41:1193, 1957.

88. Wilkinson RS Jr, et al: Electrocardiographic and pathologic features of myocardial infarction in man: a correlative study, Am J Cardiol 11:24, 1963.

89. Willich SN, et al: High-risk subgroups of patients with non–Q wave myocardial infarction based on direction and severity of ST segment deviation, Am Heart J 114:1110, 1987.

90. Wilson FN, et al: The form of the electrocardiogram in experimental myocardial infarction. IV. Additional observations on the later effects produced by ligation of the anterior descending branch of the left coronary artery, Am Heart J 10:1025, 1935.

91. Wilson FN, et al: The precordial electrocardiogram, Am Heart J 27:19, 1944.

92. Yu PNG, Stewart JM: Subendocardial myocardial infarction with special reference to the electrocardiographic changes, Am Heart J 39:862, 1950.

93. Yusuf S, et al: Factors of importance for QRS complex recovery after acute myocardial infarction, Acta Med Scand 211:157, 1982.

3

Normal-variant Q waves and related patterns

Q waves may be found normally in any of the 12 conventional ECG leads. Small *septal* q waves (Fig. 3-1), reflecting the left-to-right spread of depolarization forces in the ventricular septum, are part of the normal qR complexes seen in the left precordial leads and in I and aV_L (if the heart is electrically *horizontal*) or II, III, and aV_F (if the heart is electrically *vertical*). These normal septal q waves are less than 0.04 second in duration and are usually less than 25% of the R wave amplitude in that complex.[21]

However, Q waves of 0.04 second or more duration or of relatively deep amplitude may be found normally in aV_L, V_1, V_2, III, and aV_F (in addition to aV_R); and *positional* Q waves are found in dextrocardia, occasionally associated with left pneumothorax, and also in pectus excavatum, congenital absence of the left pericardium, and complete corrected transposition of the great arteries.

One normal variant discussed in this chapter, the early precordial transition zone pattern, is not associated with Q waves at all, but with tall right precordial R waves that may simulate posterior infarction.

Misplacement of limb leads or chest leads constitutes another positional variant that must always be excluded in the differential diagnosis of Q waves. Therefore these and other spurious causes of noninfarctional Q waves are considered first.

SPURIOUS AND ARTIFACTUAL Q WAVES

As with other clinical tests, the interpretation of apparently abnormal ECG patterns always requires excluding possible technical errors. Reversal of limb leads and improper placement of chest electrodes can both produce spurious Q waves.

Reversal of limb leads is a not infrequent cause of unexpected infarction patterns. Examples of anterolateral and inferior pseudoinfarct patterns produced by

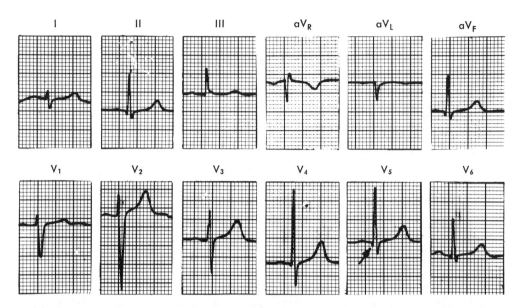

FIG. 3-1. Normal "septal" q waves. The arrow in V_5 points to a physiologic q wave related to the left-to-right orientation of the early ventricular septal activation forces. Small septal q waves are also seen in V_4, V_6, II, III, and aV_F. Lead aV_L shows a normal-variant QS pattern sometimes seen with an electrically "vertical" frontal plane QRS axis.

extremity lead reversals are shown in Fig. 3-2. Such spurious patterns can usually be easily recognized. (1) Q waves in I caused by true infarction are almost invariably associated with abnormal Q waves in the lateral precordial leads as well (V_5 and V_6). When spurious Q waves caused by lead reversal are present in the limb leads, the precordial leads will not be affected. (2) Q waves produced in the inferior leads (II, III, and aV_F) by limb reversal are generally associated with *inverted* P waves and a normal PR interval (Fig. 3-2, C).

Improper placement of the precordial leads is a more subtle source of error that can produce *poor R wave progression* patterns and sometimes actual QS waves in the right precordial leads. Thus if the right precordial chest leads are placed too high (for example, in the second or third interspace), they will overlie the base of the heart, a region of electrical negativity, and the normal precordial R wave progression may be lost.

Spurious poor R wave progression in the precordial leads is particularly common in women because of misplacement of the chest leads. A frequent technical error is placement of one or more chest electrodes *on* the left breast (instead of under it) when recording the middle and lateral precordial leads. As a result cardiac potentials from higher interspaces will be obtained, producing poor R wave progression.

Other causes of spurious Q waves include mislabeling the leads, mounting

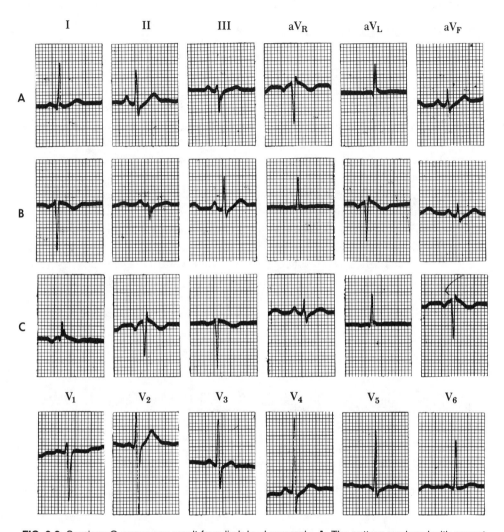

FIG. 3-2. Spurious Q waves can result from limb lead reversals. **A,** The pattern produced with correct limb lead placement. **B,** A lateral wall pseudoinfarct pattern is produced by reversal of the left and right arm electrodes. **C,** An inferior wall pseudoinfarct pattern is produced when the left and right leg electrodes are reversed. Note that the precordial leads (V_1 to V_6) *(bottom tracing)* show normal R wave progression. There is flattening of the T wave in the lateral leads (V_4 to V_6). Lead aV_L (in **A**) also shows T wave flattening. This ECG was recorded from a healthy 25-year-old man who had just eaten a large meal; the nonspecific ST-T alterations may therefore represent functional postprandial repolarization changes.

leads upside down, and inadvertently taking the ECG at fast paper speed (i.e., 50 mm/sec instead of 25 mm/sec), a technical oversight that will "stretch" normal septal q waves into large Q waves.

QS OR Qr COMPLEXES IN aV_L

When the heart is electrically *vertical,* Q waves as part of a QS (Fig. 3-1) or occasionally a Qr (Fig. 3-3) complex may appear as normal variants in aV_L, simulating the pattern of lateral wall infarction.[19,21,52]

These Q wave variants have been ascribed to positional factors.[19,21] The normal variant QS_{aV_L} is said to represent transmission of left ventricular cavity (QS) potentials to the left arm. The Qr_{aV_L} has been attributed to *backward rotation* of the cardiac apex, permitting back-of-the-heart (Qr) potentials to be transmitted to the left arm.

However, the QS pattern in aV_L cannot rigorously be considered a reflection of *ventricular* cavity potentials. The term *cavity potential* (which has been widely used in the past to explain certain unipolar patterns) should be used only to describe a complex that is at least qualitatively similar to the pattern actually recorded in the particular cardiac chamber. Left ventricular intracavity electrodes normally record a *positive* P wave followed by a QS complex with a negative T wave.[52] The normal variant QS_{aV_L}, however, is usually preceded by a *negative* P wave[19] and therefore cannot be considered exactly equivalent to a left ventricular cavity potential.

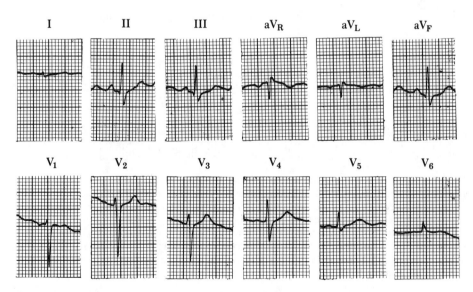

FIG. 3-3. Normal-variant Qr complex in aV_L simulating an anterior wall infarction. Lead aV_L may show noninfarctional Q waves as part of QS (Fig. 3-1) or Qr complexes when the heart is electrically vertical. Lead I and the lateral precordial leads will *not* show abnormal Q waves.

Although the QS_{aV_L} cannot be attributed to direct transmission of ventricular cavity potentials, it does resemble the pattern recorded from leads overlying the base of the heart (e.g., potentials from the left subclavian vein[5]). Similarly the Qr_{aV_L} variant resembles the pattern recorded from appropriately placed dorsal leads, although there is no evidence of actual backward rotation of the apex in such cases. However, for conceptual purposes, the QS_{aV_L} can be considered equivalent to base-of-the-heart potentials whereas the Qr_{aV_L} is equivalent to back-of-the-heart potentials.

Differential diagnosis. The positional Q waves just described can usually be readily differentiated from pathologic Q waves in lead aV_L on the basis of (1) the absence of abnormal Q waves in lead I and the lateral precordial leads and (2) the absence of marked ST-T abnormalities in lead aV_L.

Lead I and lateral precordial leads. Normal variant Q waves in aV_L are *not* accompanied by prominent (≥ 0.04 sec) Q waves in I or the lateral precordial leads.

ST-T complex. The QS or Qr variant in aV_L is usually accompanied by slight T wave inversions. However, marked ST segment elevations or deep T wave inversions (greater than 5 mm) are not seen in the normal ECG pattern.

QS COMPLEXES IN V_1 AND V_2

A QS complex is commonly present in V_1 as a normal variant. Rarely a QS complex in V_1 and V_2 is found in normal subjects (Fig. 3-4), simulating the pattern of anterior infarction.[36]

In most cases the initial forces of septal depolarization are oriented anteriorly and to the right, producing the small septal r waves usually seen in the right precordial leads. A QS complex in these leads could occur theoretically if (1)

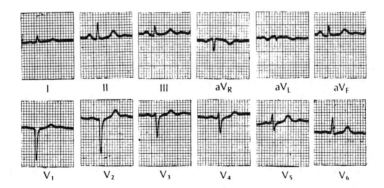

FIG. 3-4. Normal-variant QS in V_1 and V_2 from a patient who had no clinical evidence of heart disease and no cardiac pathologic condition at autopsy. Differentiation of this normal variant from actual anterior infarction may be impossible on the basis of a single tracing. (From Goldman MJ: Principles of clinical electrocardiography, ed 11, Los Altos Calif, 1982, Lange Medical Publications.)

these initial septal forces were oriented at right angles to the exploring electrodes or (2) the initial septal forces were oriented away from (at greater than right angles to) the positive poles of the right precordial leads. This normal variation in the direction of the septal depolarization vector could result from either an actual anatomic shift in the position of the septum relative to the chest leads[18] or from an intrinsic change in the balance of early depolarization forces.

If the initial septal forces were directed precisely at right angles to a right precordial lead axis, the septal forces would be recorded as an isoelectric line rather than as a positive r wave deflection.[18,19] In this way the septal r wave would be "masked," and V_1 or V_1 and V_2 could record a noninfarctional QS complex instead of the rS wave usually seen.

This masking hypothesis can be tested (Fig. 3-5) by recording a right precordial QS complex (in this case from V_{5R} in a normal subject) simultaneously with the QRS complexes in II and III. If the right precordial QS complex actually resulted from the isoelectric masking of the septal r wave, then the QS complex should commence approximately 0.02 second (duration of the normal septal r wave) after the onset of the QRS complex in other leads in which the septal forces were not masked (II and III in this case). The tracings shown in Fig. 3-5 are consistent with the masking hypothesis and suggest that in certain cases the QS complexes seen in the right precordial leads may result from similar orientation of septal forces at right angles to the exploring leads.

As mentioned previously, a right precordial QS complex might also theoretically result from the spread of early forces *away from* the right precordial leads in the absence of infarction. In such cases the septal forces would be recorded as an initial negative deflection rather than as a positive r wave or an isoelectric line, and the QS complex would commence synchronously with the QRS complexes in other leads.

Differential diagnosis. It may be difficult (and sometimes impossible) to distinguish the normal-variant QS in V_1 and V_2 from the pattern of anteroseptal infarction or fibrosis.

Physiologic QS waves normally do not extend to the left of V_2. A possible exception to this has been reported[30] in an apparently normal 22-year-old basketball player whose ECG demonstrated QS complexes in V_1 to V_3. However, in most cases a QS in V_1 to V_3 suggests either improper chest lead placement or one of the other conditions listed on p. 170. *Clinically, common pathologic causes of a QS in V_1 to V_2 or V_3 are anterior infarction, left ventricular hypertrophy, left bundle branch block, and chronic obstructive lung disease.* (See p. 170 for a complete summary of the differential diagnosis of a QS in V_1 to V_3 and p. 44 for a discussion of "poor R wave progression.")

The morphology of the QS may also help in distinguishing normal from pathologic Q waves. The normal QS in V_1 and V_2 is usually sharply inscribed, without notching or slurring (Fig. 3-4). Myocardial damage, however, some-

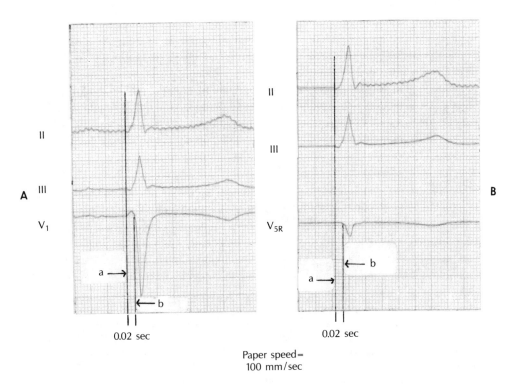

FIG. 3-5. Right precordial QS caused by the masking of septal forces in a normal subject. **A,** Leads II and III recorded synchronously with V_1. The electrical axis is vertical; note the qR complexes in II and III with small q waves of about 0.02 second duration. Lead V_1 shows an rS complex with the septal r also of about 0.02 second duration (distance between the vertical lines *a* and *b*). The onset of depolarization in all three leads is the same (line *a*). **B,** Leads II and III recorded synchronously with V_{5R}. Once again, note the small septal q waves. The onset of depolarization in all three of these leads is, likewise, shown by line *a*. Lead V_{5R} records a QS complex. However, note that the septal r wave in V_1 of **A** is not apparent in this lead. Instead, an isoelectric line is recorded in V_{5R} at the same time that the septal q waves are being inscribed in II and III. The apparent delay between the onset of depolarization in leads II and III (line *a*) and the onset of depolarization in V_{5R} (line *b*) is approximately 0.02 second in duration. Thus the isoelectric line in V_{5R} of **B** suggests that the septal r wave in V_1 of **A** is being masked, which could occur if the initial septal forces responsible for the r wave in V_1 were oriented at right angles to the axis of V_{5R}. In that case septal forces would be recorded as an isoelectric line rather than as a positive (septal r) wave.

times produces notching or slurring, especially on the initial downstroke of the QS wave (Fig. 3-6).

Finally, the normal $QS_{V_1-V_2}$ variant may be associated with a positive, isoelectric, or slightly negative T wave. The presence of marked ST deviation or deep T wave inversions (greater than 5 mm) should suggest underlying septal ischemia or right ventricular strain. Furthermore, the presence of an upright T wave in lead V_1 followed by a negative T wave in lead V_2 is always abnormal.

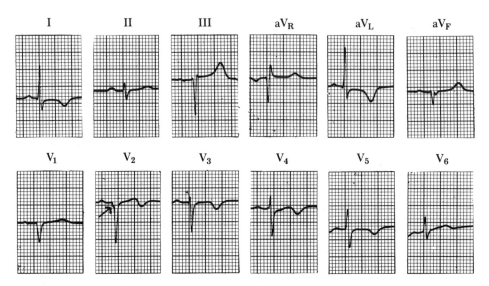

FIG. 3-6. Anteroseptal infarction. On the ECG of this 49-year-old man with coronary artery disease and angina, QS waves are present in V_1 and V_2, consistent with an anteroseptal infarction of indeterminate age. T wave inversions suggesting anterior wall ischemia appear in V_2 to V_5 and in I and aV_L. The arrow in V_2 points to characteristic notching of the initial downstroke of the QS. Downstroke notching is particularly suggestive of underlying myocardial damage. QS waves may also be seen in V_1 and V_2 as a normal variant (Fig. 3-4).

"POOR" PRECORDIAL R WAVE PROGRESSION

Using the term poor R wave progression, as commonly applied by electrocardiographers, may create some confusion, because the pattern is not clearly defined and it may have multiple etiologies.[4] Normally, as one progresses from V_1 to the middle and lateral chest leads, there is a relative increase in R wave amplitude and also in the R/S ratio. Poor R wave progression usually describes ECGs on which there are relatively small r waves (or frank QS waves) in V_1 to V_3.* Although precise criteria for this pattern have not been established, Zema et al.[64] arbitrarily required an R wave of ≤ 3 mm (0.3 mV) in V_3 and $R_{V_2} \leq R_{V_3}$.

There are multiple conditions associated with poor R wave progression. Zema et al.[64,65,67] observed it in 8% of hospitalized patients. The four most common causes in their series were (1) anterior infarction, (2) left ventricular hypertrophy, (3) chronic obstructive pulmonary disease, and (4) normal variant. Poor R wave progression can also be due to chest lead misplacement, left bundle branch block (complete or incomplete), and any of the other conditions listed on p. 170 that may be associated with actual QS waves in V_1 to V_3.

---

*The term *poor R wave progression* should not be applied when there is a prominent R wave in V_1 (i.e., R>S) with a subsequent decrease in R wave amplitude such that $R_{V_1} > R_{V_2} > R_{V_3}$. This pattern may be seen with severe right ventricular hypertrophy (Fig. 4-4), among other conditions, and has been referred to as "reversed" R wave progression.[67] However, the term "poor R wave progression" should be reserved for cases in which the R waves in V_1 to V_3 are diminutive or absent.

QS OR QR COMPLEXES IN III AND aV$_F$

The differentiation of pathologic and normal Q waves in leads III and aV$_F$ is a frequent and troublesome problem for electrocardiographers. A Q wave may be present in lead III alone or in leads III and aV$_F$ (Fig. 3-7) as a normal finding.[35]

Q$_{III}$ Wave

A Q wave in III as part of a QS, QR, or Qr type of complex is a common normal variant. The T wave in such cases is usually slightly inverted (Fig. 3-7). Lead III is a bipolar lead that represents the difference in potentials between the left leg and the left arm. A Q wave in lead III therefore simply indicates that the initial forces oriented toward the left arm (aV$_L$) are more positive (or less negative) than those oriented toward the left leg (aV$_F$).[35]

Simonson[51] reported prominent Q waves in lead III in 12% of a sample of healthy men 18 to 25 years of age and in 20% of a sample of healthy men 26 to 57 years of age.

Differential diagnosis. Criteria that have been suggested in the past for distinguishing pathologic from normal Q waves in III have not proved to be reliable. Pardee[41] originally proposed that a Q$_{III}$ be considered abnormal if it exceeded 25% of the amplitude of the R wave in any of the standard leads (provided a rightward axis was not present). Bayley[3] later suggested that a Q$_{III}$ of 0.04 second or more duration was abnormal. However, Q waves that exceed these limits are not uncommon in normal subjects. Weisbart and Simonson,[60] for example, found the upper limits of normal for the duration of the Q$_{III}$ to be as high as 0.06 second. The normal variant Q$_{III}$ usually decreases in size with inspiration secondary to the change in position of the heart (Fig. 3-8). However, pathologic Q waves in III may also decrease in size with inspiration. Therefore this maneuver cannot be used for reliable differentiation of the pathologic and normal Q$_{III}$.[5,33,50]

In summary: The diagnosis of infarction exclusively on the basis of a Q wave in III will result in an unacceptably high number of false-positive readings. Occasionally a Q$_{III}$ will be the only sign of inferior wall infarction. In such cases the diagnosis can sometimes be made with reasonable certainty if the Q$_{III}$ appears acutely and is associated with evolving ST-T changes in two or more of the inferior limb leads. However, as a general rule a Q$_{III}$ should not be considered definitely abnormal in the absence of pathologic Q waves in II and aV$_F$. In equivocal cases, as discussed below, the echocardiogram may be helpful. The utility of the vectorcardiogram (VCG) is also discussed in the next section.

Q$_{III}$ and Q$_{aV_F}$ Waves

The diagnosis of inferior wall infarction is made more difficult because prominent Q waves may also be present in both III and aV$_F$ in the absence of infarction (Fig. 3-7).

A Q$_{aV_F}$ is generally considered abnormal if it is 25% or more larger than the

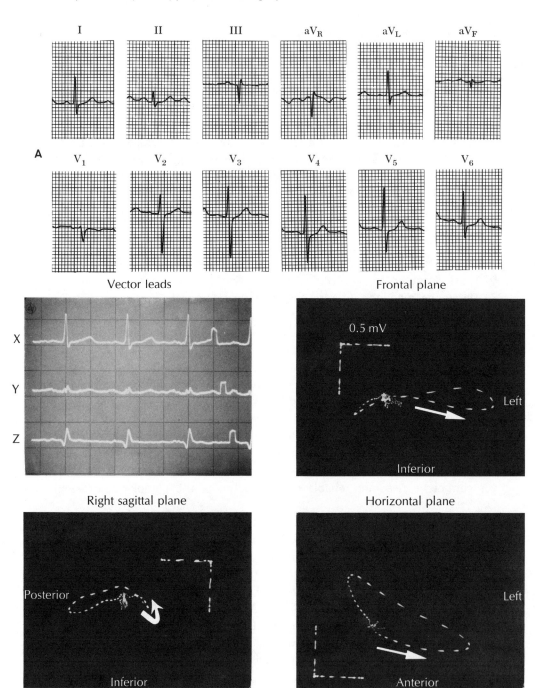

FIG. 3-7. Positional (physiologic) Q waves in leads III and aV_F. **A,** The scalar ECG of a 40-year-old man without clinical evidence of coronary disease showing Q waves in III and aV_F (or possibly a miniscule R wave in aV_F). Note the QR pattern in aV_R. **B,** Frank lead vectorcardiogram from the same patient. Note here the leftward orientation of the initial QRS forces in the frontal plane, which is in contrast to the superior orientation seen with inferior infarction. (Compare Fig. 3-9.)

III

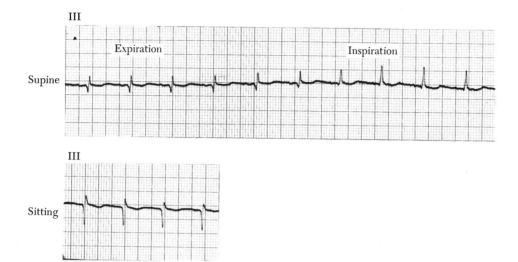

FIG. 3-8. Effect of position and respiration on the physiologic Q_{III}. Note the decreased size of this wave with inspiration and the increase with change from a supine to a sitting position. Pathologic Q waves in the inferior leads may also show positional and respiratory change. Therefore such maneuvers are not of diagnostic help.

R wave in aV_F or its duration equals or exceeds 40 msec.[21] More recently, a Q_{aV_F} exceeding 30 milliseconds has been suggested as a useful sign of inferior infarction.[59] However, Q waves meeting these criteria as part of a QS, QR, or Qr type of complex in aV_F may also be found in normal subjects. The T wave may be upright or slightly inverted in such cases.

The Q_{III} or Q_{aV_F} pattern has been attributed to positional factors.[34,48] If the apex of the heart were rotated anteriorly, electrical potentials from the posterior basal surface of the heart (i.e., QS or QR complexes) might theoretically be transmitted to the left leg. Rubin and Most[48] observed prominent Q waves in lead aV_F in patients with marked elevation of the diaphragm caused by artificial pneumoperitoneum. These physiologic Q waves were largest during expiration, when the diaphragm was most elevated. During inspiration the Q_{aV_F} diminished in size or disappeared entirely in some cases.

The normal variant Q_{aV_F} may also vary in prominence depending on the position of the patient. For example, a Q_{aV_F} that is present when the patient is supine may disappear when an ECG is taken while the patient is sitting, or in other cases (Fig. 3-8) it may become larger.[48] However, pathologic Q waves in leads III and aV_F may show a similar variability caused by respiratory and postural changes. Therefore such maneuvers cannot be used reliably to differentiate normal and pathologic Q waves in either III or aV_F.[33,48,50]

Differential diagnosis. Definitive assessment of the significance of inferior Q waves is often impossible from the ECG alone. In certain cases vectorial analysis can aid deciding whether prominent Q waves in III and aV_F are positional or

Inferior myocardial infarction

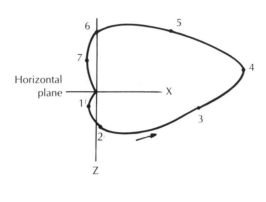

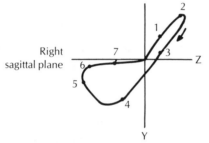

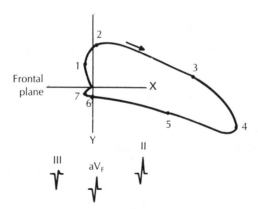

FIG. 3-9. An inferior wall infarction causes abnormal superior displacement of the initial QRS vector in the frontal and sagittal planes. Numbers on the loops indicate the position of the cardiac vector at 10 msec intervals. (Compare with Fig. 3-7, *B,* showing the vectorcardiogram associated with normal-variant inferior Q waves.) (With permission from Chou TC, et al: Clinical vectorcardiography, ed 2, New York, 1977, Grune & Stratton Inc.)

pathologic. When inferior infarction occurs, there is a primary loss of inferiorly directed depolarization forces in the frontal plane and a reciprocal gain in superiorly directed forces (Fig. 3-9). In cases of inferior infarction, therefore, the initial depolarization vector tends (although not invariably) to be displaced superiorly, producing an initial r wave in aV_R (Fig. 4-8). In other cases of inferior wall infarction, aV_R may show only a QS complex. However, a QR or Qr pattern in aV_R is not typically seen in cases of inferior infarction unless concomitant anterior wall injury is present.[20]

Positional Q waves in the inferior leads (III and aV_F), as opposed to the pathologic Q waves of infarction, reflect the orientation of initial forces horizontally and to the left rather than in a superior direction. Consequently when positional Q waves are present in the inferior leads, aV_R will usually not show an rS type of complex but may show a QS, QR, or Qr complex.[20] Fig. 3-7 shows the ECG and VCG patterns in a case of positional Q waves in leads III and aV_F. Fig. 3-9 depicts the typical VCG pattern of inferior infarction.

In summary: A large Q wave in III and aV_F in the presence of an rS (RS) complex in aV_R is usually abnormal whereas a Q_{III} or Q_{aV_F} in the presence of a QR in aV_R indicates that the Q waves may be positional. A QS in lead aV_R, however, may be present in association with either pathologic or normal variant Q waves in III and aV_F and is therefore of no diagnostic significance.

Examination of lead II may also be helpful. Prominent Q waves in II, III, and aV_F are almost always abnormal. The small septal q waves seen normally in II with an electrically vertical heart are always of less than 0.04 second duration and less than 25% the amplitude of the R wave in that lead. Q waves exceeding either of these dimensions are usually abnormal. (NOTE: Pectus excavatum may be associated with prominent but narrow Q waves in the inferior leads as an apparently normal variant.) The presence of large Q waves in II, III, and aV_F, though usually abnormal, does not necessarily indicate infarction. Other pathologic noninfarctional causes of Q waves simulating inferior infarction are listed on p. 171.

Several studies[25,53,54] suggest that the VCG may be more sensitive than the standard scalar ECG in diagnosing prior inferior infarction. For example, Stein and Simon[54] studied 31 patients with angiographic evidence of right coronary occlusion, most of whom also had inferior wall motion abnormalities. The ECG showed 0.04-second Q waves in III and aV_F in only 29% of cases. By contrast, depending on the criteria used, up to 77% of cases showed VCG evidence of prior inferior MI, without an increase in the number of false-positive diagnoses. Howard et al.,[25] in a similar study of patients with inferior wall motion abnormalities, found that the diagnostic sensitivity of the ECG was 63% compared to 81% for the VCG. The superior accuracy of VCG[53,54,62] versus traditional ECG[37,57] criteria in the diagnosis of inferior infarction was supported in a subsequent evaluation.[27] However, two later studies[23,32] have challenged the claim since they did not reveal any significant differences in the accuracy of VCG versus ECG for the diagnosis of inferior infarction in patients undergoing cardiac catheterization.

In cases of equivocal inferior lead Q waves, echocardiographic examination may be of considerable help. The presence of a segmental inferior wall motion abnormality strongly suggests underlying infarction, although its absence does not rule out this diagnosis. (See Chapter 22.)

NORMAL-VARIANT EARLY PRECORDIAL TRANSITION VERSUS POSTERIOR INFARCTION

In progressing from V_1 to the left precordial leads, there is normally a relative increase in the size of the R wave and a concomitant decrease in S wave amplitude. The lead in which the R/S ratio is 1 or greater is referred to as the *transition zone*. In most normal tracings the transition zone occurs at about the V_3 or V_4 position. Displacement of the zone to the right is known as counterclockwise rotation[61] or *early precordial transition*. Counterclockwise rotation may appear as a normal variant (Fig. 3-10) or be a nonspecific finding in abnormal conditions. For example, an early precordial transition can occur with congenital or acquired *dextroversion,* in which the left ventricle is displaced more anteriorly. Several studies[40,45,46,66] have suggested that prominent right precordial R waves, without a wide QRS, may be due to an atypical septal, right ventricular, or even left ventricular conduction disturbance.

Early precordial R wave transition, occurring as a normal variant, is sometimes confused with the pattern of posterior wall infarction, which also produces tall R waves in the right to middle precordial leads.[29,43,66]

Posterior infarction (Figs. 3-11 and 3-12) refers to infarction of the dorsal area of the heart.* The major ECG feature of posterior wall infarction is an increase in the voltage of the R waves in the right to midprecordial leads. This increase is reciprocal to a primary decrease in posteriorly directed forces. Posterior wall infarction is one cause of an R/S ratio equal to or greater than 1 in V_1 and V_2. The R waves are usually wide (0.04 sec or more) in these leads.[43] The ST-T segments in the right precordial leads may show a variable pattern, depending on the stage of infarction. In cases of acute infarction, the right to middle precordial leads typically show ST depressions reciprocal to the primary ST elevations that would be recorded by a lead placed over the dorsal aspect of the heart (Fig. 3-11). When the T waves become inverted over the posterior surface, the right to middle precordial leads show reciprocally tall positive T waves[12] (Fig. 3-12).

In most cases posterior wall infarction also involves part of the inferior or lateral walls of the left ventricle, and the ECG will also show abnormal Q waves in the appropriate leads in addition to the prominent right precordial R waves. Occasionally, however, an increase in the R/S ratio in the right precordial leads may be the major ECG indication of infarction. Huey et al.[26] reported that the

---

*As noted in Chapter 2 the precise electrocardiographic distinction between pure inferior and "true" posterior infarction is not supported by pathologic studies.

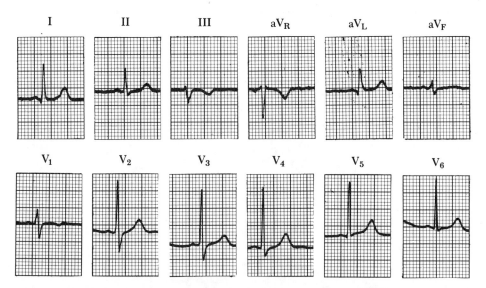

FIG. 3-10. Normal-variant early precordial transition simulating a posterior infarction. This patient, a 58-year-old woman, had no clinical evidence of heart disease. Her ECG shows an early precordial transition zone (counterclockwise rotation) with prominent R waves in the right precordial leads. This variant, especially in older patients, may be mistaken for the pattern of posterior wall infarction, which also produces tall right precordial R waves. However, posterior wall infarction is also frequently associated with the ECG signs of inferior or lateral wall ischemia (Fig. 3-12). Furthermore, QRS voltages in the lateral precordial leads are often decreased with posterior infarction (voltage drop-off pattern, Figs. 3-11 and 3-12).

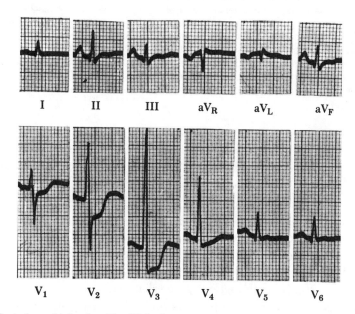

FIG. 3-11. Posterior wall infarction. The ECG of a patient with posterior wall aneurysm documented at autopsy shows prominent R waves in the right precordial leads. ST depressions in these leads do not necessarily reflect anterior wall ischemia but are probably reciprocal to primary ST elevations that would have been recorded over the posterior aneurysm. Note the marked decrease in voltage in the lateral precordial leads (voltage drop-off pattern), which is often helpful in distinguishing normal-variant right precordial R waves from the similar R waves of posterior infarction (compare with Fig. 3-10). (From Perloff JK: Circulation 30:706, 1964. By permission of the American Heart Association Inc.)

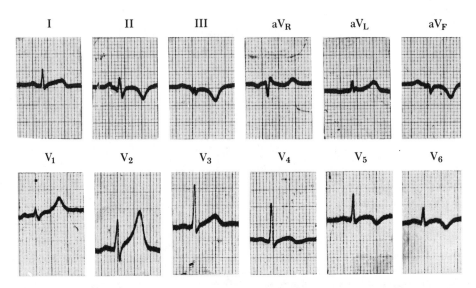

FIG. 3-12. Posteroinferior wall infarction. The ECG of a patient with evolving infarction consistent with both inferior and posterior wall damage shows Q waves in II, III, and aV_F, with T wave inversions in these leads. True posterior infarction is suggested by the relatively prominent R waves in V_1 and V_2 associated with positive T waves. These tall right precordial T waves are reciprocal to T wave negativity over the inferior and posterior surface of the heart. In addition, there are T wave inversions in V_5 and V_6 that are consistent with lateral wall ischemia. Tall R waves in the right precordial leads raise the possibility of right ventricular hypertrophy. However, the diagnosis of posterior infarction is supported by the associated Q waves in II, III, and aV_F and by tall positive T waves in the right precordial leads. Right ventricular hypertrophy does not produce abnormal Q waves in the inferior leads and is often associated with T wave inversions (strain pattern) in the right precordial leads and with right axis deviation (compare with Fig. 4-4). This tracing also shows the characteristic decrease in lateral precordial lead QRS potentials (voltage drop-off pattern), which is frequently seen with posterior infarction and probably reflects concomitant loss of lateral wall potentials (Fig. 3-11).

electrocardiographic pattern of "posterior" infarction with an R/S ratio ≥ 1 in V_1 was highly correlated with occlusion of the left circumflex coronary artery, and only rarely with right coronary artery occlusion. However, a prominent R wave in V_2 (and not V_1) occurred nearly as often with left circumflex as with right coronary occlusion. (See also Chapter 20.)

Differential diagnosis. Posterior infarction is also usually associated with a characteristic voltage "drop-off" pattern in the left precordial leads (Figs. 3-11 and 3-12). With posterior infarction the voltage typically peaks in V_3 and V_4 and then falls off abruptly in the lateral precordial leads (V_5 and V_6). This loss of leftward forces in the horizontal plane is probably caused by lateral wall extension of the infarct and is not a usual feature of normal variant counterclockwise rotation.

The tall right precordial R waves seen on the scalar ECG with posterior infarction are reflected by abnormal anterior orientation of QRS forces in the horizontal plane of the VCG. However, studies[1,22] have shown that some normal adults can show anterior displacement of the horizontal QRS forces exactly simulating the VCG pattern of posterior infarction. Ha, Kraft, and Stein[22] observed anterior duration of the QRS vector in the horizontal plane exceeding 42 and even 50 msec in several normal subjects. Similarly, other commonly used vector criteria for posterior infarction yielded false-positive diagnoses in this group of normal adults. The VCG therefore cannot be relied on to differentiate between anteriorly oriented horizontal QRS forces caused by posterior infarction and those that are normal variants. More recent criteria to distinguish normal-variant tall right precordial R waves from the pattern of posterior infarction[63,66] have yet to be prospectively validated in a large series. (The application of VCG criteria in differentiating tall right precordial R waves caused by posterior infarcts and right ventricular hypertrophy is discussed on pp. 71 and 72.)

In summary, the normal counterclockwise rotation variant and the pattern of posterior infarction can usually be distinguished on the basis of the following criteria:

1. Abnormal Q waves in the inferior or lateral precordial leads are frequently, though not invariably, seen with posterior infarction.
2. The voltage drop-off pattern in the lateral chest leads is characteristic of posterior infarction.
3. ST segment depressions in the right precordial leads are seen with acute posterior infarction, and tall positive right precordial T waves are seen with subacute or chronic posterior infarction.
4. An R/S ratio greater than 1 in lead V_1 is rarely encountered on the normal adult ECG (Fig. 15-2 shows an exception).

    The use of additional dorsal leads in diagnosing posterior infarction is of limited value in most cases, because many normal subjects will show prominent Q waves in leads reflecting the back of the heart. For example, in one study[15] about one third of normal subjects had a wide Q in lead V_9 (recorded posteriorly to the left of the spine).

The electrocardiographic differential diagnosis of posterior wall infarction, with a list of the multiple causes of tall right precordial R waves, is summarized on p. 71.

Finally, *echocardiographic* studies may be of considerable utility in the differential diagnosis of tall right precordial R waves, particularly in distinguishing normal variants from right ventricular hypertrophy, posterior infarction, or hypertrophic cardiomyopathy (Chapter 22).

DEXTROCARDIA

The ECG pattern of dextrocardia presents the appearance of extensive anterior wall infarction (Fig. 3-13). The chest leads show a progressive loss of volt-

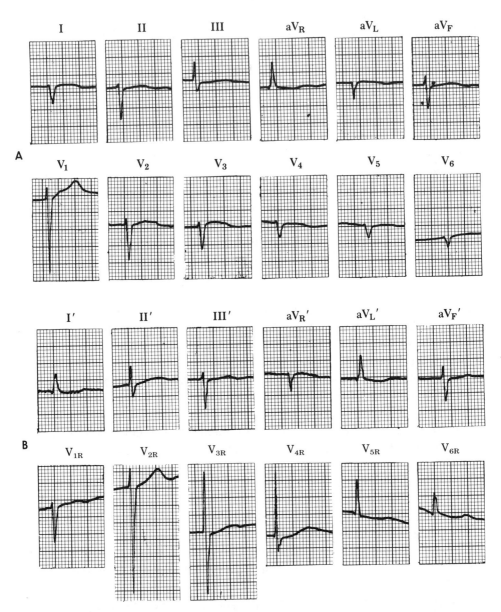

FIG. 3-13. Dextrocardia mimicking extensive anterior infarction. **A,** On the ECG of this 83-year-old woman with situs inversus totalis, the extremity leads show reversal of the usual pattern: an R wave in lead aV_R and a QS complex in aV_L. The precordial leads show a characteristic loss of normal R wave progression and a diminution of QRS voltage (in the left-sided leads). **B,** "Corrected" ECG obtained by reversing the left and right arm electrodes (leads I′, II′, etc.) and placing the precordial leads (V_{1R} to V_{6R}) over the right chest. The revised tracing now shows prominent voltage in the precordial leads, suggesting left ventricular hypertrophy. Nonspecific ST-T changes are present. The underlying rhythm in both tracings is atrial fibrillation.

age and poor R wave progression; QS waves are seen in the left precordial leads and in I and aV_L. Leads aV_R and aV_L also show a reversal of their usual patterns — aV_R reflecting left ventricular epicardial potentials with generally an upward P wave, a normal PR interval, and a positive QRS; aV_L showing the pattern usually seen in aV_R: a negative P wave, normal PR interval, and negative QRS. This reversal of the right and left arm patterns, coupled with the characteristic precordial lead pattern just described, is pathognomonic of dextrocardia and is caused entirely by the altered cardiac position. In Fig. 3-13 atrial fibrillation makes the diagnosis more challenging since the clues provided by altered P wave polarity in aV_R and aV_L are not present.

A corrected ECG can be obtained in patients with dextrocardia simply by reversing the left and right arm electrodes and recording right-sided chest leads (i.e., V_{1R} to V_{6R}) as shown in Fig. 3-13, *B*. Any underlying ECG abnormality will be more readily identified after this correction.

Dextrocardia can occur with complete situs inversus (Fig. 3-13) or as an isolated anomaly. In the former it is generally of no clinical significance unless part of Kartagener's triad, which also includes sinusitis and bronchiectasis. Isolated dextrocardia, however, is usually associated with underlying congenital cardiac anomalies.[44] The ECG in such cases will show a complicated pattern reflecting this underlying abnormality superimposed on the pattern of dextrocardia.

LEFT PNEUMOTHORAX

Marked ECG changes simulating anterior wall infarction may occur with left pneumothorax. The specific ECG changes include the following[2,8,10,16,31,58]:

1. Progressive loss of voltage in the precordial leads with poor R wave progression and sometimes actual QS complexes in the right to midprecordial leads may appear (Fig. 3-14). Occasionally there will be a virtual loss of R waves from V_1 to V_6, simulating extensive anterior wall injury.[17] This characteristic diminution of precordial voltage and loss of R wave progression will usually be apparent only when the patient is supine. When the patient with left pneumothorax sits or stands, the normal precordial R wave pattern typically reappears.[8,31] *Reappearance of the normal precordial ECG with resumption of an erect posture is pathognomonic of left pneumothorax.* Reexpansion of the collapsed lung will also normalize the ECG.

2. A rightward shift in the frontal plane QRS axis may also occur (Fig. 3-14).

3. Nonspecific T wave flattening and sometimes actual T wave inversions may appear in the precordial leads.

These ECG changes are discussed as "normal variants" because the pathologic condition is completely extracardiac and the changes are attributable en-

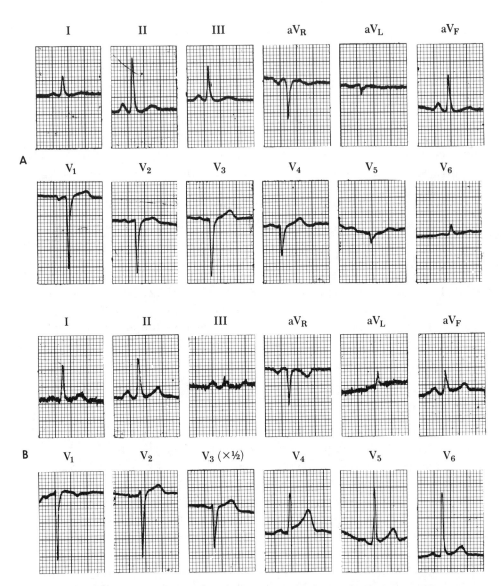

FIG. 3-14. Left pneumothorax simulating anterior wall infarction. This patient, a 73-year-old man with chronic obstructive pulmonary disease, was admitted with acute (90%) left pneumothorax. **A,** Note the classic findings on the supine ECG: loss of R wave progression in the middle to lateral precordial leads, with a progressive diminution in lateral lead voltages. These changes are the result of a rightward shift of the mediastinum, with the interposition of air between the heart and the precordial leads. **B,** Note the striking "regeneration" of precordial voltages on the postexpansion ECG. Another feature of ECGs in patients with left pneumothorax is the rightward shift of the frontal plane QRS axis. In **A** the axis is approximately +70 degrees; in **B** (postexpansion) it has shifted horizontally to about +40 degrees. There is also a marked alteration in polarity of the QRS in lead aV_L: in **A** we see a QS complex, a normal variant with electrically vertical hearts and not indicative of anterior wall infarction; in **B** a qR pattern has resulted from leftward shift of the axis. These shifts are attributable to changes in cardiac position. In addition, the postexpansion ECG shows nonspecific poor R wave progression in leads V_1 to V_3.

tirely to the shift in cardiac position and to alteration of the extracardiac electrical field by intrathoracic air.[55] Left pneumothorax may produce a marked mediastinal shift to the right. As a result the heart is moved away from the exploring electrodes on the left precordium. Furthermore, a large amount of insulatory air becomes interposed between the heart and the chest leads. These factors account for the progressive diminution in precordial voltage. A certain degree of actual anatomic clockwise rotation of the heart may also occur, accounting for the persistence of right ventricular epicardial potentials (QS and rS complexes) toward the left precordium.[2] When the patient sits or stands, the heart shifts back closer to the chest wall and these positional ECG effects are obviated. (In *right* pneumothorax the mediastinum is shifted to the left, and the pattern of decreased precordial voltages and loss of R wave progression is not seen.) Acute right ventricular dilation caused by pulmonary hypertension may also contribute to the delayed precordial transition and anterior T wave inversions in selected patients.

Clinically the patient with left pneumothorax may have acute chest pain, and the initial supine ECG may support the mistaken diagnosis of anterior wall infarction. Demonstrating the reversibility of these ECG changes when the patient sits up will not only exclude consideration of infarction but will definitively establish the diagnosis of left pneumothorax, even before the chest x-ray is obtained.

PECTUS EXCAVATUM

Pectus excavatum (funnel chest) is a congenital skeletal deformity characterized by indentation of the lower sternum. The heart is usually displaced to the left by the sternal depression.

There have been a number of reports of pseudoinfarct patterns in such patients. Dressler and Roesler[11] noted a high incidence of T wave inversions in the right to midprecordial leads. This pattern resembled the juvenile T wave pattern (described in Chapter 15) and was thought to be caused either by leftward displacement of the heart or possibly by sternal pressure on the right ventricle. Poor R wave progression in the precordial leads has also been observed in patients with pectus excavatum.[11,49]

DeOliveira, Sambhi, and Zimmerman[9] described Qr complexes (in association with negative P waves) in lead V_1 in four of 13 patients studied. They attributed this to cardiac displacement that shifted the right atrium to a position directly under V_1.

There have also been isolated reports of pectus excavatum simulating inferior and lateral wall infarction. Elisberg[13] reported the case of a patient with relatively prominent but narrow Q waves in the inferior and lateral leads. These Q waves were attributed to cardiac displacement that could theoretically shift a normally negative initial depolarization vector further from these leads. Penchas and Kenyan[42] reported a similar case with deep but narrow Q waves in I, II, aV_L, and V_4 to V_6.*

Patients with funnel chest deformity may have additional ECG and physical findings suggestive of organic heart disease. An rSr' or rSR' pattern in the right precordial leads is not uncommon, suggesting a right ventricular conduction delay.[9,13] A functional systolic murmur and on rare occasions even a benign systolic thrill may be present.[47] Hemodynamic studies in subjects with mild to moderate sternal depression have generally not revealed significant cardiac impairment, and care must be taken not to overdiagnose cardiac disease on the basis of equivocal ECG and physical findings in these patients. Pectus excavatum may be associated with mitral valve prolapse, an important cause of inferolateral ST-T changes and arrhythmias simulating ischemia (Chapter 17).[56]

CONGENITAL ABSENCE OF THE LEFT PERICARDIUM

Pseudoinfarct patterns may occur in a rare congenital anomaly characterized by either complete or partial absence of the left pericardium.[7,38,39]

In cases in which the left pericardium is completely absent, the ECG frequently shows delayed R wave progression in the precordial leads (clockwise rotation pattern), which may mistakenly suggest anteroseptal infarction. In one reported case[7] a QS complex extended to lead V_3 with a small R wave in lead V_4. The ECG also commonly shows a vertical axis or even right axis deviation. An incomplete right bundle branch block pattern may also be present. Displacement of the precordial transition zone to the left reflects the anatomic levoposition of the heart that occurs with this anomaly. Some of these patients have pectus excavatum, which can also be associated with poor precordial R wave progression and an incomplete right bundle branch block pattern.

Chest x-rays of patients with complete absence of the left pericardium typically show displacement of the heart shadow to the left, elongation of the left cardiac border, and prominence of the pulmonary artery segment. Diagnostic left pneumothorax will produce a pathognomonic pneumopericardium in cases of complete absence of the left pericardium.

One third of the patients with this anomaly have underlying congenital heart disease. However, *complete* absence of the left pericardium per se is not associated with any specific cardiac disability. On the other hand, *partial* absence of the left pericardium may be an indication for corrective surgery because of the documented risk of cardiac prolapse through the pericardial defect and death from cardiac strangulation.

---

*Epstein and Wasserburger[14] presented an unusual example of a woman 34 years of age with pectus excavatum and otherwise normal findings on physical examination. Her ECG showed abnormal Q waves in the inferior limb and lateral precordial leads with poor R wave progression in the right precordial to midprecordial leads. This combination of ECG abnormalities had not been reported previously in uncomplicated pectus excavatum, and the possibility of occult cardiac disease was not excluded in this case.

CONGENITAL CORRECTED TRANSPOSITION OF THE GREAT VESSELS

Congenital corrected transposition of the great vessels (levotransposition) is a rare abnormality characterized by inversion of the left and right ventricles with normal direction of blood flow through the lungs and systemic circuits. Thus venous blood is pumped from a right-sided chamber (anatomically resembling the left ventricle) through the pulmonary artery to the lungs. The pulmonary veins then return normally oxygenated blood to the left atrium and left-sided ventricle (anatomically resembling the right ventricle), which empties into the aorta.[44]

The ECG in cases of congenital corrected transposition may show a pattern simulating anteroseptal and sometimes inferior infarction (Fig. 3-15).[44] These pseudoinfarct patterns are caused by the inverted position of the His bundle as well as by altered orientation of the ventricular septum.[44] Normally, as described on p. 37, the ventricular septum is activated from left to right, resulting in small r waves in leads such as V_1 and small septal q waves in the lateral chest leads. With congenital corrected transposition, the reversed orientation of the conduction system results in right-to-left septal activation, with consequent QS waves in the right precordial leads (Fig. 3-15) and loss of normal lateral septal q waves. Furthermore, the septum in these cases tends to be perpendicular rather than parallel to the anterior chest wall. As a result the early ventricular depolar-

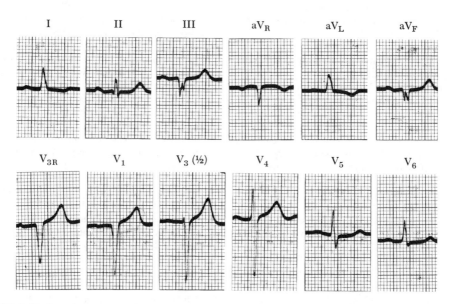

FIG. 3-15. Complete corrected transposition of the great vessels simulating anteroseptal and inferior myocardial infarction. The patient is a 38-year-old man without other associated congenital anomalies. Note the inferior Q waves, poor R wave progression in V_{3R} to V_3, and first-degree AV block. (From Gooch AS, et al: Clues to diagnosis in congenital heart disease, Philadelphia, 1969, FA Davis Co.)

ization forces may be directed superiorly and leftward, resulting in noninfarctional Q waves in one or more of the inferior limb leads (Fig. 3-15).

Most patients with this congenital abnormality have other associated cardiac abnormalities (e.g., atrioventricular valve insufficiency, ventricular septal defect, pulmonic stenosis). However, in some cases an unusual ECG simulating infarction may be the major diagnostic clue. A high percentage of patients may also have AV conduction disturbances, including complete heart block. The chest x-ray may show rounding of the left heart border and a narrow vascular pedicle. On physical examination a single, loud, second heart sound is characteristically heard.[44] Echocardiography may be helpful in confirming the altered spatial orientation of the great arteries.

REFERENCES

1. Antonin B, Roje J: Separation of strictly posterior infarction from anteriorly oriented QRS loop as "normal variation," Adv Cardiol 19:224, 1977.
2. Armen RN, Frank TV: Electrocardiographic patterns in pneumothorax, Dis Chest 15:709, 1949.
3. Bayley RH: The significance of the duration of Q_3 with respect to coronary disease, Am Heart J 18:308, 1939.
4. Bewick DJ, et al: The diagnostic utility of precordial R wave progression in the clinical electrocardiograms of male subjects, Am J Noninvas Cardiol 2:332, 1988.
5. Bing OHL, et al: Pacemaker placement by electrocardiographic monitoring, N Engl J Med 287:651, 1972.
6. Bodenheimer MM, et al: Determination of lead III Q waves significance: utility of deep inspiration, Arch Intern Med 137:437, 1977.
7. Broadbent JC et al: Congenital deficiency of the pericardium, Dis Chest 50:237, 1966.
8. Copeland RB, Omenn GS: Electrocardiogram changes suggestive of coronary artery disease in pneumothorax, Arch Intern Med 125:151, 1970.
9. DeOliveira JM, et al: The electrocardiogram in pectus excavatum, Br Heart J 20:495, 1958.
10. Diamond JR, Estes NM: ECG changes associated with iatrogenic left pneumothorax simulating anterior myocardial infarction, Am Heart J 103:303, 1982.
11. Dressler W, Roesler H: Electrocardiographic changes in funnel chest, Am Heart J 40:877, 1950.
12. Eisenstein I, et al: Electrocardiographic and vectorcardiographic diagnosis of posterior wall myocardial infarction. Significance of the T wave, Chest 88:409, 1985.
13. Elisberg EI: Electrocardiographic changes associated with pectus excavatum, Ann Intern Med 49:130, 1958.
14. Epstein M, Wasserburger RH: Electrocardiograms simulating myocardial infarction in the presence of normal coronary arteries, Vasc Dis 4:215, 1967.
15. Falsetti HL, Willson RA: QRS voltage criteria for posterior unipolar chest leads in a normal population, Dis Chest 52:695, 1967.
16. Feldman D, Silverberg C: Electrocardiographic changes in pulmonary collapse therapy. I. Artificial pneumothorax, Am Heart J 35:800, 1948.
17. Giknis FL: The electrocardiogram in spontaneous pneumothorax [Letter to the editor], JAMA 199:433, 1967.
18. Goldberger E: The differentiation of normal from abnormal Q waves, Am Heart J 30:341, 1945.
19. Goldberger E: Unipolar lead electrocardiography and vectorcardiography, ed 3, Philadelphia, 1953, Lea & Febiger.
20. Goldberger E: How to interpret electrocardiograms in terms of vectors, Springfield Ill, 1968, Charles C Thomas Publisher.
21. Goldman MJP: Principles of clinical electrocardiography, ed 12, Los Altos Calif, 1986, Lange Medical Publications.
22. Ha D, et al: The anteriorly oriented horizontal vector loop: the problem of distinction between direct posterior myocardial infarction and normal variation, Am Heart J 88:408, 1974.

23. Hill NE, et al: Comparison of optimal scalar electrocardiographic orthogonal electrocardiographic and vectorcardiographic criteria for diagnosing inferior and anterior myocardial infarction, Am J Cardiol 54:274, 1974.
24. Hoffman I, et al: Anterior conduction delay: a possible cause for prominent anterior QRS forces, J Electrocardiol 9:15, 1976.
25. Howard PF, et al: Correlation of electrocardiogram and vectorcardiogram with coronary occlusion and myocardial contraction abnormality, Am J Cardiol 38:582, 1976.
26. Huey BL, et al: A comprehensive analysis of myocardial infarction due to left circumflex coronary artery occlusion: comparison with infarction due to right coronary artery and left anterior descending artery occlusion, J Am Coll Cardiol 12:1156, 1988.
27. Hurd HP, et al: Comparative accuracy of electrocardiographic and vectorcardiographic criteria for inferior myocardial infarction, Circulation 63:1025, 1981.
28. Kulbertus HE, et al: Vectorcardiographic study of aberrant conduction. Anterior displacement of QRS: another form of intraventricular block, Br Heart J 38:549, 1976.
29. Levine HD, et al: Electrocardiogram and vectorcardiogram in myocardial infarction, Circulation 45:457, 1972.
30. Lichtman J, et al: Electrocardiogram of the athlete: alterations simulating those of organic heart disease, Arch Intern Med 132:763, 1973.
31. Littmann D: Electrocardiographic phenomena associated with spontaneous pneumothorax and mediastinal emphysema, Am J Med Sci 212:682, 1946.
32. Lui CY et al: Lack of superiority of the vectorcardiogram over the electrocardiogram in detecting inferior wall myocardial infarction regardless of time since infarction, J Electrocardiol 20:241, 1987.
33. Mimbs JW, et al: The effect of respiration on normal and abnormal Q waves: an electrocardiographic and vectorcardiographic analysis, Am Heart J 94:579, 1977.
34. Myers GB, Klein HA: The relation of unipolar limb leads to precordial and esophageal leads, Am Heart J 35:727, 1948.
35. Myers GB, Oren BG: The use of the augmented unipolar left leg lead in the differentiation of the normal from abnormal Q wave in standard lead III, Am Heart J 29:708, 1945.
36. Myers GB, et al: Normal variations in multiple precordial leads, Am Heart J 34:785, 1947.
37. Myers GB, et al: Correlation of electrocardiographic and pathologic findings in posterior infarction, Am Heart J 38:547, 1949.
38. Nasser W, et al: Congenital absence of the left pericardium, Circulation 34:100, 1966.
39. Nasser W, et al: Congenital absence of the left pericardium. Clinical electrocardiographic, radiographic, hemodynamic, and angiographic findings in six cases, Circulation 41:469, 1970.
40. Paparella N, et al: Prominent anterior QRS forces: clinical electrocardiographic and prospective study, J Electrocardiol 20:233, 1987.
41. Pardee HEB: The significance of an electrocardiogram with a large Q in lead III, Arch Intern Med 46:470, 1930.
42. Penchas S, Kenyan A: Acute myocardial infarction pattern in the ECG of a patient with funnel-chest, J Electrocardiol 2:285, 1969.
43. Perloff JK: The recognition of strictly posterior myocardial infarction by conventional scalar electrocardiography, Circulation 30:706, 1964.
44. Perloff JK: The clinical recognition of congenital heart disease, ed 3, Philadelphia, 1987, WB Saunders Co.
45. Piccolo E, et al: The anterior displacement of the QRS loop as a right ventricular conduction disturbance. Electrocardiographic and vectorcardiographic study in man, J Electrocardiol 13:267, 1980.
46. Reiffel JA, Bigger JT Jr: Pure anterior conduction delay: a variant "fascicular" defect, J Electrocardiol 11:315, 1978.
47. Reusch CS: Hemodynamic studies in pectus excavatum, Circulation 24:1143, 1961.
48. Rubin IL, Most W: Positional changes in Q_{aV_F} and the esophageal leads induced by pneumoperitoneum, Am Heart J 43:236, 1952.
49. Ruskin J, et al: Electrocardiogram and vectorcardiogram simulating myocardial infarction in patient with pectus excavatum and straight back, Am J Cardiol 21:446, 1968.
50. Shettigar UR, et al: Diagnostic value of Q-waves in inferior myocardial infarction, Am Heart J 88:170, 1974.
51. Simonson E: Differentiation between normal and abnormal in electrocardiography, St Louis, 1961, The CV Mosby Co.

52. Sodi-Pallares D: New bases of electrocardiography, St Louis, 1956, The CV Mosby Co.
53. Starr JW, et al: Vectorcardiographic criteria for the diagnosis of inferior myocardial infarction, Circulation 49:829, 1974.
54. Stein PD, Simon AP: Vectorcardiographic diagnosis of diaphragmatic myocardial infarction, Am J Cardiol 38:568, 1976.
55. Tsutsumi T, et al: Vectorcardiographic QRS loop in spontaneous pneumothorax, J Electrocardiol 20:375, 1987.
56. Udoshi MB, et al: Incidence of mitral valve prolapse in subjects with thoracic skeletal abnormalities—a prospective study, Am Heart J 97:303, 1979.
57. Walsh TJ, et al: The vectorcardiographic QRS–sE-loop findings in inferoposterior myocardial infarction, Am Heart J 63:516, 1962.
58. Walston A, et al: The electrocardiographic manifestations of spontaneous left pneumothorax, Ann Intern Med 80:375, 1974.
59. Warner R, et al: Improved electrocardiographic criteria for the diagnosis of inferior myocardial infarction, Circulation 66:422, 1982.
60. Weisbart MH, Simonson E: The diagnostic accuracy of Q_3 and related electrocardiographic items for the detection of patients with posterior wall myocardial infarction, Am Heart J 50:62, 1955.
61. Yanagisawa N: Counterclockwise rotation of the heart; correlation of electrocardiography and chest radiography and their clinical significance, J Electrocardiol 14:233, 1981.
62. Young E, Williams C: The frontal plane vectorcardiogram in old inferior myocardial infarction: criteria for diagnosis and electrocardiographic correlation, Circulation 37:604, 1968.
63. Zema MJ: Electrocardiographic tall R waves in the right precordial leads, J Electrocardiol 23:147, 1990.
64. Zema MJ, Kligfield P: Electrocardiographic poor R wave progression. I. Correlation with the Frank vectorcardiogram, J Electrocardiol 12:3, 1979.
65. Zema MJ, Kligfield P: Electrocardiographic poor R wave progression. II. Correlation with angiography, J Electrocardiol 12:11, 1979.
66. Zema MJ, Kligfield P: Electrocardiographic tall R waves in the right precordial leads: vectorcardiographic and electrocardiographic distinction of posterior myocardial infarction from prominent anterior forces in normal subjects, J Electrocardiol 17:129, 1984.
67. Zema MJ, et al: Electrocardiographic poor R wave progression. III. The normal variant, J Electrocardiol 13:135, 1980.

4 Ventricular hypertrophy and dilation patterns

Hypertrophy or dilation of the ventricular myocardium may alter the balance or orientation of initial normal depolarization forces, in some cases resulting in abnormal but noninfarctional Q waves. Such pseudoinfarct patterns may occur with left ventricular hypertrophy and dilation, right ventricular hypertrophy and dilation, and hypertrophic cardiomyopathy, including the subset of patients with idiopathic hypertrophic subaortic stenosis.

The section on right ventricular hypertrophy and dilation (right ventricular overload) is subdivided into separate discussions of pseudoinfarct patterns seen in classic right ventricular hypertrophy, in acute cor pulmonale (especially pulmonary embolism patterns), chronic cor pulmonale (especially pulmonary emphysema patterns), and arrhythmogenic right ventricular dysplasia. The last is included in this discussion as a special topic because it may be associated with poor R wave progression and T wave inversions, as well as with life-threatening ventricular arrhythmias, simulating acute coronary disease.

LEFT VENTRICULAR HYPERTROPHY

The following pseudoinfarct patterns may be seen in left ventricular hypertrophy.

1. *QS complexes in the right to middle precordial leads.* Left ventricular hypertrophy is often associated with poor R wave progression in the right to middle precordial leads (delayed precordial transition zone, clockwise rotation pattern). Not infrequently in cases of left ventricular hypertrophy the septal r wave may be completely absent, producing a QS pattern in V_1 and V_2 that mimics anteroseptal infarction.[44,51,84] In rare cases a QS complex may extend as far left as V_3 or even V_4 (Fig. 4-1) in the absence of infarction.[16,72]

2. *Prominent septal q waves.* Septal hypertrophy, occurring as a consequence of pressure or volume loads, may accentuate the physiologic septal q waves seen in the lateral chest leads and limb leads. The problem of Q waves associated with asymmetric septal hypertrophy is discussed separately later.

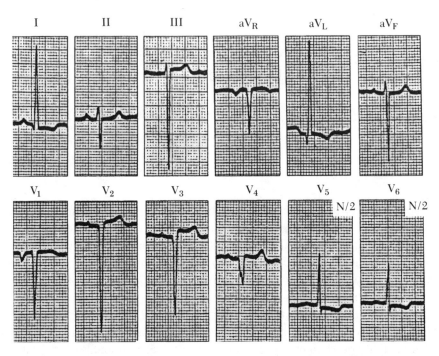

FIG. 4-1. Left ventricular hypertrophy simulating extensive anterior infarction. This patient was a 35-year-old woman with rheumatic aortic stenosis. No evidence of infarction was noted at autopsy despite the QS waves in V_1 to V_4. Prominent voltage is present with "strain" pattern in the lateral leads, and V_2 and V_3 show slight ST elevations. A prominent negative P wave in V_1 is compatible with left atrial abnormality. (From Friedman HH: Diagnostic electrocardiography and vectorcardiography, New York, 1971, McGraw-Hill Book Co. Used with permission of McGraw-Hill.)

3. *Left ventricular "strain" pattern.* The left ventricular "strain" pattern refers to a characteristic biphasic or inverted T wave pattern, usually with an asymmetric shape, in leads with a predominant R wave (Fig. 4-1). The T wave may be minimally inverted, or the inversion may exceed 5 mm in depth. Left ventricular hypertrophy may be present without the strain pattern, and conversely the strain pattern may be present without prominent voltage.[33]

The precise pathophysiology of the strain pattern remains unresolved. One speculation[6] is that the ST-T changes seen with hypertrophy are caused by relative myocardial ischemia. However, this pattern has also been attributed to a delay in epicardial repolarization resulting from increased muscle mass and not from coronary insufficiency.[67] To avoid the ambiguity of the term *strain*, some cardiologists refer more generally to "repolarization abnormalities associated with left ventricular hypertrophy."

4. *ST segment elevations in the right precordial leads.* Left ventricular hy-

pertrophy is often associated with ST segment elevations in the right precordial leads (Fig. 4-1). The T waves in such cases may also be prominent, simulating the hyperacute phase of infarction. The ST segment may be elevated as much as 5 mm or more at the J point.[51] The basis for these ST elevations is not known with certainty, although it is clear that they do not reflect acute anterior wall ischemia. Such right precordial ST elevations may reflect relatively early right ventricular repolarization occurring in the setting of delayed left ventricular activation and recovery. (See Chapter 19 for further discussion of these patterns and also of tall left precordial T waves with diastolic overload.)

Etiology of right precordial QS waves. The pathogenesis of pseudoinfarctional right precordial QS waves occurring with left ventricular hypertrophy is still uncertain. The following factors have been cited.

Incomplete left bundle branch block.[77] Incomplete left bundle branch block might disrupt the normal early septal activation responsible for the initial septal r wave in the right precordial leads.

Altered balance of depolarization forces.[2,20] The hypertrophied and dilated left ventricle may generate posteriorly directed early depolarization forces that could cancel out or overbalance the normal, anteriorly directed septal forces.

Altered spatial orientation of septal forces.[72,77] The initial depolarization forces in left ventricular hypertrophy appear to be oriented inferiorly and to have a lower point of origin than normal, resulting in initial negativity in the right precordial leads.

Anatomic clockwise rotation. Grant[20] found no evidence of actual anatomic clockwise rotation of the heart in left ventricular hypertrophy. It is therefore not likely that true cardiac rotation contributes much to the pattern of electrical rotation seen in conjunction with left ventricular hypertrophy. However, concomitant right ventricular dilation may be responsible for the delayed precordial R wave progression in some cases.

Septal fibrosis.[5] In some cases actual septal fibrosis caused by chronic scarring might cause a primary loss of septal forces in left ventricular hypertrophy. However, the right to midprecordial QS waves seen in some cases of left ventricular hypertrophy can occur in the absence of apparent septal injury.

Differential diagnosis. The differentiation of Q waves caused by pure left ventricular hypertrophy from infarctional Q waves may be difficult if not impossible at times.[44]

The major differences between the ECG patterns of left ventricular hypertrophy and infarction are as follows:

Distribution of QS waves. Right precordial QS waves caused by pure left ventricular hypertrophy never extend left of lead V_4 and only rarely as far as V_3. A QS in V_5 and V_6 indicates anterolateral infarction or one of the other conditions listed on p. 170. Furthermore, left ventricular hypertrophy is not usually a cause of abnormal Q waves in I or aV$_F$. Occasionally with left ventricular hypertrophy, relatively deep but narrow Q waves as part of QR complexes will appear in the lateral leads, reflecting associated septal hypertrophy.

ST-T changes. The ST segment elevations seen in the right precordial leads with left ventricular hypertrophy are stable over time and do not undergo the ischemic pattern of evolution seen with ST elevations caused by an acute current of injury. The presence of T wave inversions in the right precordial leads associated with QS waves usually suggests anteroseptal ischemia or right ventricular strain. T wave inversions as a rule are *not* seen in the right precordial leads (with an rS configuration) in uncomplicated left ventricular hypertrophy.

This comparison of the ECG patterns of left ventricular hypertrophy and infarction is at best a guideline for differential diagnosis and not a set of rigid criteria. However, it is important to recognize that right to midprecordial QS complexes, deep T wave inversions in the *left* precordial leads, and ST elevations in the *right* precordial leads may be secondary to pure left ventricular hypertrophy in the absence of infarction.

Vectorcardiographic diagnosis of anterior myocardial infarction with left ventricular hypertrophy. The problems of differentiating left ventricular hypertrophy from anterior myocardial infarction using the scalar ECG also afflict vectorcardiographic diagnosis.[24,28,58] Normally the initial 20 msec QRS forces are oriented anteriorly in the horizontal (transverse) plane. These initial anterior depolarization forces give rise to the initial positive (r) waves in the right precordial leads. As described in the preceding section, pure left ventricular hypertrophy may produce a loss of these normal anterior forces in the absence of infarction. For example, in one study[77] of patients with left ventricular hypertrophy caused by aortic valve disease (with no arteriographic evidence of coronary involvement), vector criteria for anterior myocardial infarction were present in 46% of cases. Furthermore, in 13% of cases there was total absence of anterior forces in the horizontal plane caused by uncomplicated left ventricular hypertrophy. Therefore the authors suggested that the vectorcardiographic diagnosis of anterior myocardial infarction *not* be made on the basis of a loss of anterior forces if evidence of left ventricular hypertrophy is also present (transverse plane QRS magnitude greater than 1.8 mV). Another notable finding was that 14% of cases of pure left ventricular hypertrophy in this series also met vector criteria for inferior wall myocardial infarction.

RIGHT VENTRICULAR OVERLOAD/DYSFUNCTION

This section explores pseudoinfarct patterns seen in conjunction with four syndromes that are associated with right ventricular enlargement or dysfunction:

1. Right ventricular hypertrophy
2. Acute cor pulmonale (pulmonary embolism)
3. Chronic cor pulmonale (pulmonary emphysema)
4. Arrhythmogenic right ventricular dysplasia

The first three syndromes are secondary to underlying right ventricular over-load (pressure or volume overload or both). These patterns are obviously not mutually exclusive. Patients with cor pulmonale, especially in the late stages, may develop the classic ECG pattern of right ventricular hypertrophy. However, important distinctions among these three groups of patterns make it useful to consider them separately. For example, recognition of the classic $S_I Q_{III}$ pattern may be critical in making the diagnosis of acute pulmonary embolism. Similarly, a diagnosis of chronic obstructive pulmonary disease can often be suggested on the basis of the ECG tracing alone when poor R wave progression and low volt-age with a vertical or rightward electrical axis coexist.

The fourth syndrome, arrhythmogenic right ventricular dysplasia, is a rare type of cardiomyopathy that may be associated with prominent precordial T wave inversions simulating anterior ischemia or infarction.

Right Ventricular Hypertrophy

Right ventricular hypertrophy may be the cause of anterior or posterior wall pseudoinfarct patterns. The following pseudoinfarct patterns may be seen:

1. *QR (qR, Qr) complexes in the right precordial leads simulating an-teroseptal infarction* (Fig. 4-2). The same right precordial Q wave pattern may be seen with acute right ventricular strain secondary to pulmonary embolism (Fig. 4-3).
2. *QS waves in the lateral precordial leads (V_4 to V_6) and in I and aV_L mim-icking anterolateral infarction* (Fig. 4-4).
3. *Tall, wide, right precordial R waves suggesting posterior infarction* (Fig. 4-4).
4. *Deep T wave inversions in the right precordial leads (right ventricular strain pattern) mimicking anteroseptal infarction* (Fig. 4-5). These T wave inversions sometimes have a coved plane (p. 278) or symmetric ap-pearance that is morphologically indistinguishable from the T wave inver-sions seen with actual infarction (Fig. 14-4).

Etiology. The QR (qR, Qr) pattern seen in the right precordial leads with right ventricular hypertrophy has been interpreted in several ways. It has been attributed to a marked clockwise rotation of the heart, causing the right precor-dial leads to face the posterior surface of the heart,[18] or to a disturbance in the normal left-to-right orientation of early septal depolarization forces.[14] Sodi-Pal-lares, Bisteni, and Hermann[68] correlated these QR complexes in the right pre-cordial leads with right atrial dilation. In experimental conditions associated with right atrial dilation in dogs they found that leads placed over the enlarged right atrium recorded a QR type of complex. The QR complex of right ventricu-

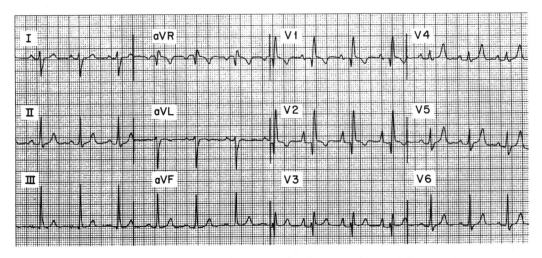

FIG. 4-2. Right ventricular hypertrophy simulating an anteroseptal infarct with QR complexes in V_1 and V_2. The patient, a 60-year-old woman, had a large ostium secundum atrial septal defect (pulmonary-systemic flow ratio, 4.6/1; pulmonary artery pressure, 49/23 mm Hg; pulmonary vascular resistance, 195 dyne sec cm^{-5}). Note also the right axis deviation, right ventricular conduction delay, and right atrial enlargement patterns.

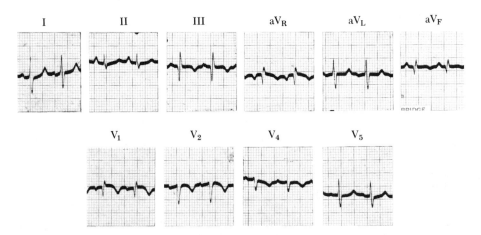

FIG. 4-3. Acute cor pulmonale secondary to pulmonary embolism simulating inferior and anterior infarction. This tracing exemplifies the classic pseudoinfarct patterns sometimes seen: an $S_I Q_{III} T_{III}$, a QR in V_1 with poor R wave progression in the right precordial leads (clockwise rotation), and right ventricular strain T wave inversions (in V_1 to V_4). Sinus tachycardia is also present. The $S_I Q_{III}$ pattern is usually associated with a QR or QS complex, but not an rS, in aV_R. Furthermore, acute cor pulmonale per se does not cause abnormal Q waves in II (only in III and aV_F).

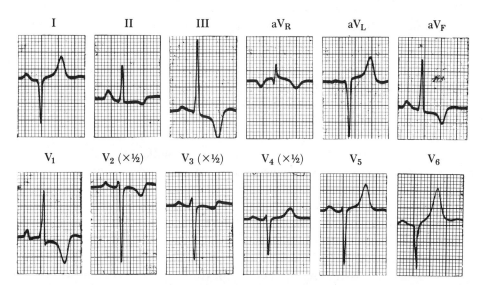

FIG. 4-4. Right ventricular hypertrophy simulating anterolateral infarction. This patient is a 33-year-old woman with tetralogy of Fallot 20 years after undergoing a Blalock-Taussig operation. Right ventricular hypertrophy is evidenced by the tall R wave in V_1, marked right axis deviation, and right ventricular strain T wave inversions in V_1 to V_3, II, III, and aV_F. The peaked P wave in V_1 indicates right atrial enlargement (P pulmonale). "Reversed" R wave progression in the precordial leads is sometimes seen with right ventricular hypertrophy. In extreme cases an actual QS complex may be present in the lateral leads (I, aV_L, and V_6 here). The absence of lateral depolarization forces is due to a marked preponderance of right ventricular forces and not to primary loss of left ventricular potentials seen with infarction.

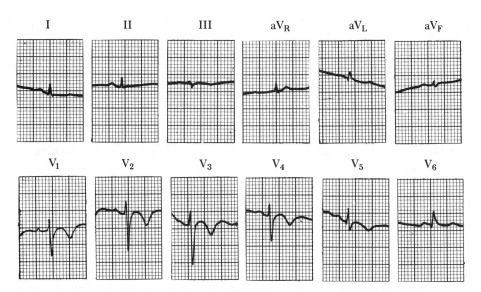

FIG. 4-5. Right ventricular strain secondary to interstitial pulmonary disease simulating anteroseptal infarction. The patient was a 62-year-old woman with diffuse pulmonary carcinomatosis. Her ECG shows poor R wave progression in the precordial leads (clockwise rotation pattern) and deep symmetric T wave inversions in V_1 to V_5. Low voltage is also present. At autopsy the heart showed right ventricular hypertrophy and dilation without evidence of infarction. The pattern of poor R wave progression with deep T wave inversions caused by right ventricular strain may be seen in both cor pulmonale (acute and chronic) and anteroseptal infarction. Differentiation of these two conditions cannot be made on the basis of electrocardiographic criteria alone. However, it is important to recognize that right ventricular overload patterns like this can completely mimic the pattern of anterior wall ischemia.

lar hypertrophy therefore may reflect epicardial potentials transmitted from the dilated right atrium. Similar patterns may be seen in acute and chronic cor pulmonale, which are also associated with dilation of the right atrium. Wide QR waves are also seen in some patients with Ebstein's anomaly of the tricuspid valve (p. 118), another syndrome characterized by right atrial dilation (Fig. 5-13). The association of noninfarctional right precordial QR waves with right atrial enlargement has been confirmed in a two-dimensional echocardiographic study.[60]

The QS complexes sometimes seen in the lateral leads in patients with right ventricular hypertrophy are caused by a reversal in the normal balance of ventricular forces. Normally the depolarization forces generated by the left ventricle are dominant, so that tall R waves are seen in the left precordial leads and deep S waves are seen over the right precordium. If the right ventricle becomes sufficiently hypertrophied, this vectorial balance can be completely reversed and the right ventricular forces will dominate the left. In such cases tall wide R waves will be seen in the right precordial leads and deep wide QS (or rS) complexes in the left precordial leads and also in I and aV_L.

The deep T wave inversions seen with right ventricular hypertrophy (in the right and middle precordial leads) are called "strain" T waves and are analogous to the left ventricular strain pattern seen in leads with a positive QRS complex in some cases of left ventricular hypertrophy. As mentioned earlier, the precise cause of this pattern and the possible role that actual ventricular ischemia plays in generating these strain T wave inversions have not been elucidated. However, right ventricular strain T wave inversions do have a different significance from the identical T wave pattern that can be produced in the right precordial leads by anterior ischemia and infarction. The term *strain T wave* is only a descriptive label for separating these morphologically similar patterns (p. 64).

Differential diagnosis of right ventricular hypertrophy versus anterior wall infarction. The differentiation of right ventricular hypertrophy from anteroseptal and anterolateral infarction is usually not difficult. The QR pattern seen in the right precordial leads with right ventricular hypertrophy rarely extends beyond V_2 or V_3 and is usually associated with right axis deviation. Similarly, the QS complexes occasionally seen in the left precordial leads with right ventricular hypertrophy are invariably accompanied by right axis deviation (usually marked). A similar pattern of lateral QS waves and right axis deviation can also occur with anterolateral myocardial infarction. The differential diagnosis of right ventricular hypertrophy and anterior infarction is shown in Figs. 4-2 and 4-6.

Differential diagnosis of right ventricular hypertrophy versus posterior infarction. The presence of tall R waves in the right precordial leads is a feature of both right ventricular hypertrophy and posterior wall infarction and may occasionally lead to diagnostic confusion.[45]

The ECG pattern of posterior wall myocardial infarction was described earlier, in the section on normal variant early precordial transition (p. 50). The tall

I   II   III   aV~R~   aV~L~   aV~F~

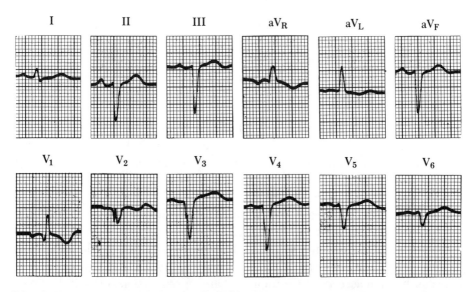

V~1~   V~2~   V~3~   V~4~   V~5~   V~6~

FIG. 4-6. Massive anterior wall infarction. The ECG of this 64-year-old man with a history of previous infarction shows extensive loss of anterior wall depolarization forces. The terminal R wave in lead V~1~ suggests underlying right bundle branch block. Left axis deviation is also present, consistent with left anterior hemiblock. Therefore a bifascicular block is present. A similar pattern with QR complexes in the right precordial leads and poor R wave progression across the precordium can be produced by right ventricular hypertrophy without infarction (Fig. 4-10). However, in such cases right axis deviation is usually present.

right precordial R waves in both right ventricular hypertrophy and posterior myocardial infarction result from a change in the vectorial balance of depolarization forces.[45] In right ventricular hypertrophy there is an actual increase in muscle mass; therefore anterior forces are directly augmented while posteriorly oriented forces remain constant. In cases of posterior myocardial infarction, however, anterior forces remain constant and posterior forces are diminished. The net result in both cases is an increase in the magnitude of anterior forces in the horizontal plane, which is reflected by the tall R waves seen in the right precordial leads.

Differentiation of these two ECG patterns based on scalar or vectorcardiographic criteria is not always possible.[45] The following general guidelines may be helpful:

Frontal plane axis. In general, the presence of right axis deviation with tall right precordial R waves suggests right ventricular hypertrophy. Mathur and Levine[45] found that the mean frontal plane QRS axis was between +75 degrees and +220 degrees in about two thirds of their cases of right ventricular hypertrophy as compared with those findings in only 5% of cases of posterior myocardial infarction. Conversely, 80% of cases of posterior myocardial infarction showed an axis between +74 degrees and −110 degrees as compared with only 28% of cases of right ventricular hypertrophy.

Q waves. Posterior myocardial infarction, as mentioned in Chapter 3, is most often associated with abnormal Q waves in the inferior limb leads or lateral precordial leads. Marked right ventricular hypertrophy, as previously noted, may also produce abnormal Q waves in the lateral precordial leads but is *not* generally associated with abnormal Q waves in the inferior limb leads (II, III, and aV_F).

Additional leads. The use of extra leads such as V_{3R} and V_{4R} may be very helpful. With right ventricular hypertrophy these leads often show a virtually pathognomonic QR or qR pattern, as described previously. However, Rs (RS, rS) patterns may be seen with either right ventricular hypertrophy or posterior myocardial infarction.

The differential features of posterior myocardial infarction and right ventricular hypertrophy are shown in Figs. 3-12 and 4-4.

The echocardiogram may provide important data to help in the differential diagnosis of prominent anterior forces. Right ventricular enlargement may be indicated by increased right ventricular chamber dimensions or wall thickness. Posterior wall infarction usually produces abnormal left ventricular posterior wall movement.[29] (See also Chapter 22.)

Acute Cor Pulmonale (Pulmonary Embolism)

Acute cor pulmonale secondary to pulmonary embolism and other causes may produce any of the following pseudoinfarct patterns either singly or in combination*:

1. $S_IQ_{III}T_{III}$ *pattern of McGinn and White*[46] (Figs. 4-3 and 4-7). This pattern consists of an S wave in lead I (as part of an RS or rS complex) and a Q wave in lead III and sometimes in aV_F (as part of a qR, QR, or Qr complex) with T wave inversions in one or more of the inferior leads. In addition, the inferior limb leads may show slight ST segment elevation. The combination of Q waves in III and aV_F with ST-T changes may simulate the pattern of acute inferior infarction.

2. *Deep T wave inversions in the right to midprecordial leads* (Figs. 4-3 and 4-5). These right ventricular strain T wave inversions often have a classic coved plane or symmetric morphology that is indistinguishable from the patterns seen with true infarction.

3. *qR (QR) complexes in the right precordial leads* (Fig. 4-3). Acute right ventricular strain is also sometimes associated with qR (QR) complexes in the right precordial leads (V_{3R}, V_1, and V_2). ST segment elevations and T wave inversions may also occur in these leads, suggesting acute or evolving anteroseptal infarction.

4. *Poor R wave progression in the precordial leads* (Figs. 4-3 and 4-5). Both acute and chronic cor pulmonale can produce a marked delay in normal

---

*References 8, 12, 46, 47, 65, 70, 71, 80.

precordial R wave progression (clockwise rotation pattern). An rS or RS type of complex may be present as far left as V_4 or V_5, or even V_6, simulating loss of anterior forces caused by ischemic damage.

These pseudoinfarct patterns reflect marked right ventricular overload and are generally seen with more extensive obstruction of the pulmonary artery system.[70] However, even with massive pulmonary obstruction the ECG is notoriously deceptive and may show little more than minor or nonspecific changes, or may even be normal.[81] In one series of 50 patients with angiographically documented acute pulmonary embolism,[73] the classic S_IQ_{III} pattern was noted in only 5 cases (10%), each of which involved severe pulmonary obstruction. Similarly, in the subsequent Urokinase–Pulmonary Embolism Trial,[8] the S_IQ_{III} pattern was seen in only 14 of the 132 patients who had had ECGs recorded prior to therapy; and subgroup analysis showed this pattern to have occurred in 11 of 90 patients (12%) *without* prior cardiac or pulmonary disease. Delayed R wave progression in the right precordial leads may be a more subtle sign of acute right ventricular dilation.[65] The other patterns seen with acute pulmonary embolism (e.g., right axis shift and right bundle branch block) are discussed in the section on differential diagnosis (p. 75). The frequency of the various ECG findings with pulmonary embolism is presented in Table 4-1. These findings may also be seen with acute or subacute cor pulmonale due to other causes such as extensive pneumonitis or diffuse pulmonary carcinomatosis[37] (Fig. 4-5).

Etiology. The S_IQ_{III} pattern, the right precordial qR (QR) waves, and the delayed precordial QRS transition zone pattern sometimes seen with acute cor pulmonale are all probably caused primarily by acute right-sided dilation. Massive pulmonary obstruction produces both right ventricular and right atrial dilation. Consequently, leads as far left as V_5 or even V_6 may still reflect potentials from the dilated and anteriorly displaced right ventricle and record an rS or RS complex.

The cause of right precordial qR (QR) complexes was discussed in the preceding section on right ventricular hypertrophy. The right precordial QR complexes seen in acute cor pulmonale probably also reflect epicardial potentials from leads overlying the dilated right atrium. Transmission of these QR potentials inferiorly may account for the S_IQ_{III} pattern (with Q waves sometimes in lead aV_F).[86] It has also been suggested that the Q waves seen in the inferior limb leads as part of this pattern of acute cor pulmonale reflect back-of-the-heart potentials that are transmitted inferiorly because of altered cardiac position.[18]

Whereas the Q waves seen with acute right ventricular strain are attributable entirely to positional factors, the ST-T changes seen with acute right ventricular overload probably reflect actual ischemia.[70,86] Acute pulmonary embolism may be associated with both hypoxemia and decreased cardiac output. At the same time, right ventricular dilation increases myocardial oxygen require-

TABLE 4-1. Electrocardiographic findings with acute pulmonary embolism: patients without prior cardiac or pulmonary disease*

Electrocardiogram	Massive pulmonary embolism (%) (50 patients)	Submassive pulmonary embolism (%) (40 patients)	Massive/submassive pulmonary embolism (%) (90 patients)
Normal	6	23	13
P pulmonale	6	5	6
QRS abnormalities			
Right axis deviation†	8	5	7
Left axis deviation‡	4	10	7
Clockwise rotation (V_5)§	10	3	7
Incomplete right bundle block	8	3	6
Complete right bundle block	8	10	9
$S_I Q_{III} T_{III}$	18	5	12
Primary ST segment and T wave abnormalities			
ST depression (not reciprocal)	28	23	26
ST elevation	18	13	16
T wave inversion‖	46	38	42

*Some patients had more than one abnormality. The prevalence of none of these findings differed significantly between patients with massive and submassive pulmonary embolism. Massive embolism was defined angiographically by obstruction or filling defects involving two or more lobar pulmonary arteries or their equivalent. Submassive embolism was defined as obstruction or filling defects in at least one pulmonary artery.
†Mean frontal plane QRS axis >90 degrees.
‡Mean frontal plane QRS axis ≥−30 degrees.
§Transition zone (R = S).
‖In any lead except aV_R, aV_L, III, or V_1.
Adapted from Stein PD, et al: Prog Cardiovasc Dis 17:247, 1975.

ments in accord with Laplace's law.[70] The net result is relative right and left ventricular ischemia. Massive pulmonary embolism is also frequently accompanied by hypotension and shock, which further exacerbate cardiac ischemia. The resulting right ventricular ischemia probably accounts for the ST elevations and T wave inversions that may be seen in the right precordial and inferior leads.

Pulmonary embolism is also sometimes associated with the ECG features of left ventricular subendocardial ischemia (Fig. 4-7). Dack et al.[11] found evidence at autopsy to confirm diffuse left ventricular subendocardial ischemia in patients with massive pulmonary embolism and diffuse ST depressions.

By way of summary: In describing the ST-T changes associated with acute cor pulmonale the term *pseudoinfarct pattern* must be carefully qualified since these repolarization abnormalities probably reflect some degree of actual right

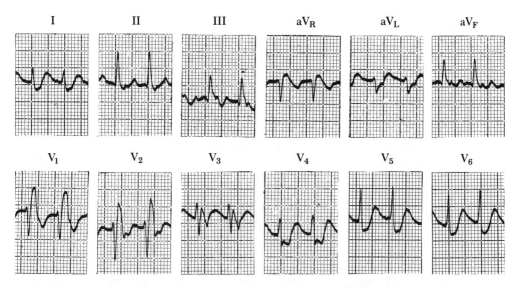

FIG. 4-7. Acute pulmonary embolism simulating acute inferior wall infarction. This tracing of a patient with pulmonary embolism shows the classic $S_I Q_{III} T_{III}$ pattern with ST elevation and terminal T wave inversion in III. It also shows sinus tachycardia, right bundle branch block, and deep ST depressions in V_4 to V_6, I, and aV_L, with reciprocal ST elevation in aV_R. The pattern of ST depression in the lateral precordial leads is consistent with left ventricular ischemia. The combination of ECG findings seen here is highly suggestive, though not diagnostic, of acute pulmonary embolism.

and left ventricular ischemia. However, the term *pseudoinfarct* is appropriate because these right ventricular "strain" patterns have a very different pathologic and clinical significance from the similar patterns produced by actual anterior and inferior infarction. Furthermore, the right precordial and inferior Q waves seen with acute cor pulmonale are functional and do not signify myocardial damage.

Differential diagnosis. The guidelines presented next are suggested for differentiating the patterns seen with acute cor pulmonale from those seen with myocardial infarction.

$S_I Q_{III} T_{III}$ *versus actual inferior wall infarction.* Differentiation between inferior wall infarction and acute cor pulmonale may be difficult if not impossible on the basis of a single tracing. However, in many cases these two conditions can be distinguished on the basis of the patterns seen in aV_R and II.

Acute cor pulmonale does not produce abnormal Q waves in II; by contrast, inferior infarction, sometimes but not invariably is associated with a significant Q_{II}.

In cases of inferior wall infarction, as noted earlier, the initial depolarization forces are oriented superiorly because of a primary loss of inferior wall potentials. Lead aV_R frequently shows an initial r wave as part of an rS (RS) complex in such cases. In pulmonary embolism the Q waves in III and aV_F are positional and not secondary to a loss of inferior wall forces. The initial depolarization vector in these cases is generally oriented horizontally and to the left, while the terminal forces in the frontal plane are directed upward and to the right. Lead aV_R therefore typically shows a qR or QR pattern with acute cor pulmonale and not an rS.[19,26]

As a general rule, therefore, prominent Q waves in the inferior leads suggest inferior wall injury when aV_R shows an rS type of pattern whereas a QR pattern in aV_R associated with the $S_IQ_{III}T_{III}$ pattern is characteristic of positional changes secondary to acute cor pulmonale (Figs. 4-7 and 4-8).

Furthermore, the ST segment elevations and T wave inversions seen in the inferior leads as part of the $S_IQ_{III}T_{III}$ pattern are usually of relatively small amplitude. For example, the inferior lead T wave inversions rarely if ever exceed 5 mm (0.5 mV), in contrast to the more marked ST-T deviations frequently seen with acute inferior wall myocardial infarction.

QR in the right precordial leads due to acute cor pulmonale versus anteroseptal infarction. QR complexes associated with acute cor pulmonale generally do not extend beyond V_2. More extensive Q waves are sometimes but not invariably seen with anterior infarction (Fig. 4-9).

Right precordial T wave inversions and poor R wave progression due to acute cor pulmonale. These may be indistinguishable from the pattern of anterior infarction. Right ventricular "strain" T wave inversions also often have a

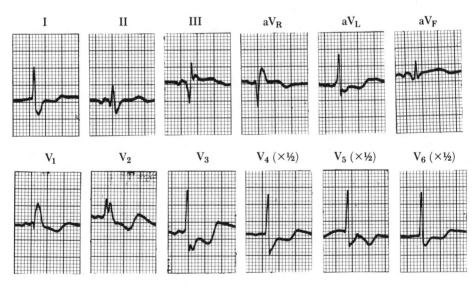

FIG. 4-8. Inferior wall infarction with right bundle branch block. Note the initial r wave (rSr' complex) in aV_R reciprocal to the inferior Q waves. Acute pulmonary embolism sometimes produces a similar pattern, with right bundle branch block and inferior Q waves. However, acute cor pulmonale does not produce a pathologic Q wave in II. Furthermore, the $S_IQ_{III}T_{III}$ is associated with an initial Q wave in aV_R (horizontal orientation of early QRS forces), not an r wave, as is often seen with inferior infarction due to the superior orientation of early QRS forces. Ectopic atrial rhythm is also present in this case.

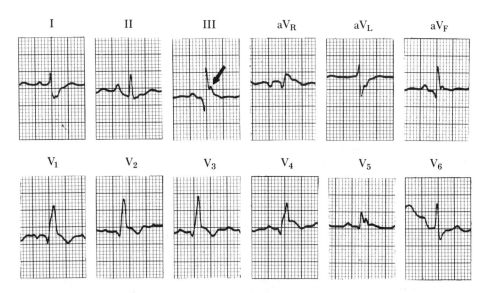

FIG. 4-9. Anterior and inferior infarct patterns with right bundle branch block. Prominent Q waves are seen in V_1 to V_5 with ST elevations consistent with acute anterior myocardial infarction. In addition, there are significant Q waves in III and aV_F from a prior inferior infarct. A similar pattern is sometimes seen with acute cor pulmonale. However, the right precordial QR complexes with acute cor pulmonale do not usually extend to the left of V_2. Also note the wide terminal R wave in III (*arrow*) caused by the right bundle branch block, simulating J point elevation.

classic "coved plane" or symmetric "coronary" morphology (Figs. 4-5 and 14-4). Poor R wave progression is a nonspecific finding that may occur as a normal variant or with any of the conditions listed on p. 170. Two of the most important pathologic causes of poor right precordial R wave progression are anterior infarction and acute cor pulmonale. The sudden appearance of T wave inversions in the right to middle precordial leads with poor R wave progression should always suggest acute cor pulmonale. In general, all the pseudoinfarct patterns seen with acute cor pulmonale tend to evolve more rapidly and more transiently (often within hours) than the Q waves and ST-T alterations seen with actual infarction.[26] In the Urokinase–Pulmonary Embolism Trial the S_IQ_{III} pattern had disappeared within 5 or 6 days of pulmonary angiography in all of the 11 patients with this sign who did not have known prior cardiac and pulmonary disease.[8,71]

In addition to the pseudoinfarct patterns just described, pulmonary embolism may be associated with any of the following ECG changes (see also Table 4-1):

1. Axis shifts
   a. Acute right axis shift with or without the classic S_IQ_{III} pattern
   b. Acute left axis deviation, possibly caused by transient left anterior hemiblock[36]

2. Conduction disturbances
   a. Right bundle branch block (complete or incomplete)
   b. First-degree AV block
3. Subendocardial ischemia pattern with deep ST depressions in the precordial leads
4. P pulmonale
5. Arrhythmias
   a. Sinus tachycardia
   b. Atrial arrhythmias, especially atrial flutter or fibrillation
   c. Ventricular ectopy

As expected, ECG evidence of actual right ventricular *hypertrophy* (tall R in V_1) is very uncommon with acute pulmonary embolism.[8,71] Indeed, probable or definitive evidence of right ventricular hypertrophy (tall R in V_1 with right axis deviation) in a patient with pulmonary thromboembolic disease should point to recurrent embolization leading to subacute or chronic cor pulmonale.[49,55]

To summarize: Q waves and ST-T changes simulating inferior or anterior wall myocardial infarction may occur in association with acute cor pulmonale. Recognition of these pseudoinfarct variants is essential because of the clinical importance of distinguishing acute cor pulmonale from myocardial infarction. In addition to nuclear lung scans, the echocardiogram may be a useful test for differentiating acute cor pulmonale due to pulmonary embolism from myocardial infarction. For example, Kasper et al.[27] reported a dilated right ventricle in 42% and a dilated pulmonary artery in 77% of patients with pulmonary embolism.

Chronic Cor Pulmonale (Pulmonary Emphysema)

The following pseudoinfarct patterns may be seen in association with pulmonary emphysema.

1. *Anterior wall infarct patterns* (Figs. 4-10 to 4-12). Poor precordial R wave progression (delayed precordial transition zone, clockwise rotation) is a characteristic finding in patients with emphysema. In such cases a QS complex may extend to V_3 and V_4 in the absence of infarction.[51,52,54] In rarer cases a noninfarctional QS complex may extend to the lateral precordial leads (Fig. 4-10). The T waves in the anterior precordial leads may be upright, flat, or deeply inverted (as part of a right ventricular strain pattern).
2. *Inferior wall infarct pattern* (Fig. 4-11). In rare cases chronic cor pulmonale may be associated with noninfarctional QS complexes in II, III, and aV_F.[32,34] One case report[3] described QR complexes in all three inferior leads in a patient with no clinical history of infarction. (Chronic cor pulmonale due to recurrent pulmonary emboli may also be associated with the $S_I Q_{III} T_{III}$ [described on p. 72].)

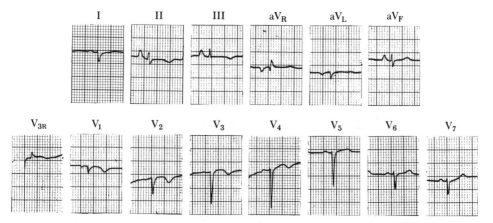

FIG. 4-10. Cor pulmonale simulating extensive anterior infarction. This patient, a 58-year-old woman with a long history of chronic cor pulmonale, had suffered an acute exacerbation of symptoms. There was no clinical history of ischemic heart disease. Her ECG shows extreme clockwise rotation in the precordial leads, with an rS complex in V_7. The qR in V_{3R} and the marked right axis deviation are indicators of underlying right ventricular hypertrophy. T wave inversions in the right precordial leads are consistent with right ventricular strain. Note the P pulmonale (in II) and the low voltage. Although an underlying infarct cannot be ruled out with certainty in this case, the pattern shown here is compatible with a diagnosis of severe chronic cor pulmonale in the absence of coronary disease.

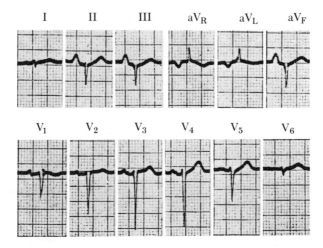

FIG. 4-11. Chronic cor pulmonale simulating anterior and inferior wall infarction. This ECG of a 57-year-old man shows poor R wave progression across the entire precordium (extreme clockwise rotation) plus QS waves in III and aV_F and an rS in II. P pulmonale is present, with a markedly superior mean frontal plane QRS axis (−90 degrees). At autopsy there was no evidence of infarction. Cor pulmonale (acute or chronic) frequently mimics the pattern of anterior infarction. Rarely, however, does chronic cor simulate the pattern of both anterior and inferior necrosis. In such cases there is no way to exclude the diagnosis of infarction on the basis of the ECG findings alone. (From Lipman BS, et al: Clinical scalar electrocardiography, ed 6, Chicago, 1972, Year Book Medical Publishers Inc. Used with permission.)

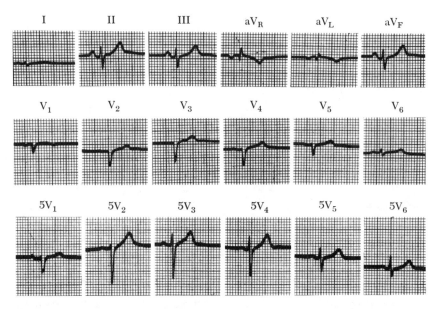

FIG. 4-12. Pulmonary emphysema simulating anterior infarction in a 58-year-old man with no clinical evidence of coronary disease. Note the relative normalization of R wave progression with placement of the chest leads on interspace below their usual position ($5V_1$, $5V_2$, etc.) (From Chou TC: In Fisch C [editor]: Complex electrocardiography, Philadelphia, 1973, FA Davis Co, vol 1).

3. *Other pseudoinfarct patterns.* In advanced cor pulmonale the ECG pattern of right ventricular hypertrophy may be present, with tall right precordial R waves and marked right axis deviation. In such cases any of the pseudoinfarct patterns just described in the section on right ventricular hypertrophy may also be present (e.g., QR complexes in the right precordial leads and QS complexes in the left precordial leads and in aV_L and I).

In addition, any of the patterns that are associated with acute cor pulmonale ($S_I Q_{III} T_{III}$, right ventricular strain) may appear. Littmann[34] estimated the prevalence of pseudoinfarct patterns in patients with pulmonary emphysema at 2% to 3%.

Besides these pseudoinfarct patterns, pulmonary emphysema is commonly though not invariably associated with two other important ECG patterns: low voltage and P pulmonale.[34,69,78]

Etiology. The pseudoinfarct patterns just described probably result from a number of factors, including changes in cardiac position and rotation, right ventricular overload, and pulmonary hyperaeration.

In patients with emphysema the diaphragm is low and the heart is displaced inferiorly. If placed in their usual positions, the precordial leads therefore will tend to overlie the base of the heart. The base of the heart is a region of electrical negativity, accounting in part for the pattern of poor R wave progression.[60] (An analogous "loss of anterior wall forces" occurs in normal subjects when the chest leads are inadvertently placed too high; see the section on spurious causes of Q waves, p. 38). The pattern of marked clockwise rotation can sometimes be normalized in patients with emphysema simply by recording the chest leads an interspace lower than usual[78] (Fig. 4-12).

The pattern of clockwise rotation and poor R wave progression may also be partly caused by actual anatomic rotation of the heart on its long axis. Such clockwise rotation would tend to bring the right ventricle more anteriorly, so that leads overlying the left midprecordium might still record right ventricular epicardial (QS or rS) types of complexes.[67] Littmann,[34] however, observed no objective radiographic or autopsy evidence for actual anatomic rotation of the heart in this manner. Right ventricular hypertrophy and dilation associated with chronic cor pulmonale would also tend to displace the right ventricle anteriorly, thus contributing to the pattern of clockwise rotation.

The cause of the QS waves occasionally seen in emphysema in II, III, and aV_F is not clear. The QS pattern in these leads is associated with a markedly superior frontal plane QRS axis. In such cases the mean cardiac vector is oriented at about −90 degrees in the frontal plane, and leads aV_R and aV_L typically show nearly identical patterns (negative P wave followed by a qR complex), as seen in Fig. 4-11.

The significance of superior axis deviation in emphysema is still unsettled. Rosenbaum, Elizari, and Lazzari[61] considered this unusual pattern to be a variant of the common type of left axis deviation caused by left anterior hemiblock. However, in most cases of classic left anterior hemiblock associated with coronary artery disease or other causes, the QRS axis generally does not exceed −80 degrees. The superior axis seen with emphysema is typically about −90 degrees, a finding that suggests different or additional etiologic factors. Grant[21] proposed that the hyperaerated lungs might produce verticalization of cardiac potentials. Spodick[69] suggested the existence of an "axis illusion" phenomenon; the mean QRS forces in chronic cor pulmonale appear to be oriented posteriorly, and theoretically a slight shift in cardiac rotation could result in the projection of this posterior vector either superiorly or inferiorly in the frontal plane.

Differential diagnosis. The problem of differentiating chronic cor pulmonale from myocardial infarction is a frequent ECG dilemma. When poor R wave progression is found in patients with emphysema, it is usually impossible to rule out underlying infarction absolutely. Similarly, when a QS complex is present in II, III, and aV_F in these patients, inferior wall infarction cannot be excluded with certainty. However, it is important not to overdiagnose coronary disease in these cases and to recognize that infarction patterns (particularly poor precordial R wave progression) are common findings in uncomplicated emphysema.

The presence of chronic cor pulmonale can often be inferred from the ECG by the combination of low voltage, P pulmonale, and poor R wave progression. A vertical or rightward QRS axis is usually present. Loss of normal R wave progression with a left axis deviation is more suggestive of underlying coronary disease.[50] As already mentioned, a marked superior (left) axis is sometimes seen in uncomplicated chronic cor pulmonale.

In cases of poor R wave progression in the precordial leads it may be useful to record the chest leads an interspace lower than usual for the reasons described earlier. Normalization of precordial R wave progression following this maneuver suggests that the clockwise rotation pattern in such cases is caused by emphysema alone (Fig. 4-12). In one study[22] with a relatively small sample size (16 patients) the amplitude of the R wave in V_3 recorded one interspace lower than usual was found to be diagnostically useful. An R wave ≤ 0.5 mm suggested infarction, while an R wave ≥ 3.5 mm suggested emphysema (Fig. 4-12). R waves of intermediate amplitude were nondiagnostic.

Finally, the ST-T wave configuration may also help in differentiating these patterns. Deep T wave inversions in the right precordial leads may be found in both anterior wall infarction and right ventricular strain. However, marked ST elevations are not a feature of chronic cor pulmonale, and the sequence of ST elevation followed by T wave inversion is virtually pathognomonic of myocardial infarction.

Arrhythmogenic Right Ventricular Dysplasia

Arrhythmogenic right ventricular dysplasia (ARVD) is a specific form of cardiomyopathy that primarily affects the right ventricle.* The right ventricular musculature is partially or sometimes completely replaced by fatty and fibrous tissue. Uhl's anomaly (parchment right ventricle) is generally considered to be the most extreme form of right ventricular dysplasia. The descriptor "arrhythmogenic" is applied to patients with this cardiomyopathy because of the high frequency of ventricular tachycardia (usually with a left bundle branch block morphology) that may lead to syncope or sudden death (Fig. 4-13). Patients may also present with asymptomatic cardiomegaly or right-sided congestive failure.

The electrocardiogram in patients with ARVD often shows precordial T wave inversions that may extend out to V_4 or even V_6, thus mimicking anterior wall ischemia or infarction. Incomplete (and more rarely complete) right bundle branch block may present, as may P pulmonale. Postexcitation waves, also called *epsilon waves,* may appear as small undulations in the ST segment (Fig. 4-13). They probably correlate with delayed ventricular potentials and are thought to be related to the increased susceptibility to ventricular tachycardia.

Diagnosis is supported by echocardiographic or angiographic documentation of regional or global right ventricular wall motion disorders. High-grade ventricular arrhythmias not responding to empirical antiarrhythmic therapy may require surgical intervention (ventriculotomy). The pathogenesis of ARVD is unknown. Presumably, the precordial T wave inversions reflect delayed or abnormal repolarization of the right ventricle. There is a male predominance, and familial cases are well described.

---

*References 13, 38, 39, 53, 62, 74.

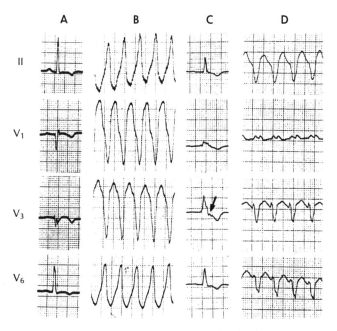

FIG. 4-13. Arrhythmogenic right ventricular dysplasia simulating anterior wall infarction in a 44-year-old man. **A** (1966), Note the minor right ventricular conduction delay with poor R wave progression and the anterior T wave inversions on the resting ECG. **B** (1969), Ventricular tachycardia with a left bundle branch block pattern. **C** (1982), A more prominent ventricular conduction disturbance. The arrow in V_3 indicates a delayed (so-called "epsilon") potential. **D** (1982), Ventricular tachycardia with a right bundle branch block morphology. (From Higuchi S, et al: Am Heart J 108:1363, 1984).

HYPERTROPHIC CARDIOMYOPATHY

The term hypertrophic cardiomyopathy describes a disorder characterized by predominant overgrowth of the ventricular septum sometimes with secondary subaortic and more rarely subpulmonic obstruction.

Observations over the past few decades[7,15,43] have broadened our understanding of this cardiomyopathy and have demonstrated that classic *idiopathic hypertrophic subaortic stenosis* (IHSS) constitutes only one manifestation of a spectrum usually associated with primary asymmetric septal hypertrophy. Patients with such hypertrophy, often inherited as an autosomal dominant trait, fall into a number of clinical groups: (1) those with latent septal hypertrophy, identifiable at echocardiographic examination, who are otherwise without symptoms, (2) those with septal hypertrophy and symptoms related to ventricular outflow obstruction (IHSS), (3) those with symptoms but *without* evidence of outflow obstruction (cardiac symptoms in this group have been attributed to ventricular hypertrophy and decreased left ventricular compliance[23]), and (4) those with or without symptoms who are identified as having predominant *apical hypertrophic cardiomyopathy.*

ECGs of patients with hypertrophic cardiomyopathy (with or without outflow obstruction) may show a variety of patterns. In some cases the ECG is completely normal. In others the classic pattern of left ventricular hypertrophy is seen. An important subset of patients with this cardiomyopathy have prominent noninfarctional Q waves. *Indeed, hypertrophic cardiopathy is one of the most important causes of pseudoinfarct patterns and may be associated with noninfarctional Q waves in any of the standard leads. In addition, ST-T patterns simulating those of acute or evolving myocardial infarction may be present.* The following simulators have been encountered[*]:

1. *Anteroseptal infarction pattern,* with QS waves in the right to midprecordial leads (V_1 to V_4) identical to the pseudoinfarctional QS waves sometimes seen with concentric left ventricular hypertrophy, described earlier (Figs. 4-14 and 4-15)
2. *Anterolateral infarction pattern,* with abnormal Q waves (as part of a QS or QR complex or a W-shaped QS complex) in the left precordial leads and also in I and aV_L (Figs. 4-16, 4-17, and 4-18, *B*)
3. *Inferior wall infarction pattern,* with abnormal Q waves (as part of a QS, QR, or Qr complex or a W-shaped QS complex) in one or more of II, III, and aV_F (Fig. 4-19)
4. *Posterior wall infarction pattern,* with tall R waves in the right precordial leads, usually associated with abnormal Q waves in the inferior or lateral precordial leads (Figs. 4-17 and 4-18, *B*); this pattern also mimics that of right ventricular hypertrophy
5. *Deep T wave inversions* (Fig. 4-20); a subset of patients with nonobstructive hypertrophic cardiomyopathy has been described with predominant *apical* location of the septal hypertrophy; this variant is referred to as apical hypertrophic cardiomyopathy, or Yamaguchi's syndrome[85]

    The initial Japanese reports of this syndrome[63,85] called attention to the deep precordial T wave inversions, exceeding 10 mm (1 mV) in some cases ("giant T wave negativity"). Subsequent communications from North America[35,41,43,79] have confirmed this variant.

    In a follow-up of patients studied for 1 to 22 years after the initial diagnosis, Webb et al.[79] reported giant T wave inversions in 14 of 26 cases. The inverted T waves sometimes became more prominent with time and were typically most apparent in V_3 to V_5 (usually V_4). A direct correlation between their magnitude and noninvasive measurements of apical wall thickness or left ventricular mass was not observed.[79] The mechanism of

---

[*]References 4, 15, 30, 57, 59, 63, 83, 85.

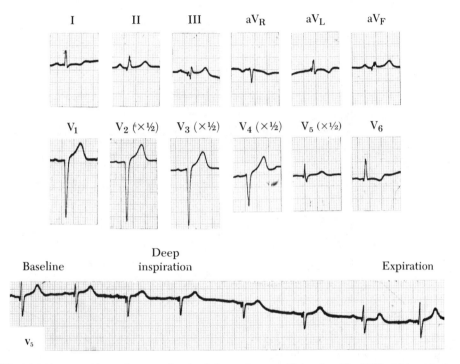

FIG. 4-14. Hypertrophic cardiomyopathy simulating anteroseptal infarction. The ECG of this patient, a 27-year-old man, shows poor R wave progression in the right to middle precordial leads with minuscule r waves in V_3 and V_4. Voltage in the precordial leads is increased, consistent with left ventricular hypertrophy, and the T wave inversions in I, aV_L, and V_6 are consistent with a left ventricular strain pattern. Small q waves appear in II, aV_F, and V_5 to V_6. Lead III shows bizarre notched Qr complexes. The strip at the bottom illustrates the effect of deep inspiration on the QRS morphology in V_5: with normal respiration a qRS is present whereas with deep inspiration a qrS appears. This marked change in QRS morphology is probably caused by the shift in cardiac (and therefore septal) orientation that occurs with deep inspiration.

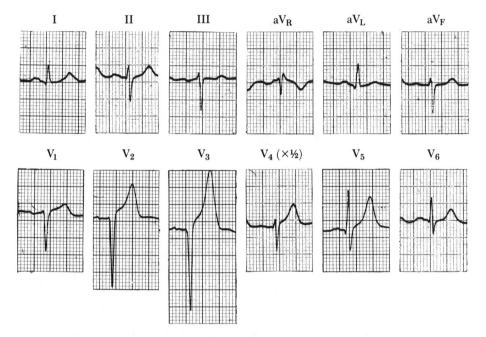

FIG. 4-15. Hypertrophic cardiomyopathy simulating acute anteroseptal infarction. On the ECG of this 40-year-old man, the precordial leads show poor R wave progression, with QS complexes in V_1 to V_3. Tall positive T waves with a high ST takeoff are also present in the right precordial leads, simulating the hyperacute phase of infarction (see Fig. 18-3, A). This ECG also shows left axis deviation and left atrial abnormality (wide notched P waves in I and II).

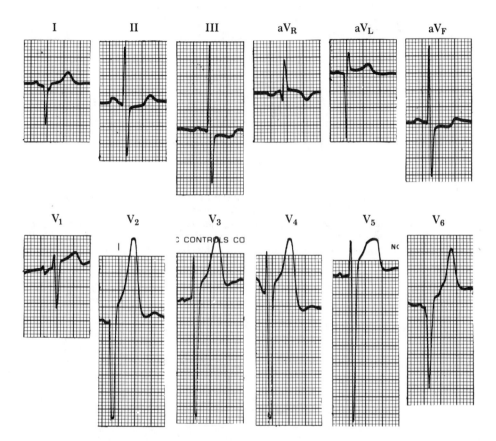

FIG. 4-16. Hypertrophic cardiomyopathy simulating anterolateral infarction in a 19-year-old man. Prominent Q waves are present in leads I, aV$_L$, and V$_6$. The voltage is markedly increased, and right axis deviation is present. In addition, the precordial leads show vaulting T waves with a high ST take-off mimicking the hyperacute phase of infarction (see Fig. 18-3, *A*). Borderline wide P waves in II and V$_1$ suggest left atrial abnormality. Nonspecific ST-T changes are seen in leads II, III, and aV$_F$.

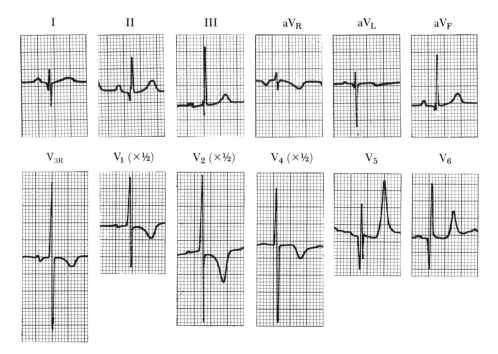

FIG. 4-17. Hypertrophic cardiomyopathy simulating posterolateral infarction. Note the bizarre narrow T waves in the lateral precordial leads. Deeply inverted T waves are also noted in V_{3R} and V_4, along with right axis deviation. The patient (a 7-year-old boy) died suddenly 1 year after this tracing was obtained. At autopsy his heart showed marked septal and biventricular hypertrophy. The significance of the tall peaked T waves in these leads was not clear. Hyperkalemia was not present.

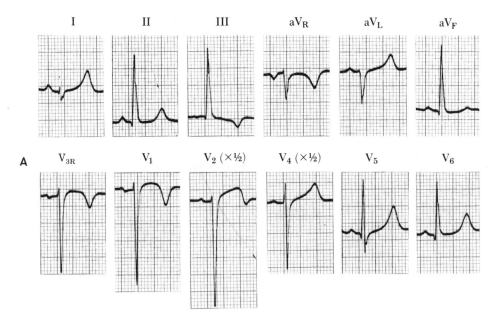

FIG. 4-18. For legend see opposite page.

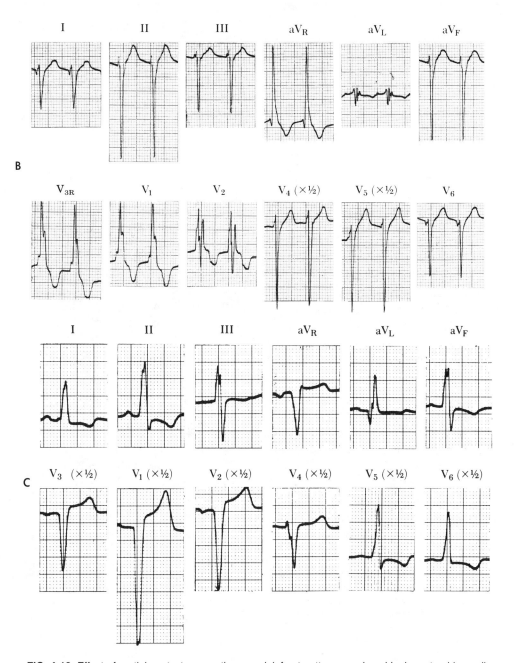

FIG. 4-18. Effect of partial septectomy on the pseudoinfarct patterns produced by hypertrophic cardiomyopathy. **A,** Preoperative ECG of a 13-year-old boy showing increased precordial voltage and poor R wave progression consistent with left ventricular hypertrophy. Prominent coved T wave inversions are present in V_{3R} and V_2, but their significance is not clear. They may indicate right ventricular strain or actual anterior ischemia, both of which could have exaggerated the normal juvenile pattern of right precordial T wave inversions. The frontal plane QRS axis is +90 degrees. **B,** ECG obtained 2 days after resection of a portion of the hypertrophied septal tissue. Note the bizarre right ventricular conduction disturbance, resembling right bundle branch block; however, there are deep QS waves in V_6, and a qrS in I simulates lateral wall infarction. Extreme axis deviation is also present (+240 degrees or -120 degrees), with a supraventricular tachycardia. **C,** ECG taken 5 years after **B.** Notice the left bundle branch block pattern, with an electrical axis of +30 degrees. Pseudoinfarctional QS waves are present in V_1 to V_3. In addition, a deep Q wave is present in aV_L. ST elevations and prominent T waves in the right precordial leads are commonly seen with left bundle branch block or left ventricular hypertrophy and should not be confused with the hyperacute T waves of infarction. (Compare with Figs. 18-2, *A,* and 18-3, *A.*)

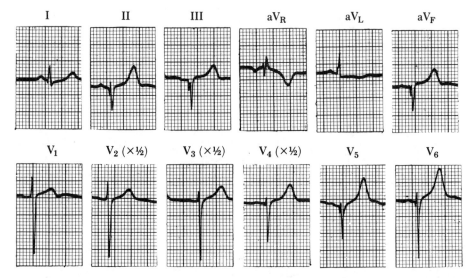

FIG. 4-19. Hypertrophic cardiomyopathy simulating inferolateral infarction. This 11-year-old girl had a family history of hypertrophic cardiomyopathy. (The ECG of her father is shown in Fig. 4-14). Note the W-shaped QS waves and qrS complexes in the inferior and lateral precordial leads. These are virtually diagnostic of hypertrophic cardiomyopathy in patients in this age group. Leads showing abnormal Q waves (II, III, aV$_F$, V$_5$, and V$_6$) all have positive T waves. Pathologic septal Q waves, as part of QS or Qr complexes, seen with hypertrophic cardiomyopathy are characteristically associated with upright T waves, in contrast to the pattern seen with infarction (in which abnormal Q waves are frequently though not always associated with *inverted* T waves).

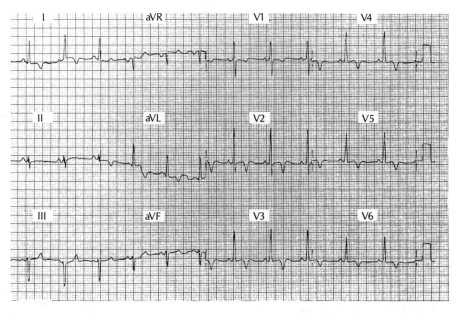

FIG. 4-20. Apical variant of hypertrophic cardiomyopathy in a 39-year-old white man. Note the prominent anterior T wave inversions, which are a characteristic feature of this syndrome. There are also tall R waves in V_1. Left axis deviation is present.

such T wave abnormalities is not certain but may relate to abnormal repolarization patterns of the hypertrophic muscle or to actual ischemia.

6. *ST-T changes simulating the hyperacute phase of infarction* (Chapter 8)

This pattern is characterized by tall positive T waves with or without the ST elevations of early infarction (Figs. 18-1 to 18-5). A similar pattern of tall positive T waves, sometimes with marked ST elevations, occurs in patients with hypertrophic cardiomyopathy (Figs. 4-15 to 4-17) in which the T waves are usually most prominent in the right or left precordial leads and are broad based (Figs. 4-15 and 4-16).

The repolarization voltages with hypertrophic cardiomyopathy, evidenced by tall positive T waves, are roughly proportional to the increased amplitude of the depolarization (QRS) voltages seen in these cases. As a rule the T waves with hypertrophic cardiomyopathy are upright in leads showing prominent pathologic Q waves (specifically, QS or Qr waves where the Q exceeds the R amplitude).[17] This discordance of the QRS and T wave axes is analogous to the discordant QRS and T wave axes of the classic left ventricular "strain" pattern. With left ventricular hypertrophy and strain, tall R waves (reflecting positive free wall depolarization forces) are associated with negative T waves. With hypertrophic cardiomyopathy the deep Q waves (reflecting negative septal forces) are associated with tall upright T waves. Conversely, in some cases of hypertrophic cardiomyopathy a possible "septal strain" pattern may be seen in leads that face the hypertrophied septum (V_1 and V_2) and record tall R waves with T wave inversions (Fig. 4-17). (An alternative explanation would be the presence of an intraventricular conduction disturbance causing secondary ST-T changes.)

On the basis of a single tracing, the tall positive T waves seen with hypertrophic cardiomyopathy may be indistinguishable from the pattern of hyperacute infarction. However, the ST-T complex of hypertrophic cardiomyopathy is usually stable over time. In contrast, the hyperacute T waves of infarction are generally followed within 24 hours by the more familiar ST-T changes of evolving infarction (e.g., ST segment lability and deep T wave inversions).

Q Waves With Hypertrophic Cardiomyopathy

The abnormal noninfarctional Q waves just described are an important diagnostic finding with hypertrophic cardiomyopathy. In Frank and Braunwald's series of patients with classic idiopathic hypertrophic subaortic stenosis,[15] Q waves were noted in 56% of 123 cases. Savage et al.[64] reported prominent Q waves in 28 of 68 patients (41%) with obstructive cardiomyopathy and 16 of 66 patients (24%) with nonobstructive cardiomyopathy. The actual prevalence of pseudoinfarctional Q waves in unselected patients with hypertrophic cardiomyopathy is probably lower. Abnormal Q waves may be observed in both children and adults with this syndrome, but are rare in patients past the age of 60 years.[82] There have also been reports suggesting an association between hypertrophic cardiomyopathy and Friedreich's ataxia (p. 151).

These pseudoinfarct Q waves have not been consistently correlated with any significant echocardiographic, hemodynamic, or prognostic parameter.[15,64] In some cases they regress spontaneously with time. In other instances new Q waves appear during the course of observation.[15] Wigle and Baron[83] reported several cases in which abnormal Q waves disappeared or diminished in size immediately following surgical incision of the left side of the hypertrophied septum (left septal myotomy). In some of these cases the deep abnormal Q waves previously present in the lateral precordial leads were replaced postoperatively by tall R waves typical of the pattern seen with concentric left ventricular hypertrophy. The abrupt appearance of tall R waves in leads formerly showing deep Q waves suggests that this pattern of free wall hypertrophy had been masked preoperatively by the preponderant septal forces.[83] The striking effects of partial septectomy on the ECG pattern of one patient with hypertrophic cardiomyopathy are shown serially in Fig. 4-18.

The morphology of the pseudoinfarctional Q waves in hypertrophic cardiomyopathy is variable. In some cases the Q waves are sharply inscribed and pointed (lancelike), as shown in Fig. 4-17. In other cases the Q waves may be notched or slurred and sometimes have a bizarre W-shape (Fig. 4-19).

Etiology. The pathogenesis of these striking pseudoinfarct patterns in patients with hypertrophic cardiomyopathy is a subject of some controversy. One of the earliest and most attractive explanations for them was proposed by Braudo, Wigle, and Keith.[4] They ascribed the Q waves directly to an increase in septal musculature, resulting in exaggeration of the normal electrical forces generated by the ventricular septum. Normally the initial forces of septal depolarization spread from left to right, producing a small septal r wave usually seen in V_1. Reciprocally, these early septal forces are directed away from the left precordial leads, which accounts for the normal septal q waves seen in the left precordial leads and usually in one or more of the limb leads as part of a qR type of complex. Such normal septal q waves are of short duration (usually about 0.02 sec) and relatively low amplitude (less than 25% of the succeeding R wave in that lead).

Massive septal hypertrophy would be expected to augment both the magnitude and the duration of these septal forces, accounting for the deep Q waves that may appear in the lateral or inferior leads and also for the tall right precordial R waves in some patients with hypertrophic cardiomyopathy. If the septal forces were of sufficient magnitude, they might completely overbalance the forces generated by the left ventricular free wall, producing an entirely negative QS complex or W-shaped complex in the left precordial or inferior limb leads (Fig. 4-19). As mentioned previously, hypertrophic cardiomyopathy may also be associated with deep QS waves in the right precordial leads, simulating the pattern of anteroseptal infarction. Wigle and Baron[83] speculated that these right precordial QS complexes might reflect predominant posteroseptal hypertrophy, resulting in a preponderance of dorsally directed depolarization forces. Alternatively these right precordial QS waves could reflect hypertrophy of the left ventricular free wall.

Left ventricular free wall hypertrophy can occur in patients with hypertrophic cardiomyopathy from at least two possible mechanisms: in some cases there may be hypertrophy of the left ventricle secondary to subaortic obstruction; in others the myopathic process appears to extend to involve the free wall as well as the septum. Theoretically, if sufficient hypertrophy of the free wall occurs for either reason, the posteriorly and laterally directed depolarization forces generated by the hypertrophied left ventricle might reach the critical magnitude required to overbalance the anterior and rightward forces of the septum. This concept of an evolving balance between septal and free wall depolarization forces may also help to account for the changing ECG patterns observed over time in some patients with hypertrophic cardiomyopathy (e.g., the appearance or regression of Q waves).[4]

The pseudoinfarctional Q waves of hypertrophic cardiomyopathy may, however, be the product of more than a simple augmentation of septal forces caused by the "bulk effect" of muscular hypertrophy. Indeed, van Dam, Roos, and Durrer,[75] using intramural electrodes in patients with hypertrophic cardiomyopathy, failed to document any increase in the voltage of septal forces. Subsequent echocardiographic studies[31,36,40,48] have failed to define consistent correlations between the location or degree of septal, left ventricular free wall, or right ventricular hypertrophy and the presence of Q waves. Lemery et al.[31] reported that the *ratio* of upper anterior septal to mean right ventricular wall thickness was significantly greater in patients with abnormal Q waves than in those without. If this preliminary finding is confirmed, it will lend credence to the notion that Q waves in hypertrophic cardiomyopathy may be associated with an altered balance of early depolarization forces.

Other explanations for these unusual ECG patterns have focused on the possibility of altered myocardial activation.

Histologic examination of the septal tissue of patients with hypertrophic cardiomyopathy typically reveals massive myocardial hypertrophy with the individual fibers arrayed in an unusual manner. In some areas the fibers are grouped in concentric rings, producing a whorl-like appearance.[76] This bizarre microscopic architecture may form the structural basis for the altered depolarization pathways that have been postulated to occur in hypertrophic cardiomyopathy. Coyne,[10] for example, suggested that altered transseptal conduction pathways might account for the remarkable variety of ECG patterns encountered in this cardiomyopathy.

An additional factor that may also play a role in the pathogenesis of Q waves with hypertrophic cardiomyopathy is premature septal activation,[83] analogous to the preexcitation phenomenon seen with the Wolff-Parkinson-White syndrome. Snellen,[66] for example, documented early activation of the anterior paraseptal basal region in one case. An association between hypertrophic cardiomyopathy and the classic Wolff-Parkinson-White syndrome has been observed. The complete Wolff-Parkinson-White triad was noted in 4 of 124 patients in Frank and Braunwald's series,[15] in which 11 other patients manifested two components of the syndrome. Pseudoinfarctional Q waves are a well-recognized feature of Wolff-Parkinson-White patterns (and are described in detail in Chapter 5). However, most cases of hypertrophic cardiomyopathy with pseudoinfarctional Q waves are not associated with the classic pattern of preexcitation or other evidence of gross conduction disturbances on the conventional ECG recording.

In a study of septal and ventricular activation in patients with classic hypertrophic cardiomyopathy, van Dam, Roos, and Durrer[75] noted a delay in subendocardial activation and suggested that irregular activation of the inner layers of the left ventricle might account for the unusual Q waves. However, the exact mechanism of Q wave pathogenesis in such cases remains obscure.

The pseudoinfarct Q waves of hypertrophic cardiomyopathy may decrease in amplitude during atrial pacing, supporting the general concept that these abnormal depolarization forces are related to an abnormality in early septal activation.[9]

In summary: Two principal, though not mutually exclusive, factors have been cited to account for the Q waves in hypertrophic cardiomyopathy. They are primary septal hypertrophy and altered ventricular activation.

Differential diagnosis. The differential diagnosis of hypertrophic cardiomyopathy versus coronary artery disease poses a number of problems. ECGs of patients with hypertrophic cardiomyopathy not only frequently show the picture of infarction (including Q waves and ST-T alterations), but such patients also often have angina and a systolic murmur, mimicking the clinical presentation of atherosclerotic heart disease with papillary muscle dysfunction.[58] Patients with hypertrophic cardiomyopathy may also show prominent ST depressions during exercise testing (see Fig. 13-5).

As a general rule, the diagnosis of hypertrophic cardiomyopathy should always be considered (especially in the younger patient) when any of the ECG patterns just described are encountered. Deep lancelike Q waves are particularly suggestive but not diagnostic of hypertrophic cardiomyopathy. Relatively deep septal Q waves are sometimes observed in any condition that produces generalized left ventricular (including septal) hypertrophy. In pediatric patients deep, narrow, septal Q waves are sometimes observed in ventricular septal defects, patent ductus arteriosus, and other conditions causing left ventricular volume overloading.[56] Prominent septal Q waves are also sometimes seen in patients with left ventricular hypertrophy due to volume or pressure overload (p. 63). Deep narrow Q waves in the inferior limb or lateral precordial leads are also commonly seen with Duchenne muscular dystrophy (p. 143).

As mentioned earlier, some cases of hypertrophic cardiomyopathy may present with wide, notched, or W-shaped Q waves that are morphologically indistinguishable from the irregular Q waves produced by actual myocardial injury. In such instances the polarity of the T wave may provide an important clue to the differential diagnosis of these deep Q waves.[17] The QS, QR, or W-shaped complexes of hypertrophic cardiomyopathy are ordinarily associated with upright (positive) T waves. This pattern of Q wave–T wave axis discordance in hypertrophic cardiomyopathy was just described. The deep Q waves seen with infarction may also be associated with positive T waves. However, the deep T wave inversions commonly seen in leads with infarctional Q waves are not a feature of hypertrophic cardiomyopathy.

(Coronary artery disease and hypertrophic cardiomyopathy may coexist in the same patient. Theoretically, a septal infarct in such cases might result in a decrease in the size of pathologic Q waves caused by prior septal hypertrophy.[17] Such paradoxical diminution in Q wave amplitude with septal infarction in hypertrophic cardiomyopathy has not been reported as yet.)

Finally, it should be emphasized that patients with unexplained Q waves or T wave inversions should undergo careful two-dimensional echocardiographic studies to exclude the possibility of a hypertrophic cardiomyopathy variant.

In summary: Hypertrophic cardiomyopathy and myocardial infarction are two pathologic conditions with similar ECG manifestations produced by diametrically opposed mechanisms. The abnormal Q waves of hypertrophic cardiomyopathy are associated with an apparent *increase* in the magnitude and duration of septal depolarization forces. By contrast, the Q waves associated with myocardial infarction or other types of myocardial injury (e.g., myocarditis, amyloidosis, and cardiac tumor) reflect a primary *loss* of depolarization forces. These examples illustrate how the same electrocardiographic "phenotype" (Q waves) can be associated with markedly different electrophysiologic "genotypes" (hypertrophy vs. myocardial destruction).

REFERENCES

1. Alfonso F, et al: Clinical significance of giant negative T waves in hypertrophic cardiomyopathy, J Am Coll Cardiol 15:965, 1990.
2. Benchimol AB, Schlesinger P: Electrocardiographic changes in a case of left ventricular and septal hypertrophy resembling anterior myocardial infarction, Circulation 1:970, 1950.
3. Bernreiter M: Cor pulmonale simulating myocardial infarction, Dis Chest 37:573, 1960.
4. Braudo M, et al: A distinctive electrocardiogram in muscular subaortic stenosis due to ventricular septal hypertrophy, Am J Cardiol 14:599, 1964.
5. Cabrera E, Gaxiola A: Diagnostic contribution of vectorcardiogram in hemodynamic overloading of the heart, Am Heart J 60:296, 1960.
6. Caskey TD, Estes EH Jr: Deviation of the S-T segment: a review, Am J Med 36:424, 1964.
7. Clark CE, et al: Familial prevalence and genetic transmission of idiopathic hypertrophic subaortic stenosis, N Engl J Med 289:709, 1973.

8. Clinical and electrocardiographic observations. In Sasahara RA, et al (editors): The Urokinase–Pulmonary Embolism Trial, Circulation 47(suppl II):60. 1973.
9. Cosio FG, et al: The Q waves of hypertrophic cardiomyopathy: an electrophysiologic study, N Engl J Med 302:96, 1980.
10. Coyne JJ: New concepts of intramural myocardial conduction in hypertrophic obstructive cardiomyopathy, Br Heart J 30:546, 1968.
11. Dack S, et al: Acute coronary insufficiency due to pulmonary embolism, Am J Med 7:464, 1949.
12. Eliaser M, Giansiracusa F: The electrocardiographic diagnosis of acute cor pulmonale, Am Heart J 43:533, 1952.
13. Fontaine G, et al: Dysplasie ventriculaire droite arythmogène et maladie de Uhl, Arch Mal Coeur 75:361, 1982.
14. Fowler NO, et al: The Q wave in precordial electrocardiograms overlying the hypertrophied right ventricle: intracavity leads, Circulation 5:441, 1952.
15. Frank S, Braunwald E: Idiopathic hypertrophic subaortic stenosis: clinical analysis of 126 patients with emphasis on the natural history, Circulation 37:759, 1968.
16. Friedman HH: Diagnostic electrocardiography and vectorcardiography, New York, 1971, McGraw-Hill Book Co.
17. Goldberger AL: Q wave T wave vector discordance in hypertrophic cardiomyopathy: septal hypertrophy and strain pattern, Br Heart J 42:201, 1979.
18. Goldberger E: Unipolar lead electrocardiography and vectorcardiography, ed 3, Philadelphia, 1953, Lea & Febiger.
19. Goldberger E: How to interpret electrocardiograms in terms of vectors, Springfield Ill, 1968, Charles C Thomas Publisher.
20. Grant RP: The relationship between the anatomic position of the heart and the electrocardiogram: a criticism of "unipolar" electrocardiography, Circulation 7:890, 1953.
21. Grant RP: Left axis deviation: an electrocardiographic-pathologic correlation study, Circulation 14:233, 1956.
22. Hart GJ, et al: Diagnosis of old anterior myocardial infarction in emphysema with poor R wave progression in anterior chest leads, Br Heart J 45:522, 1981.
23. Henry WL, et al: Asymmetric septal hypertrophy (ASH): the unifying link in the IHSS disease spectrum, Circulation 47:827, 1973.
24. Hugenholtz PG, et al: Recognition of anterior wall infarction in patients with left ventricular hypertrophy, Circulation 27:386, 1963.
25. Iida K, et al: Diurnal changes of giant negative T wave in patients with hypertrophic cardiomyopathy, Clin Cardiol 13:272, 1990.
26. Karlen W, Wolff L: The vectorcardiogram in pulmonary embolism. II, Am Heart J 51:839, 1956.
27. Kasper W, et al: Echocardiographic findings in patients with proved pulmonary embolism, Am Heart J 112:1284, 1986.
28. Kini PM, et al: Electrocardiographic differentiation between left ventricular hypertrophy and anterior myocardial infarction, Circulation 42:875, 1970.
29. Kramer NE, et al: Differentiation of posterior myocardial infarction from right ventricular hypertrophy and normal anterior loop by echocardiography, Circulation 58:1057, 1978.
30. Leachman RD, Leatherman LL: Idiopathic hypertrophic subaortic stenosis, Cardiovasc Res Cen Bull 7:9, 1968.
31. Lemery R, et al: Q waves in hypertrophic cardiomyopathy in relation to the distribution and severity of right and left ventricular hypertrophy, J Am Coll Cardiol 16:368, 1990.
32. Lipman BS, et al: Clinical scalar electrocardiography, ed 7, Chicago, 1984, Year Book Medical Publishers Inc.
33. Littmann D: Ventricular strain and ventricular hypertrophy, N Engl J Med 241:363, 1949.
34. Littmann D: The electrocardiographic findings in pulmonary emphysema, Am J Cardiol 5:339, 1960.
35. Louie EK, Maron BJ: Apical hypertrophic cardiomyopathy: clinical and two-dimensional echocardiographic assessment, Ann Intern Med 106:663, 1987.
36. Lynch RE, et al: Leftward shift of frontal plane QRS axis as a frequent manifestation of acute pulmonary embolism, Chest 61:443, 1972.
37. Mack I, et al: Acute cor pulmonale in the absence of pulmonary embolism, Am Heart J 39:664, 1950.
38. Manyari DE: Arrhythmogenic right ventricular dysplasia: a generalized cardiomyopathy, Circulation 68:251, 1983.
39. Marcus FI, et al: Right ventricular dysplasia: a report of 24 cases, Circulation 65:384, 1982.

40. Maron BJ: Q waves in hypertrophic cardiomyopathy: a reassessment, J Am Coll Cardiol 16:375, 1990.

41. Maron BJ, et al: Hypertrophic cardiomyopathy with ventricular septal hypertrophy localized to the apical region of the left ventricle (apical hypertrophic cardiomyopathy), Am J Cardiol 49:1838, 1982.

42. Maron BJ, et al: Relation of electrocardiographic abnormalities and patterns of left ventricular hypertrophy identified by 2-dimensional echocardiography in patients with hypertrophic cardiomyopathy, Am J Cardiol 51:189, 1983.

43. Maron BJ, et al: Hypertrophic cardiomyopathy: interrelations of clinical manifestations, pathophysiology, and therapy. I, II, N Engl J Med 316:780, 844, 1987.

44. Master AM, et al: Electrocardiographic patterns simulating coronary occlusion in patients with chronic rheumatic cardiovascular disease, Am Heart J 54:50, 1957.

45. Mathur VS, Levine HD: Vectorcardiographic differentiation between right ventricular hypertrophy and posterobasal myocardial infarction, Circulation 42:833, 1970.

46. McGinn S, White PD: Acute cor pulmonale resulting from pulmonary embolism: its clinical recognition, JAMA 104:1473, 1935.

47. McIntyre KM, et al: Relation of the electrocardiogram to hemodynamic alterations in pulmonary embolism, Am J Cardiol 30:205, 1972.

48. Mori H, et al: Pattern of myocardial hypertrophy as a possible determinant of abnormal Q waves in hypertrophic cardiomyopathy, Jpn Circ J 47:513, 1983.

49. Moser KM, et al: Chronic thrombotic obstruction of major pulmonary arteries: results of thromboarterectomy in 15 patients, Ann Intern Med 99:299, 1983.

50. Murata K, et al: QS- and QR-pattern in leads V_3 and V_4: electrocardiographic and pathologic correlation of 41 cases, including 25 cases without myocardial infarction, Jpn Circ J 27:259, 1963.

51. Myers GB: QRS-T patterns in multiple precordial leads that may be mistaken for myocardial infarction. I. Left ventricular hypertrophy and dilatation, Circulation 1:844, 1950.

52. Myers GB: QRS-T patterns in multiple precordial leads that may be mistaken for myocardial infarction. II. Right ventricular hypertrophy and dilatation, Circulation 1:860, 1950.

53. Navo A, et al: Electrovectorcardiographic study of negative T waves on precordial leads in arrhythmogenic right ventricular dysplasia: relationship with right ventricular volumes, J Electrocardiol 21:239, 1988.

54. Oram S, Davies P: The electrocardiogram in cor pulmonale, Prog Cardiovasc Dis 9:341, 1967.

55. Owen WR, et al: Unrecognized emboli to the lungs with subsequent cor pulmonale, N Engl J Med 249:919, 1953.

56. Perloff JK: The clinical recognition of congenital heart disease, ed 3, Philadelphia, 1987, WB Saunders Co.

57. Peter RH, et al: Subaortic stenosis simulating coronary disease, Arch Intern Med 121:564, 1968.

58. Phillips HR, et al: Evaluation of vectorcardiographic criteria for the diagnosis of myocardial infarction in the presence of left ventricular hypertrophy, Circulation 53:235, 1976.

59. Prescott R, et al: Electrocardiographic changes in hypertrophic subaortic stenosis which simulate myocardial infarction, Am Heart J 66:42, 1963.

60. Reeves WC, et al: Two-dimensional echocardiographic assessment of electrocardiographic criteria for right atrial enlargement, Circulation 64:387, 1981.

61. Rosenbaum MB et al: The hemiblocks, Oldsmar Fla, 1970, Tampa Tracings.

62. Ruder MA, et al: Arrhythmogenic right ventricular dysplasia in a family, Am J Cardiol 56:799, 1985.

63. Sakamoto T, et al: Giant negative T-wave inversion as a manifestation of asymptomatic apical hypertrophy (AAH) of the left ventricle: echocardiographic and ultrasonocardiotomographic study, Jpn Heart J 17:611, 1976.

64. Savage DD, et al: Electrocardiographic findings in patients with obstructive and nonobstructive hypertrophic cardiomyopathy, Circulation 58:402, 1978.

65. Smith M, Ray CT: Electrocardiographic signs of early right ventricular enlargement in acute pulmonary embolism, Chest 58:205, 1970.

66. Snellen HA: Discussion. In Westenholme GEW, O'Connor M (editors): Cardiomyopathies, London, 1964, J & A Churchill Ltd.

67. Sodi-Pallares D: New bases of electrocardiography, St Louis, 1956, The CV Mosby Co.
68. Sodi-Pallares D, et al: Some views on the significance of qR and QR type complexes in right precordial leads in the absence of myocardial infarction, Am Heart J 43:716, 1952.
69. Spodick DH: Electrocardiographic studies in pulmonary disease. I. Electrocardiographic abnormalities in diffuse lung disease, Circulation 20:1067, 1959.
70. Spodick DH: Electrocardiographic responses to pulmonary embolism: mechanisms and sources of variability, Am J Cardiol 30:695, 1972.
71. Stein PD, et al: The electrocardiogram in acute pulmonary embolism, Prog Cardiovasc Dis 17:247, 1975.
72. Surawicz B, et al: QS- and QR-pattern in leads V_3 and V_4 in absence of myocardial infarction: electrocardiographic and vectorcardiographic study, Circulation 12:391, 1955.
73. Szucs MM, et al: Diagnostic sensitivity of laboratory findings in acute pulmonary embolism, Ann Intern Med 74:161, 1971.
74. Thiene G, et al: Right ventricular cardiomyopathy and sudden death in young people, N Engl J Med 318:129, 1988.
75. van Dam RT, et al: Electrical activation of ventricles and interventricular septum in hypertrophic obstructive cardiomyopathy, Br Heart j 34:100, 1972.
76. Van Noorden SV, et al: Hypertrophic obstructive cardiomyopathy: a histological, histochemical, and ultrastructural study of biopsy material, Cardiovasc Res 5:118, 1971.
77. Wallace AG, et al: The vectorcardiogram in left ventricular hypertrophy: a study using the Frank lead system, Am Heart J 63:466, 1962.
78. Wasserburger RH, et al: The electrocardiographic pentalogy of pulmonary emphysema. A correlation of roentgenographic findings and pulmonary function studies, Circulation 20:831, 1959.
79. Webb JG, et al: Apical hypertrophic cardiomyopathy: clinical follow-up and diagnostic correlates, J Am Coll Cardiol 15:83, 1990.
80. Weber DM, Phillips JH: A reevaluation of electrocardiographic changes accompanying acute pulmonary embolism, Am J Med Sci 251:381, 1966.
81. Wenger NK, et al: Massive acute pulmonary embolism: deceivingly nonspecific manifestations, Am J Cardiol 29:296, 1972.
82. Whiting RD, et al: Idiopathic hypertrophic subaortic stenosis in the elderly, N Engl J Med 285:196, 1971.
83. Wigle ED, Baron RH: The electrocardiogram in muscular subaortic stenosis: effect of a left septal incision and right bundle branch block, Circulation 34:585, 1966.
84. Wilson FN, et al: The precordial electrocardiogram, Am Heart J 27:19, 1944.
85. Yamaguchi H, et al: Hypertrophic nonobstructive cardiomyopathy with giant negative T waves (apical hypertrophy): ventriculographic and echocardiographic features in 30 patients, Am J Cardiol 44:401, 1979.
86. Zuckermann R, et al: Electropathology of acute cor pulmonale, Am Heart J 40:805, 1950.

Altered ventricular conduction patterns

An alteration in the intrinsic pathway of ventricular activation can change the orientation of initial depolarization forces, sometimes producing Q waves in the absence of infarction. Pseudoinfarctional Q waves caused by altered ventricular conduction can occur with all of the following conditions: (1) left bundle branch block, (2) left anterior hemiblock, (3) artificial ventricular pacemakers, (4) right bundle branch block, and (5) Wolff-Parkinson-White preexcitation.

LEFT BUNDLE BRANCH BLOCK

The interpretation of left bundle branch block patterns poses a double-edged problem: left bundle branch block not only frequently mimics but also commonly masks underlying infarction. In this section attention is focused both on the recognition of left bundle branch block pseudoinfarct patterns and on the diagnosis of myocardial infarction in the presence of left bundle branch block. Several pseudoinfarct patterns occur with left bundle branch block.

1. *Anterior wall infarct patterns* (Fig. 5-1). Poor R wave progression or actual QS complexes are commonly seen in the right to middle precordial leads associated with uncomplicated left bundle branch block. In other cases there may be a diminution in R wave amplitude from V_1 to the midprecordial leads in the absence of septal infarction.[53] In rarer instances a noninfarctional QS complex may extend from V_1 as far left as V_5 or V_6 (Fig. 5-1).[43,53] Noninfarctional Q waves may also be present in aV_L.

In most cases left bundle branch block causes a loss of normal septal r waves in the right precordial leads. Occasionally rS complexes may be seen in V_1 and V_2 with left bundle branch block. These unexpected initial positive forces in the right chest leads may reflect early right ventricular depolarization forces and may actually mask the Q waves of anteroseptal myocardial infarction in some cases.

2. *Inferior wall infarct patterns.* Noninfarctional QS waves are occasionally seen in III and aV_F with left bundle branch block. Some investigators[19,30] have even asserted that QS complexes in all three inferior leads (II, III, and aV_F)

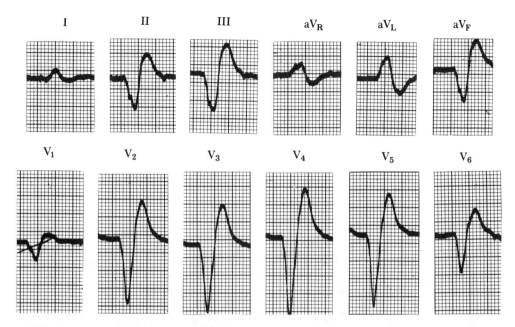

FIG. 5-1. Left bundle branch block simulating extensive anterior and inferior wall infarction in a 73-year-old man with chronic pulmonary disease and rheumatic aortic stenosis. At autopsy the heart was massively hypertrophied and dilated (total weight, 850 g). There was no evidence of myocardial infarction. This tracing exemplifies the problem of diagnosing infarction in the presence of left bundle branch block: as a general rule, with left bundle branch block, QS waves in the anterior precordial or inferior limb leads should not be interpreted as signs of infarction. (Compare this with Fig. 5-3, in which the diagnosis of infarction can be made in the presence of left bundle branch block.) (From Scott RC: Am Heart J 70:691, 1965.)

with left bundle branch block are diagnostic of underlying infarction. However, there are a number of autopsy-documented cases of QS waves in II, III, and aV_F *without* infarction (Fig. 5-1).[43,61] In several reported cases of intermittent left bundle branch block, QS waves in all three inferior leads were present only in the aberrantly conducted beats.[57] Conversely, in other cases left bundle branch block masked the Q waves of true inferior wall infarction.[26,39]

3. *Secondary ST-T changes.* The terms *primary* and *secondary* ST-T wave changes[2,56] are of central importance in electrocardiography. A primary repolarization change—seen, for example, with ischemia or electrolyte imbalance—reflects actual changes in myocardial action potentials. These changes may be regional or diffuse and are related to alterations in action potential duration or contour or to changes in the resting membrane potential. By contrast, ST-T changes may also occur when the sequence of ventricular activation is altered *without* any disturbance in the electrical properties of the myocardial cells. Such *secondary* repolarization changes are seen in a variety of settings, including left and right bundle branch block and Wolff-Parkinson-White preexcitation syndrome.

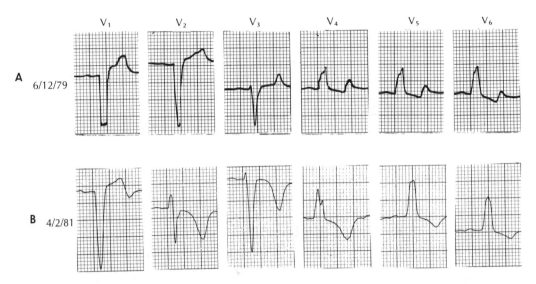

FIG. 5-2. A, Typical left bundle branch block pattern: poor R wave progression in the right precordial leads and discordance of the QRS and ST-T vectors (reflected by ST elevation in the right precordial leads and ST depression and T wave inversion in the left precordial leads). **B,** Subsequent ECG showing the development of primary T wave inversions in V$_1$ to V$_3$ caused by anterior ischemia and possible infarction.

Secondary ST-T changes result in a characteristic *discordance* of the QRS and T wave vectors. Thus, with left bundle branch block, leads that show tall R waves usually have a negative T wave whereas leads with a predominantly negative QRS (e.g., the right precordial leads) usually have a positive T wave (Fig. 5-2, *A*). These secondary ST-T changes are important for two reasons. First, they may simulate ischemic repolarization changes. Second, when infarction and left bundle branch occur together, the primary ST-T changes of ischemia may be masked by the secondary changes and this will decrease the sensitivity of the ECG (Chapter 20).

Occasionally, primary ischemic ST-T changes can be detected superimposed on the left bundle branch block pattern. The following patterns should suggest the diagnosis of ischemia or infarction:

    a. *ST segment elevation in leads with a predominant R wave.* In the presence of uncomplicated left bundle branch block, the ST segment is usually isoelectric or depressed in leads with an R or Rs type of complex, reflecting the secondary repolarization abnormality (Fig. 5-2, *A*).

    b. *T wave inversions in the right to middle precordial leads or in other leads with a predominantly negative QRS.* In the presence of uncomplicated left bundle branch block, the expected discordance of QRS and ST-T vectors causes positive T waves in leads with rS or QS complexes. The effects of anterior and inferior wall ischemia on left bundle branch block patterns are shown in Figs. 5-2, *B*, and 5-3.

I	II	III	aV_R	aV_L	aV_F

V_1	V_2	V_3	V_4	V_5	V_6

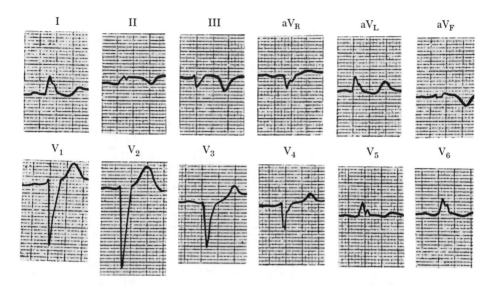

FIG. 5-3. Left bundle branch block with a recent infarction. Note the coved appearance of primary T wave inversions in leads II, III, and aV_F caused by a recent inferior wall infarction. These T waves are relatively symmetric with slight ST elevation. In most cases primary ischemic ST-T changes are masked by secondary repolarization changes associated with left bundle branch block.

Finally, the morphology of the ST-T changes may be of some aid. The secondary ST-T changes with left bundle branch block have a characteristic morphology in leads with a predominant R wave. The ST segment and T wave in such cases are actually inseparable. The ST segment begins to slope obliquely downward, melding into the T wave. A negative T wave is inscribed, and the ascending limb of the T wave rises back to the baseline at a more acute angle, giving the entire ST-T complex a triangular appearance (Fig. 5-2, *A*, lead V_6). In contrast, T wave inversions caused by ischemia may have a more symmetric appearance, with an upwardly bowed ST segment[54] (Figs. 5-2, *B*, and 5-3).

4. *ST elevations simulating acute infarction.*[8,43]The ST segment may be markedly elevated (10 mm or more at the J point) in leads with a QS or rS complex in uncomplicated left bundle branch block. This spurious "current of injury" pattern has a convex shape opposite to the T wave inversions and ST depressions seen in the lateral precordial leads (Fig. 5-1). In such cases the T wave in leads with an elevated ST segment often has a tall vaulting appearance, simulating the T wave prominence seen during the *hyperacute* phase of myocardial infarction (p. 341). This combination of ST elevations and tall positive T waves with left bundle branch block is one of the most common and most frequently misinterpreted pseudoinfarct patterns in clinical practice.

Fig. 5-1 is a striking example of the pseudoinfarctional patterns seen with left bundle branch block. In addition to QS complexes in the inferior limb leads,

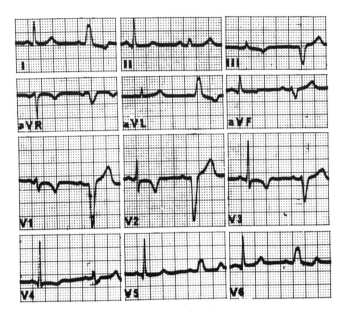

FIG. 5-4. Intermittent left bundle branch block in a patient without clinical evidence of heart disease, including a normal coronary arteriogram. In each panel the first beat shows normal conduction and the second shows left bundle branch block. Note the prominent T wave inversions in the normally conducted beats, most marked in V_1 to V_4. The mechanism of these T wave changes with intermittent left bundle branch block is not known. (From Rosenbaum MB, et al: Am J Cardiol 50:213, 1982.)

there is complete loss of R wave progression in the precordial leads. Furthermore, the ST segments have a high takeoff in both the precordial and inferior leads.

The pathogenesis of these right precordial ST elevations is not certain. One possible explanation is that they reflect relatively early repolarization of the right ventricle in the setting of delayed left ventricular activation and recovery (pp. 203 and 204). As a result, the ST vector would be shifted anteriorly and rightward.

5. *T wave inversions with intermittent left bundle branch block.* Patients with intermittent left bundle branch block may also show deep T wave inversions in the right and middle precordial leads in normally conducted beats.[16, 21, 51] The T wave inversions are typically deepest in V_1 to V_4, with a symmetric or coved appearance (Fig. 5-4). Occasionally they also appear in the limb leads.

The pathogenesis of these right precordial T wave inversions with intermittent left bundle branch block is uncertain. Some of the patients studied had coronary disease with presumed anteroseptal ischemia. In other cases there was no evidence of coronary disease. Rather, it was suggested that the T wave inversions might be functional repolarization changes related to the abnormal pattern of depolarization in the preceding left bundle branch block beats.[16,21] Anterior T wave inversions have also been reported following right ventricular pacing (which causes a left bundle branch block pattern).[15] These postpacemaker T wave changes are described in Chapter 17.

Etiology of Q waves. The pseudoinfarct Q waves with left bundle branch block are caused by a reversal in the normal pattern of septal depolarization described earlier. Normally the left side of the septum is activated first (by a ramification of the left bundle branch), and the initial septal forces are oriented from left to right, producing an initial r wave in the right precordial leads. With left bundle branch block, septal depolarization spreads from right to left. Consequently the initial septal r wave is lost and noninfarctional QS complexes may appear in the right to middle precordial and occasionally inferior limb leads. Sometimes, as mentioned earlier, these QS complexes may extend across the entire precordium in the absence of infarction. This is probably caused by concomitant right ventricular dilation, which would allow the midprecordial to lateral precordial leads to face the right ventricular epicardium and record QS (or rS) types of potentials. The reversal of septal activation seen with left bundle branch block also results in an RS type of complex in left ventricular cavity leads rather than the normal QS cavity pattern described in Chapter 2.

Differential diagnosis. Considerable attention has been directed to the problem of diagnosing myocardial infarction in the presence of left bundle branch block.* No attempt is made here to review the numerous and sometimes conflicting diagnostic criteria suggested by different authors. The present discussion is intended to highlight the major problems of diagnosing and localizing infarcts with the ECG in the presence of left bundle branch block and to provide practical guidelines.

Left ventricular free wall infarction with left bundle branch block. Infarction of the left ventricular free wall ordinarily results in abnormal Q waves in the midprecordial to lateral precordial leads (and appropriate limb leads). However, with left bundle branch block the initial septal depolarization forces are directed from right to left. These leftward forces produce an initial R wave in the midprecordial to lateral precordial leads, masking the loss of potentials (Q waves) caused by the infarction.[54] Therefore *left ventricular free wall infarction by itself will not usually produce diagnostic Q waves in the presence of left bundle branch block.* Can pure free wall infarction be determined in the presence of left bundle branch block? Sodi-Pallares et al.[54] and others have suggested that when transmural infarction of the left ventricular free wall occurs in association with left bundle branch block the potentials of the left ventricular cavity (RS potentials) will be transmitted to epicardial leads. Therefore the presence of RS complexes instead of predominant R waves in the lateral precordial leads has been suggested as a sign of free wall infarction with left bundle branch block. However, delayed R wave progression with left precordial RS complexes also oc-

---

*References 1, 4, 8, 9, 14, 18, 19, 29, 30, 32, 39, 41, 44, 46, 54, 59, 60, 62.

curs in the presence of uncomplicated left bundle branch block, and this pattern cannot be considered a specific indicator of free wall infarction.

Septal infarction with left bundle branch block. In contrast to the diagnosis of free wall infarction with left bundle branch block, the diagnosis of underlying septal infarction can sometimes be made even in the presence of the conduction disorder.[54] As discussed previously, with uncomplicated left bundle branch block the early septal forces of depolarization are directed to the left. If enough of the septum is infarcted to eliminate these initial leftward septal forces, abnormal QR, QRS, or qrS types of complexes may appear in the midprecordial to lateral precordial leads in conjunction with the left bundle branch block pattern[54] (Figs. 5-5 and 5-6). Infarction involving both the free wall and the septum will also produce abnormal Q waves (usually as part of the QRS or QrS types of complexes) in the midprecordial to lateral precordial leads. These initial Q waves may reflect posterior and superior forces from the spared basal portion of the septum.[54]

Small q waves (0.03 sec or less), however, may be seen in I and V_5 to V_6 with uncomplicated left bundle branch block.[44] Wide 0.04-second Q waves in one or more of these leads are a more reliable sign of underlying infarction. For example, wide Q waves (as part of QR complexes) in V_6, particularly with an R wave in V_1, appear to be a specific, though relatively insensitive, marker of anterior infarction.[59]

The presence of Q waves in the lateral chest leads indicating septal infarc-

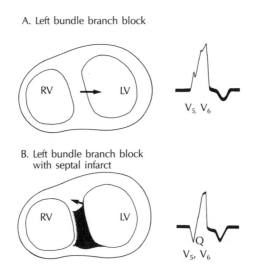

A. Left bundle branch block

RV → LV

$V_{5,}\ V_6$

B. Left bundle branch block with septal infarct

RV   LV

Q

$V_5,\ V_6$

FIG. 5-5. A, With uncomplicated left bundle branch block, early septal forces are directed to the left. Therefore no Q waves will be seen in V_5 and V_6. **B,** With left bundle branch block complicated by anteroseptal infarction, early septal forces may be directed posteriorly and rightward. Therefore prominent Q waves may appear in V_5 and V_6 as a paradoxical marker of septal infarction. (Adapted from Lipman BS, et al: Clinical scalar electrocardiography, ed 6, Chicago, 1973, Year Book Medical Publishers Inc.)

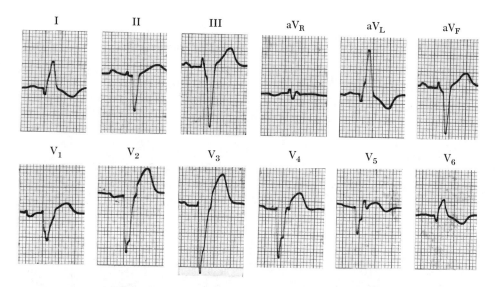

FIG. 5-6. Anterior wall infarction with left bundle branch block. This patient had sustained a prior extensive anterior myocardial infarct. Note the presence of QR complexes in I, aV$_L$, V$_5$, and V$_6$. Such complexes in lateral leads with left bundle branch block can paradoxically indicate infarction of the ventricular septum. (See text.)

tion with left bundle branch block is an example of the *false localization* of infarction by the ECG (p. 25). Fig. 5-7 is a dramatic illustration of this. The ECG showed alternating bundle branch block. When right bundle branch block was present, definite evidence of anteroseptal infarction with right and middle precordial Q waves appeared (Fig. 5-7, *A*). When left bundle branch block supervened, pathologic Q waves were apparent only in V$_6$ and the evidence of infarction was actually masked in the right chest leads (Fig. 5-7, *B*).

Another pattern that has been described as indicative of septal infarction with left bundle branch block is the presence of an rS complex in V$_1$, with progressive loss of R wave voltage in the right to middle precordial leads (Fig. 5-7, *B*). The initial r wave in V$_1$ may represent early right ventricular depolarization forces that have been unmasked by loss of septal potentials. This pattern is of limited diagnostic value (unless associated with lateral QR waves) because it also occurs with uncomplicated left bundle branch block.[53]

Acute infarction with left bundle branch block. Occasionally the diagnosis of an acute infarction can be made in patients with underlying left bundle branch block on the basis of the typical ischemic ST-T changes on serial tracings. The presence of deep symmetric coronary or coved T wave inversions is particularly helpful.[54] ST elevations in leads with a predominant R wave (as opposed to QS or rS waves) are also strongly suggestive of ischemia.[10,59] However, these primary ischemic ST-T patterns are often masked by the secondary repolarization abnormalities associated with left bundle branch block. Furthermore, although

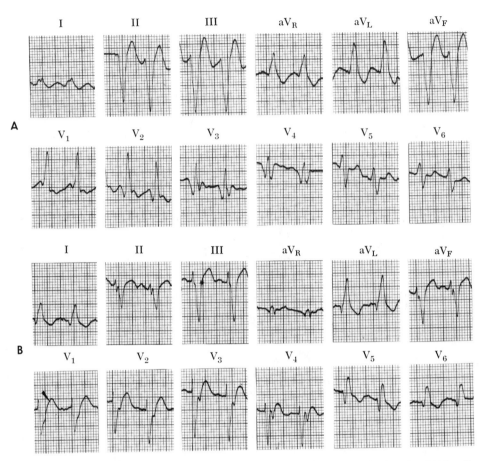

FIG. 5-7. Alternating bundle branch block with underlying anterior infarction. **A,** Note the right bundle branch block pattern with left anterior hemiblock and prominent Q waves in V_1 to V_4 consistent with underlying anteroseptal and anterior infarction. **B,** Tracing obtained several hours later. Notice now that a left bundle branch block pattern appears with prominent Q waves in I, aV_L, and V_6, suggesting an exclusively lateral infarction. In addition, R waves are now seen in the right precordial leads. These tracings illustrate how lateral Q waves with left bundle branch block can reflect septal infarction. (See text for details.) A supraventricular tachycardia is present on both ECGs.

a positive T wave in leads with a tall (concordant) R wave may be a marker of ischemia, the specificity of this finding is limited.[59]

A number of other signs of underlying infarction with left bundle branch block have been proposed.[59] These include notching of the ascending limb of an rS complex in the mid-precordial leads (Cabrera's sign)[9] and notching of the ascending limb of the R wave in V_6 (Chapman's sign).[14] However, there may be a surprising degree of interobserver variability in identifying these signs. Furthermore, the sensitivity of both signs is low, despite the fact that their specificity may approach 90%.[59]

The following points summarize the differential diagnosis of left bundle branch block versus myocardial infarction:

1. A QS pattern, poor R wave progression, or loss of R waves in the anterior precordial leads or a QS pattern in II, III, aV_F, or aV_L may occur with uncomplicated left bundle branch block.
2. Left bundle branch block characteristically masks the Q waves of lateral and free wall infarction. Left bundle branch block may also mask the Q waves of inferior or anteroseptal infarction.
3. ST segment elevations with tall positive T waves are frequently seen in the right precordial leads with uncomplicated left bundle branch block. Similarly, secondary T wave inversions are characteristically seen in the lateral precordial leads. However, the appearance of ST elevations in the lateral leads, or deep coronary or coved plane T wave inversions in any lead, suggests underlying ischemia. Close attention therefore should be paid to serial ST-T changes.[59]
4. The presence of QR complexes in I, V_5, or V_6, or in II, III, and aV_F with left bundle branch block strongly suggests underlying infarction.

HEMIBLOCKS (FASCICULAR BLOCKS)

The left bundle branch bifurcates into two major divisions (fascicles): the left anterior (superior) branch and the left posterior (inferior) branch. The term *hemiblock* refers to a conduction delay or block in either of these fascicles. Experimental and clinical data have shown that the major ECG change produced by a hemiblock, in contrast to a full left or right bundle branch block, is a marked shift in the frontal plane QRS axis with only slight widening of the QRS duration. Specifically, according to the criteria of Rosenbaum, Elizari, and Lazzari,[49] left anterior hemiblock is recognized by a frontal plane axis of -45 degrees or more, usually with qR patterns in I and aV_L and rS complexes in II, III, and aV_F. Left posterior hemiblock shifts the frontal plane QRS axis to the right ($+120$ degrees or more), usually with qR patterns in II, III, and aV_F and rS waves in I and aV_L. The diagnosis of left posterior hemiblock requires exclusion of more common causes of right axis deviation such as right ventricular hypertrophy, lateral wall infarction, normal variant, and emphysema.

The recent literature contains somewhat contradictory claims regarding the effects of hemiblocks on the ECG pattern of infarction. This section focuses on two key questions: (1) Can hemiblock patterns, like other ventricular conduction disturbances, mimic infarct patterns? (2) Can hemiblocks, like left bundle branch block and Wolff-Parkinson-White preexcitation, also mask the diagnostic Q waves of infarction?

Left anterior hemiblock, like full left bundle branch block, may both obscure and mimic the pattern of infarction in certain cases. Rosenbaum, Elizari, and Lazzari[49] first described pseudoinfarctional qRS or qrS complexes in the right

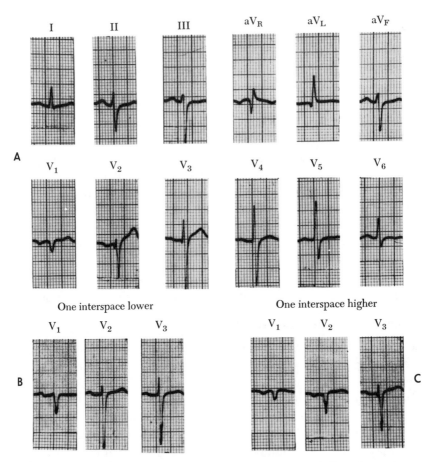

FIG. 5-8. Left anterior hemiblock simulating an anteroseptal infarction. **A,** Note the small q waves in the right precordial leads as part of a qrS pattern. **B,** Normal R wave progression with V_1 to V_3 recorded one interspace lower than usual. **C,** Q waves more evident with leads recorded one interspace higher. (From McHenry PL, et al: Am Heart J 81:498, 1971.)

precordial leads in some cases of left anterior hemiblock. Similar patterns were subsequently described by McHenry et al.[40] These right precordial q waves that may simulate the pattern of anteroseptal infarction are typically of short duration (0.02 sec) in V_1 and V_2 or V_3 (Fig. 5-8). They are usually most evident in leads placed above the usual chest positions (e.g., in the third intercostal space). Conversely, leads placed below the conventional precordial levels (the fifth intercostal space) do not show these Q waves (Fig. 5-8). Rosenbaum, Elizari, and Lazzari[49] suggested that these q waves reflect selective activation of the posteroinferior wall of the left ventricle by the left posterior fascicle in the presence of left anterior hemiblock. In such cases the early septal and left ventricular depolarization forces would be oriented inferiorly and dorsally, explaining the appearance of small q waves in high but not lower precordial leads.

However, in none of the reported cases of left anterior hemiblock simulating anteroseptal infarction has there been pathologic proof of the absence of actual septal injury. Until such confirmation is available, the significance of small right precordial q waves associated with left anterior hemiblock must remain speculative.

Actual QS complexes (in contrast to these qRS waves) in the right precordial leads are *not* a feature of uncomplicated left anterior hemiblock. There is one case report[22] of a patient with mitral stenosis whose scalar ECG showed left axis deviation and QS complexes in V_1 to V_3. Normal R wave progression was recorded when the chest leads were placed one interspace lower than normal. A vectorcardiogram showed normal anterior forces in the horizontal plane. The authors attributed the right precordial QS waves in this case to the left anterior hemiblock pattern. However, until more substantive proof is available, actual QS complexes in the right chest leads should not be ascribed to left anterior hemiblock. Furthermore, in reported cases of intermittent left anterior hemiblock, R wave progression in the early precordial leads was unaffected.[49]

Left anterior hemiblock will occasionally hide the diagnosis of inferior wall infarction. The inferior orientation of the initial QRS forces caused by the hemiblock may mask the inferior Q waves, with resultant rS complexes in II, III, and aV_F.[3,17,37,48,49] Sometimes the combination of left anterior hemiblock and inferior wall infarction will produce qrS complexes in the inferior limb leads, with the initial q wave the residual of the infarct and the minuscule r wave the result of the hemiblock.

There are also several published cases in which the Q waves of anteroseptal infarction appeared to be masked by left anterior hemiblock.[3,17] The mechanism for this apparently paradoxical increase in early right precordial forces is uncertain. However, in most cases left anterior hemiblock does not obscure the diagnostic Q waves of anteroseptal infarction and, as just noted, may actually result in small right precordial q waves simulating this pattern.

Finally, left anterior hemiblock may be associated with secondary ST-T changes suggestive of ischemia.[36,48] Secondary ST-T changes (described on p. 101) are alterations in repolarization produced entirely by changes in the sequence of ventricular activation. With left anterior hemiblock there is a characteristic discordance of the QRS and T wave vectors, with the QRS vector oriented to the left in the frontal plane and the T wave vector oriented inferiorly. As a result of these secondary ST-T changes, the T waves with left anterior hemiblock are usually slightly inverted in I and aV_L, sometimes simulating primary ischemic changes. Furthermore, the displacement of the T wave vector inferiorly with left anterior hemiblock may occasionally mask primary inferior ischemic ST-T changes. Conversely, the presence of T wave inversions in II,

III, and aV_F with left anterior hemiblock should suggest the possibility of primary inferior ischemia.[36]*

Left posterior hemiblock, in contrast to left anterior hemiblock, does not significantly affect the diagnosis of infarction. Leachman, Angelini, and Lufschanowski[37] described cases of anterolateral infarction in which the superimposition of left posterior hemiblock caused small r waves in I and aV_L in place of the Q waves. However, in these cases the precordial leads continued to show unequivocal evidence of the lateral infarct and were not affected by the left posterior hemiblock pattern.

In summary, the hemiblocks may have the following major effects on the ECG diagnosis of infarction:

1. Left anterior hemiblock may mimic the pattern of anteroseptal infarction, producing qRS or qrS types of complexes in the right precordial leads, with q waves of short duration (for example, 0.02 sec). Normal R wave progression in such cases can be restored by recording the right precordial leads one interspace lower than normal. Actual QS complexes in the right precordial leads should not be attributed to left anterior hemiblock.

2. Left anterior hemiblock may mask the pattern of inferior infarction by producing rS complexes in the inferior limb leads.

3. The secondary ST-T changes of left anterior hemiblock (with slight T wave inversions in leads I and aV_L) may simulate anterolateral ischemia and may also shift the T wave vector toward leads II, III, and aV_F, masking primary inferior wall ischemia.

4. Left posterior hemiblock generally will not mask or mimic the pattern of infarction.

PACEMAKER PATTERNS

Electronic pacemaker stimulation of either the right ventricular endocardium or epicardium usually produces the ECG pattern of complete left bundle branch block, and this may simulate the pattern of anterior or inferior wall infarction (Fig. 5-9).

Pacemaker stimulation of the endocardial surface of the right ventricular apex typically produces the ECG pattern of complete left bundle branch block with left axis deviation. Occasionally, in cases of extreme left axis deviation, QS deflections will appear in V_1 to V_6 with right ventricular apical pacing.[11] Right ventricular pacing can also induce QS waves in II, III, and aV_F. Right ventricu-

---

*Notice that with a normal horizontal QRS axis (e.g., an axis as negative as 0 degrees or even −30 degrees in some cases), the T wave and QRS vectors are normally *concordant*. Consequently the T wave vector will also point to the left, with resultant T wave inversions in III and aV_F. However, with marked left axis deviation (greater than −45 degrees) caused by left anterior hemiblock, the QRS and T wave vectors are characteristically discordant because of the secondary repolarization changes. In such cases positive T waves in III and aV_F can be expected.

I   II   III   aV$_R$ aV$_L$ aV$_F$

V$_1$ V$_2$ V$_3$ V$_4$ V$_5$ V$_6$

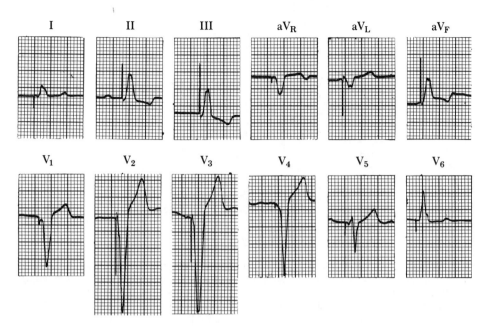

FIG. 5-9. Pacemaker pattern simulating an anterior wall infarction. Electronic pacing from the endocardium of the right ventricle usually produces a left bundle branch block pattern. Each QRS on this tracing is preceded by a positive or negative pacemaker spike. The precordial leads show poor R wave progression. Pacemakers not only can *mimic* the ECG appearance of an infarct, they also can *mask* it.

lar outflow tract pacing may be associated with noninfarctional QR-type complexes in I and aV$_L$. However, as described below, QR complexes in the precordial (or inferior limb) leads strongly suggest underlying infarction.[6,7]

Pacemaker stimulation of the left ventricle typically produces the pattern of complete right bundle branch block. In some cases of endocardial pacing at the left ventricular apex, an unusual pattern of R waves in V$_1$ and aV$_R$ with QS waves in all the other leads has been reported.[11]

Castellanos et al.[12] described the so-called St-qR pattern associated with underlying anteroseptal infarction in patients with right ventricular pacemakers. This sign is characterized by a qR or QR type of complex in the midprecordial to lateral precordial leads following the pacemaker stimulus (St) spike (Fig. 5-10). The pattern, which is highly specific for underlying infarction, is analogous to the left precordial QR complexes described earlier in connection with left bundle branch block complicated by septal infarction.

Paced beats, like left bundle branch block or Wolff-Parkinson-White beats, often mask the ST-T changes of true infarction. In such cases the diagnosis can sometimes be made on the basis of clinical signs, enzyme changes, or echocardiographic or radionuclide imaging or by temporarily inhibiting the pacemaker and observing the intrinsic beats.[13] Occasionally primary ST-T changes (e.g.,

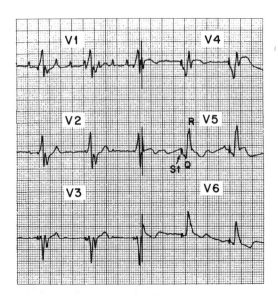

FIG. 5-10. Right ventricular pacing with a chronic extensive anterior wall infarct. Note the so-called St-qR pattern in V_5 and V_6 with the pacemaker stimulus (*St*) followed by a qR wave. This is analogous to the left precordial qR (or QR) complexes seen in some cases of left bundle branch block complicated by anteroseptal infarction (Figs. 5-6 and 5-7,*B*). The underlying rhythm is coarse atrial flutter. Another example of the St-qR pattern can be seen in Fig. 5-11.

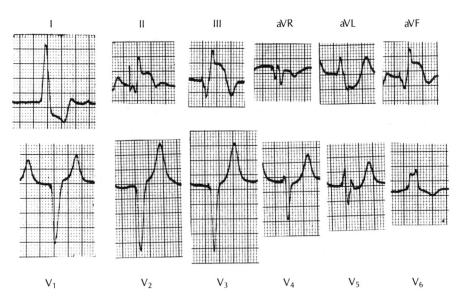

FIG. 5-11. Ventricular pacing during an acute inferior wall infarction. Note the QR waves in II, III, and aV_F associated with ST elevations. (From Barold SS, et al: Chest 69:232, 1976.)

ST elevations) will be apparent with acute ischemia or infarction, superimposed on the pacemaker pattern (Fig. 5-11).

The *postpacemaker pattern* is characterized by deep noninfarctional T wave inversions following artificial pacemaking. It is discussed separately on p. 308. An excellent review of the electrocardiographic diagnosis of infarction during ventricular pacing has been provided by Barold et al.[7]

RIGHT BUNDLE BRANCH BLOCK

Right bundle branch block (complete or incomplete) can simulate anteroseptal or inferior or posterior wall infarction. Pseudoinfarct patterns also may occur with Ebstein's anomaly of the tricuspid valve associated with a right ventricular conduction delay. In addition, secondary T wave inversions due to right bundle branch block may at times simulate ischemia.

Right bundle branch block simulating anteroseptal or inferior wall infarction. Noninfarctional QR (qR) complexes may occur in the right precordial leads and sometimes in III and aV_F (Fig. 4-7) with right bundle branch block. Horan et al.[30] noted Q waves in 10 of 40 cases of right bundle branch block without pathologic evidence of infarction. This pattern was particularly common with acute right ventricular overload (Fig. 4-7). (The possible mechanism of these pseudoinfarctional Q waves in the right precordial or inferior leads with acute cor pulmonale [pulmonary embolism] is described in Chapter 4.)

Theoretically a QR complex with right bundle branch block might also arise if the septal forces that normally produce the initial r wave in the right precordial leads were directed at right angles to these leads. Normally the right precordial leads with right bundle branch block show an rSr' (or equivalent) pattern. If the septal forces responsible for the initial r wave were oriented perpendicular to the right precordial leads, the initial r wave would be masked and the rSr' complex would be converted to a Qr pattern.

Another potential mechanism for the appearance of noninfarctional QR complexes with right bundle branch block has been suggested, namely, focal septal block.[25] The early left-to-right septal forces responsible for the right precordial septal r waves are thought to be activated by a septal ramification of the left bundle branch system. A local block in these septal fibers in the presence of concomitant right bundle branch block could also theoretically produce the pseudoinfarct patterns just described.

The QR complexes seen in the right precordial or inferior limb leads differ in several respects from the Q waves of actual infarction:

With pure right bundle branch block the right precordial QR waves rarely extend beyond V_2.

With anterior infarction and right bundle branch block, Q waves are often seen in the midprecordial to lateral precordial leads as well (see Fig. 4-6).

Although right bundle branch block may be associated with noninfarctional QR complexes in III and aV_F, it does not generally produce a significant Q wave

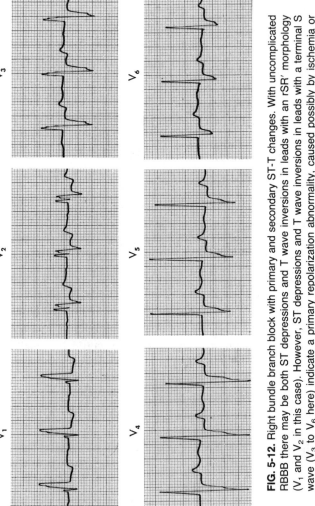

FIG. 5-12. Right bundle branch block with primary and secondary ST-T changes. With uncomplicated RBBB there may be both ST depressions and T wave inversions in leads with an rSR' morphology (V$_1$ and V$_2$ in this case). However, ST depressions and T wave inversions in leads with a terminal S wave (V$_3$ to V$_6$ here) indicate a primary repolarization abnormality, caused possibly by ischemia or other factors (e.g., digitalis effect).

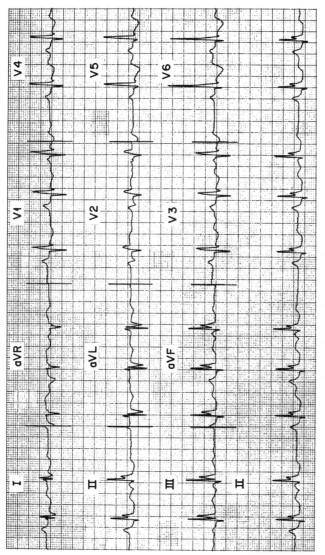

FIG. 5-13.—Ebstein's anomaly of the tricuspid valve simulating anterior and inferior wall infarcts. This tracing from a 48-year-old woman shows sinus rhythm with first-degree AV block and frequent premature atrial beats. There are anterior and inferior Q waves. Note also the prominent P waves as well as the borderline right axis deviation and right ventricular conduction disturbance. The characteristic "splintered" appearance of the QRS can be best seen in II, III, aV_F, and aV_L.

in II. Therefore the presence of QR complexes in II, III, and aV$_F$ suggests inferior wall infarction (see Fig. 4-8).

The Q waves in uncomplicated right bundle branch block are usually sharply inscribed, without notching or slurring. Myocardial infarction often but not always deforms the initial depolarization forces to produce a characteristically notched or W-shaped Q wave (see Fig. 4-6).

When intermittent right bundle branch block complicates actual anterior wall infarction, the Q waves in the right precordial leads (as part of the QR type of complexes) may become more prominent.[50] Such "right bundle branch block–dependent Q waves" may lead to the mistaken impression of reinfarction. The mechanism of Q wave enhancement in this setting is unknown.

Right bundle branch block simulating posterior wall infarction. Right bundle branch block occasionally produces tall notched R waves in the right precordial leads (Fig. 4-17, *B*) instead of the classic rSR′ or rsR′ morphologies. These tall right precordial R waves may simulate the pattern of pure posterior wall infarction described earlier. Problems differentiating uncomplicated right bundle branch block from posterior wall myocardial infarction are most likely to arise when considering the ECGs of older patients that show a right bundle branch block pattern with tall right precordial R waves and no pathologic Q waves in any of the standard leads. In such cases there is no certain means of either excluding or substantiating the presence of underlying posterior infarction. However, Q waves in the lateral or inferior limb leads in conjunction with tall right precordial R waves strongly suggest posterolateral or posteroinferior infarction.

Ebstein's anomaly of the tricuspid valve. Pseudoinfarct patterns may occur with Ebstein's anomaly in association with right ventricular conduction delays (Fig. 5-13) or the Type B Wolff-Parkinson-White pattern (next page). Ebstein's anomaly is characterized by displacement of fused and malformed portions of the tricuspid valve into the right ventricular cavity.[35,45]

The electrocardiogram may show a variety of abnormalities. Prominent, sometimes giant, P waves due to right atrial enlargement are generally seen. A wide QRS caused by a right ventricular conduction delay is usually present as well. However, the QRS often has an atypical morphology rather than the shape of the classic right bundle branch block pattern described earlier in this chapter. In particular, the QRS may appear splintered with the suggestion of a "second QRS" attached to the initial part of the waveform (Fig. 5-11). This pattern has been attributed to a conduction abnormality in the atrialized right ventricle.[45]

Frank Q waves as part of wide QR or Qr complexes may be seen in the right precordial to midprecordial leads (V$_1$-V$_4$) with inverted T waves, simulating anterior wall infarction (Fig. 5-13). In one large series[24] this pseudoinfarct pattern was noted in 16 of 55 patients (29%), excluding patients with the Type B Wolff-Parkinson-White syndrome. Rarely a Qr-type complex may appear in III and aV$_F$, simulating inferior wall infarction (Fig. 5-13).

The precise etiology of the noninfarction Q waves with Ebstein's anomaly is not certain. They have variably been attributed to right atrial dilation (p. 67), altered ventricular activation, and septal fibrosis.[24,35,45]

In summary: The combination of markedly prominent P waves with wide QR waves in V_1 to V_4 in a child or young adult with unexplained cardiomegaly (with or without cyanosis) is a relatively specific though not highly sensitive sign of Ebstein's anomaly of the tricuspid valve.

Secondary T wave inversions. Right bundle branch block also characteristically produces secondary T wave inversions in the right precordial to midprecordial leads (Fig. 4-17, *B*), simulating primary ischemic repolarization changes. These right precordial T wave inversions seen in leads with an rSR' or equivalent complex are analogous to the secondary T wave inversions in the left precordial leads with left bundle branch block (p. 102). Of clinical note, the secondary T wave inversions with right bundle branch block occur *only* in leads with a terminal R' wave (reflecting the right ventricular conduction delay). T wave inversions in leads with a qRS or RS type of complex most likely represent primary repolarization changes (Fig. 5-12).

WOLFF-PARKINSON-WHITE PATTERN

The Wolff-Parkinson-White (WPW) pattern, produced by ventricular preexcitation, is characterized by a distinctive ECG triad: a short PR interval, a widened QRS, and a delta wave (slurring or notching on the initial deflection of the QRS waveform). The WPW pattern is significant primarily because of the associated supraventricular tachyarrhythmias. Familiarity with this syndrome is also essential for the clinician because, like the left bundle branch block patterns just described, it may both mimic[52] and mask the ECG patterns of myocardial infarction.

The WPW pattern results from premature excitation of part of the ventricular muscle by way of an accessory AV pathway (bundle of Kent). The bypass tract is variably inserted in different individuals.[38,42] Preexcitation may occur at the lateral free wall or left posterior free wall of the left ventricle, the posterior septal or paraseptal region, the right ventricular free wall, or the anteroseptal or right anterior paraseptal region.

The surface ECG will vary depending on the initial site of activation, as summarized in Fig. 5-14.[38] Preexcitation of the lateral or posterior free walls of the left ventricle produces the classic Type A pattern (Fig. 5-15), characterized by tall right precordial R waves mimicking those of right bundle branch block. By contrast, preexcitation of the anteroseptal region produces QS waves in the right precordial leads (the Type B variant, which superficially resembles a left bundle branch block pattern) (Fig. 5-16). The earlier literature[23] sometimes refers to a "Type C" pattern characterized by QS or QR complexes in the left precordial leads (Fig. 5-17). This is actually a variant of the Type A pattern resulting from the lateral free wall bypass tract. Prominent Q waves caused by nega-

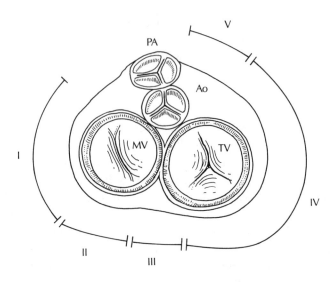

Region	Negative delta wave	QRS axis in frontal plane	R>S
I	I and/or aV_L; sometimes V_6	Normal	V_1 to V_3
II	II, III, and aV_F	−75 to +75	V_1
III	II, III, and aV_F	0 to −90	V_2 to V_4
IV	aV_R; sometimes II, III, and aV_F	Normal	V_3 to V_5
V	V_1 and V_2	Normal	V_3 to V_5

FIG. 5-14. Cross-sectional diagram of the heart (back-to-front view) showing the five major anatomic sites of preexcitation: left lateral free wall *(I)*, left posterior free wall *(II)*, posterior septal or paraseptal *(III)*, right free wall *(IV)*, and anteroseptal or paraseptal *(V)*. The following are also shown: *MV,* mitral valve; *TV,* tricuspid valve; *Ao,* aorta; *PA,* pulmonary artery. (Modified from Lindsay BD, et al: Am J Cardiol 59:1093, 1987.)

tive delta waves in the inferior limb leads may be associated with a posterior free wall, posterior septal, or paraseptal bypass tract (Fig. 5-14).

Alteration of ventricular activation can create a number of patterns simulating myocardial ischemia or infarction. The following specific pseudoinfarct patterns may appear:

1. *Anteroseptal infarct* (Fig. 5-16). The QS complexes seen in the right precordial leads with the classic Type B pattern may simulate septal infarction or left bundle branch block. Furthermore, the negative delta waves seen on the downstroke of the QS in these leads simulate the notching or slurring sometimes produced by myocardial injury.

2. *Inferior wall infarct* (Figs. 5-15 and 5-16). Q waves in the inferior limb leads may occur with either the classic Type A or the classic Type B pattern. Leads II, III, and aV_F may all show QS, QR (Qr), or W-shaped complexes.[20,27,31,61]

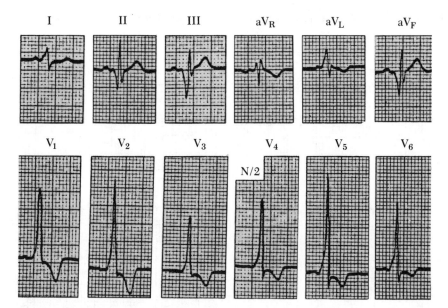

FIG. 5-15. Wolff-Parkinson-White pattern (Type A) simulating inferior and posterior wall infarction. Note the diagnostic triad: widening of the QRS, a shortened PR interval, and delta waves. The aberrant pattern produces secondary changes (seen in V_1 to V_6), which must be distinguished from primary ischemic T wave inversions. Also, note that precordial voltages are not indicative of ventricular hypertrophy in the presence of Wolff-Parkinson-White. (From Friedman HH: Diagnostic electrocardiography and vectorcardiography, New York, 1971, McGraw-Hill Book Co. Used with permission of McGraw-Hill.)

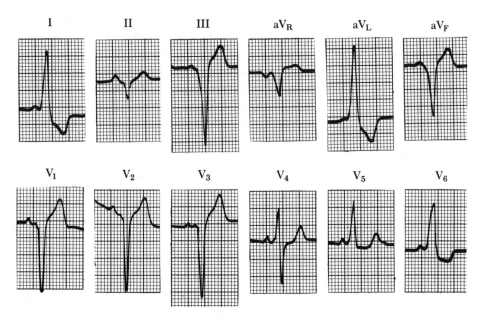

FIG. 5-16. Wolff-Parkinson-White pattern (Type B) simulating anterior and inferior infarction. The ECG of this patient, a 40-year-old man with a history of recurrent supraventricular tachyarrhythmias, shows noninfarctional QS complexes in II, III, aV_F, and V_1 to V_3. Note also the typical features of WPW (enumerated in Fig. 5-15).

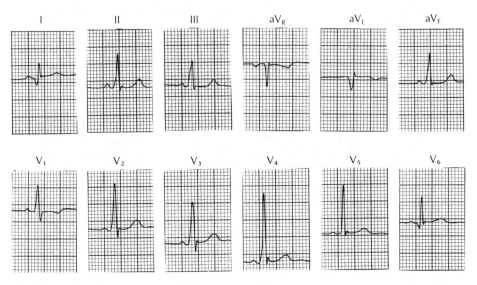

FIG. 5-17. Wolff-Parkinson-White pattern simulating posterolateral infarction. Preexcitation of the lateral wall of the left ventricle has caused negative delta waves in I, aV_L, and V_6 and positive delta waves in V_1. This has been called Type C WPW preexcitation.

3. *Posterior wall infarct* (Figs. 5-15 and 5-17). The tall wide R waves in the right precordial leads with the Type A pattern may simulate posterior wall injury or right ventricular hypertrophy.

4. *Anterolateral infarct* (Fig. 5-17). Wide Q waves in I and aV_L, and sometimes in the left precordial leads (V_5 and V_6), may occur with preexcitation of the left ventricular free wall. Tall R waves are seen in V_1.

5. *ST-T changes.* In addition to Q wave patterns, the Wolff-Parkinson-White pattern can produce secondary ST-T changes. The QRS and T wave vectors are characteristically discordant. Thus, in general, the T waves are negative in leads with a positive QRS complex.[54] These inverted T waves have a morphology similar to that of the T wave inversions seen with left bundle branch block. Spontaneous benign changes in the T waves may also occur with WPW and may be difficult to distinguish from the primary T wave changes of true ischemia.[63]

6. *False-positive exercise test.* Exercise-tolerance tests are unreliable in patients with WPW because of the marked lability of the ST-T complex (p. 263).

Etiology. The pseudoinfarct patterns seen with WPW are caused entirely by an alteration in the depolarization process. For example, Q waves in II, III, and aV_F result from anomalous spread of initial forces superiorly. Similarly, the right precordial QS waves seen with the Type B pattern are a consequence of the premature right-to-left spread of forces. Finally, the Q waves in the lateral precordial leads with the Type C pattern reflect premature activation of the left ventricular free wall and the resultant spread of initial forces anteriorly and to the right. The anomalous depolarization process, in turn, produces the secondary ST-T changes described previously, with discordance of the QRS and T wave vectors.

Differential diagnosis. The key points in the differential diagnosis of Wolff-Parkinson-White and myocardial infarction can be summarized as follows:

1. WPW patterns may mimic the patterns of anteroseptal, anterolateral, inferior, and posterior infarction. However, the diagnosis of preexcitation during sinus rhythm can usually be readily confirmed on the basis of a shortened PR interval, widened QRS, and delta wave. In equivocal cases, atrial pacing, vagal maneuvers, or intravenous adenosine may unmask this triad more definitively.

2. The characteristic Q waves of infarction will be masked by WPW, and the ischemic ST-T changes frequently concealed by the secondary repolarization alterations of preexcitation.* In such cases, underlying infarction may be diagnosed with certainty only from normally conducted complexes. Occasionally, diagnostic ischemic ST-T changes will be superimposed on the WPW pattern.[54,63] (The problem of false-positive ST-T changes during exercise testing with the WPW syndrome is discussed in Chapter 13. Refer to Chapter 22 for information on the use of ancillary tests in diagnosing ischemia or infarction with ventricular conduction abnormalities.)

---

*References 27, 33, 47, 54, 55, 58, 63.

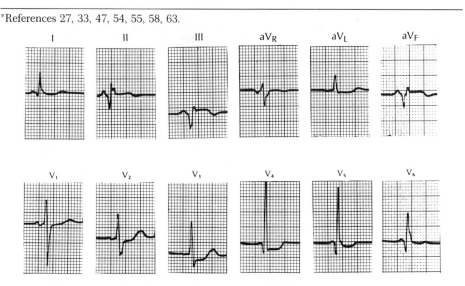

FIG. 5-18. Prior inferolateral infarction with a short PR interval. Note the primary T wave inversions in the inferior limb leads associated with Q waves. Lown-Ganong-Levine preexcitation cannot be excluded. Compare this with Figs. 5-15 and 5-16, showing the pseudoinfarct pattern of Wolff-Parkinson-White syndrome and the characteristic Q wave–T wave vector discordance.

3. The pseudoinfarct Q waves (as part of Qr or QS complexes) seen in the inferior limb leads with WPW are almost invariably associated with positive or isoelectric T waves[27] (Figs. 5-15 and 5-16). This characteristic Q wave–T wave vector discordance results from the secondary changes due to altered ventricular activation. As a corollary, the presence of T wave inversions with anterior or inferior lead Q waves and short PR intervals is strongly suggestive, though not pathognomonic, of underlying ischemia (Fig. 5-18).

REFERENCES

1. Abben R, et al: Evaluation of criteria for diagnosis of myocardial infarction: study of 256 patients with intermittent left bundle branch block, Chest 75:575, 1979.
2. Abildskov JA, et al: The primary T wave: a new electrocardiographic waveform, Am Heart J 81:242, 1971.
3. Altieri P, Schaal S: Inferior and anteroseptal myocardial infarction concealed by transient left anterior hemiblock, J Electrocardiol 6:257, 1973.
4. Baragan J, et al: Bloc complet de la branche gauche et infarctus du myocarde (étude anatomo-électrique de 48 observations), Arch Mal Coeur 56:445, 1963.
5. Barold SS, et al: Diagnosis of inferior wall myocardial infarction during right ventricular apical pacing, Chest 69:232, 1976.
6. Barold SS, et al: Electrocardiographic diagnosis of myocardial infarction in patients with transvenous pacemakers, J Electrocardiol 9:99, 1976.
7. Barold SS, et al: Electrocardiographic diagnosis of myocardial infarction during ventricular pacing, Cardiol Clin 5:403, 1987.
8. Bensoain-Santander M, Gomez-Ebensperguer G: Electrocardiographic diagnosis of myocardial infarction in cases of complete left bundle branch block, Am Heart J 60:886, 1960.
9. Cabrera E, Friedland C: La onda de activacion ventricular en el bluqueo de rama izquierda con infarcto: un nuevo signo electrocardiografico, Arch Inst Cardiol Mex 23:441, 1953.
10. Cannon A, et al: ST-segment changes during transmural myocardial ischemia in chronic left bundle branch block, Am J Cardiol 64:1216, 1989.
11. Castellanos A Jr, et al: The electrocardiogram in patients with pacemakers, Prog Cardiovasc Dis 13:190, 1970.
12. Castellanos A Jr, et al: St-qR pattern: new sign for diagnosis of anterior myocardial infarction during right ventricular pacing, Br Heart J 35:1161, 1973.
13. Center S, et al: The diagnosis of acute myocardial infarction in patients with permanent pacemakers, Arch Intern Med 127:932, 1971.
14. Chapman MG, Pearce ML: Electrocardiographic diagnosis of myocardial infarction in the presence of left bundle branch block, Circulation 16:558, 1957.
15. Chatterjee K, et al: Electrocardiographic changes subsequent to artificial ventricular depolarization, Br Heart J 31:770, 1969.
16. Denes P, et al: A characteristic precordial repolarization abnormality with intermittent left bundle-branch block, Ann Intern Med 89:55, 1978.
17. Dhingra RC, et al: Left anterior hemiblock concealing diaphragmatic infarction and simulating anteroseptal infarction, Chest 67:713, 1975.
18. Doucet P, et al: A vectorcardiographic and electrocardiographic study of left bundle branch block with myocardial infarction, Am J Cardiol 17:171, 1966.
19. Dressler W, et al: The electrocardiographic signs of myocardial infarction in the presence of bundle branch block. I. Myocardial infarction with left bundle branch block, Am Heart J 39:217, 1950.
20. Eichert H: Wolff-Parkinson-White syndrome simulating myocardial infarction, Ann Intern Med 21:907, 1944.
21. Engel TR, et al: T-wave abnormalities of intermittent left bundle-branch block, Ann Intern Med 89:204, 1978.
22. Farnham DJ, Shah PM: Left anterior hemiblock simulating anteroseptal myocardial infarction, Am Heart J 92:363, 1976.

23. Ferrer MI: Preexcitation syndrome: mechanism and treatment, Cardiovasc Clin 2:128, 1970.
24. Follath F, Hallidie-Smith KA: Unusual electrocardiographic changes in Ebstein's anomaly, Br Heart J 34:513, 1972.
25. Gambetta M, Childers RW: Rate-dependent right precordial Q waves: "septal focal block," Am J Cardiol 32:196, 1973.
26. Gilchrist IC, et al: Left bundle branch block eliminates Q waves of inferior infarction: confirmation by ventriculography, Am J Noninvas Cardiol 1:206, 1987.
27. Goldberger AL: Pseudo-infarct patterns in the Wolff-Parkinson-White syndrome: importance of Q wave–T wave vector discordance, J Electrocardiol 13:115, 1980.
28. Grayzel J: Electrocardiographic criteria in the differential diagnosis of pre-excitation (Wolff-Parkinson-White syndrome) and arteriosclerotic heart disease, N Engl J Med 259:369, 1958.
29. Hands ME, et al: Electrocardiographic diagnosis of myocardial infarction in the presence of complete left bundle branch block, Am Heart J 116:23, 1988.
30. Horan LG, et al: The significance of diagnostic Q waves in the presence of bundle branch block, Chest 58:214, 1970.
31. Kariv I: Wolff-Parkinson-White syndrome simulating myocardial infarction, Am Heart J 55:406, 1958.
32. Kindwall KE, et al: Predictive accuracy of criteria for chronic myocardial infarction in pacing-induced left bundle branch block, Am J Cardiol 57:1255, 1986.
33. Kistin AD, Robb GP: Modification of the electrocardiogram of myocardial infarction by anomalous atrioventricular excitation (Wolff-Parkinson-White syndrome), Am Heart J 37:249, 1949.
34. Kulbertus HE, de Leval-Rutten F: Vectorcardiographic study of QRS in patients with transvenous pacemakers and myocardial infarction, J Electrocardial 7:27, 1974.
35. Kumar AE, et al: Ebstein's anomaly: clinical profile and natural history, Am J Cardiol 28:84, 1971.
36. Lasser RP: T-wave changes secondary to left anterior hemiblock as shown by study of intermittent and alternating patterns, J Electrocardiol 9:147, 1976.
37. Leachman RD, et al: Electrocardiographic signs of infarction masked by coexistent contralateral hemiblock, Chest 62:542, 1972.
38. Lindsay BE, et al: Concordance of distinguishing electrocardiographic features during sinus rhythm with the location of accessory pathways in the Wolff-Parkinson-White syndrome, Am J Cardiol 59:1093, 1987.
39. Luy G, et al: Intermittent left bundle branch block, Am Heart J 85:332, 1973.
40. McHenry PL, et al: Right precordial qrS pattern due to left anterior hemiblock, Am Heart J 81:498, 1971.
41. Meyer P: L'intérêt du complexe électrocardiographique initial en W dans infarctus antéro-septaux compliqués de bloc de branche gauche ou de tracés de prédominance ventriculaire gauche, Arch Mal Coeur 58:259, 1965.
42. Milstein S, et al: An algorithm for the electrocardiographic localization of accessory pathways in the Wolff-Parkinson-White syndrome, PACE 10:555, 1987.
43. Myers GB: QRS-T patterns in multiple precordial leads that may be mistaken for myocardial infarction. III. Bundle branch block, Circulation 2:60, 1950.
44. Norris RJ, Scott RC: Diagnostic signs of myocardial infarction in the presence of complete left bundle-branch block [Abstract], Circulation 24:1007, 1961.
45. Perloff JK: The clinical recognition of congenital heart disease, ed 3, Philadelphia, 1987, WB Saunders Co.
46. Rhoads DV, et al: The electrocardiogram in the presence of myocardial infarction and intraventricular block of the left bundle branch type: a clinical-pathologic study, Am Heart J 62:735, 1961.
47. Rinzler SH, Travell J: The electrocardiographic diagnosis of acute myocardial infarction in the presence of Wolff-Parkinson-White syndrome, Am J Med 3:106, 1947.
48. Rosenbaum MB, et al: Five cases of intermittent left anterior hemiblock, Am J Cardiol 24:1, 1969.
49. Rosenbaum MB, et al: The hemiblocks, Oldsmar Fla, 1970, Tampa Tracings.
50. Rosenbaum MB, et al: Abnormal Q waves in right sided chest leads provoked by onset of right bundle-branch block in patients with anteroseptal infarction, Br Heart J 47:227, 1982.
51. Rosenbaum MB, et al: Electrotonic modulation of the T wave and cardiac memory, Am J Cardiol 50:213, 1982.
52. Ruskin JN, et al: Abnormal Q waves in Wolff-Parkinson-White syndrome: inci-

dence and clinical significance, JAMA 235:2727, 1976.

53. Scott RC: Left bundle branch block: a clinical assessment. II, Am Heart J 70:691, 1965.

54. Sodi-Pallares D, et al: Electrocardiographic diagnosis of myocardial infarction in the presence of bundle branch block (right and left), ventricular premature beats, and Wolff-Parkinson-White syndrome, Prog Cardiovasc Dis 6:107, 1963.

55. Stein I, Wroblewski F: Myocardial infarction in Wolff-Parkinson-White syndrome, Am Heart J 42:624, 1951.

56. Surawicz B: The pathogenesis and clinical significance of primary T-wave abnormalities. In Schlant RD, Hurst JW (editors): Advances in electrocardiography, New York, 1972, Grune & Stratton Inc.

57. Timmis GC, et al: Reassessment of Q waves in left bundle branch block, J Electrocardiol 9:109, 1976.

58. Verani MS, et al: Myocardial infarction associated with Wolff-Parkinson-White syndrome, Am Heart J 83:684, 1972.

59. Wackers FJT: The diagnosis of myocardial infarction in the presence of left bundle branch block, Cardiol Clin 5:393, 1987.

60. Warembourg H, et al: Le diagnostic électrocardiographique de l'infarctus du myocarde chez les malades porteurs d'un bloc complet de la branche gauche, Ann Cardiol Angeiol 23:501, 1974.

61. Wasserburger RH, et al: Noninfarctional QS_{II,III,aV_F} complexes as seen in the Wolff-Parkinson-White syndrome syndrome and left bundle branch block, Am Heart J 64:617, 1962.

62. Wilson FN, et al: The electrocardiographic diagnosis of myocardial infarction complicated by bundle branch block, Arch Inst Cardiol Mex 14:201, 1945.

63. Wolff L, Richman JL: The diagnosis of myocardial infarction in patients with anomalous atrioventricular excitation (Wolff-Parkinson-White syndrome), Am Heart J 45:545, 1953.

64. Zoneraich O, Zoneraich S: Pacemaker vectorcardiography in patients with myocardial infarction and intraventricular conduction defect, J Electrocardiol 4:1, 1971.

6

Noninfarctional myocardial injury: acute myocardial injury patterns

Pathologic Q waves are not specific for myocardial infarction. Recall that the Q waves of infarction signify a loss of myocardial forces caused by ischemic cell injury. However, severe but *noninfarctional ischemia* may also cause transient Q waves; and *nonischemic myocardial injury* that causes myocardial damage may produce abnormal Q waves that are indistinguishable from the Q waves of infarction. The noninfarctional causes of myocardial injury that have been reported to produce abnormal Q waves are discussed here and in Chapter 7.

This chapter discusses pseudoinfarctional Q waves associated with *acute* myocardial injury, including acute myocarditis, reversible ischemia, other metabolic perturbations (e.g., hyperkalemia), and traumatic noncoronary injury to the myocardium. Pseudoinfarctional Q waves associated with *chronic* myocardial injury, including those conditions that cause the replacement of functional myocardium with electrically inert tissue or material (e.g., amyloid, tumor, fibrosis), are discussed in Chapter 7.

ACUTE MYOCARDITIS

Acute myocardial inflammation may be caused by any type of infectious agent (viral, bacterial, rickettsial, spirochetal).[74] In other cases, such as giant cell myocarditis or Fiedler's myocarditis, the exact cause of the cardiac inflammatory process is not known but presumably may be due to infectious, immune, or toxic factors.

There is no specific electrocardiographic pattern diagnostic of acute myocarditis. Commonly associated abnormalities[74] include arrhythmias, AV conduction disturbances, bundle branch block, and nonspecific ST-T changes. Low voltage is frequently found during the acute process. In rarer instances ST-T changes and sometimes pathologic Q waves simulating acute transmural infarction may occur (Figs. 6-1 and 6-2). Pseudoinfarct patterns have been found with idiopathic or viral myocarditis,* Fiedler's myocarditis,[32] giant cell myo-

---

*References 14, 21, 29, 36, 47, 51, 52.

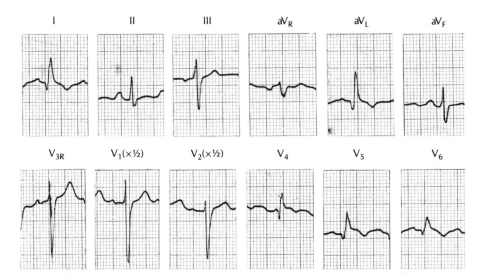

FIG. 6-1. Viral myocarditis simulating anterolateral infarction. This patient was a 14-year-old boy with a fatal type of influenza (Maryland strain, type B) and myocarditis. The tracing shown was recorded 2 weeks before his sudden death. Note the pathologic Q waves in I, aV$_L$, and V$_4$ to V$_6$, with elevated ST segments and terminal T wave inversions in those leads. The pattern is consistent with an evolving anterolateral infarct. In addition, the QRS duration is slightly prolonged. Autopsy revealed diffuse myocardial fibrosis, especially in the lateral portion of the left ventricle. There was no microscopic evidence of acute inflammation, and the coronary arteries were all normal.

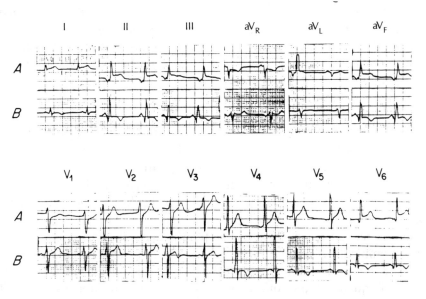

FIG. 6-2. Probable acute viral myocarditis simulating an inferolateral wall infarct in a 23-year-old man with chest pain. The admission ECG, **A**, shows ST elevations in I, II, III, aV$_F$, and V$_4$ to V$_6$, with reciprocal ST depressions in aV$_R$. An ectopic atrial or junctional rhythm is present. Five days later, **B**, note the Q waves that have evolved in the inferior leads and the inferolateral T wave inversions. Sinus rhythm is now present. (Courtesy WM Abelmann, MD.)

carditis,[15] and acute chagasic myocarditis.[63] Ainger et al.[1] noted infarct patterns in 10 of 47 cases of neonatal rubella myocarditis. The ECGs in these cases showed abnormal Q waves, abnormal ST-T changes, or both, that were suggestive of an evolving myocardial necrosis secondary to the viral inflammatory process.

Miklozek et al.[51] reported on 10 adult patients initially diagnosed as having acute myocardial infarction who were subsequently found to have acute viral myocarditis. Diagnostic confusion can easily arise in such cases because myocarditis may cause not only ST elevations and Q waves but also an increase in the CK-MB isoenzyme fraction, positive technetium pyrophosphate scans, and regional wall motion abnormalities.

Abnormal Q waves with bacterial myocarditis are relatively rare. Infarct patterns have been described in children with diphtheritic myocarditis.[17] Isolated case reports have described Q wave infarct patterns with acute gummatous (syphilitic) myocarditis,[60] myocardial abscess caused by melioidosis,[8] and acute bacterial myocarditis with mixed flora following dentoalveolar infection[54] and childbirth.[23]

The pattern of acute diffuse myocardial infarction has also been described in a case report of fatal sodium azide ingestion.[42] At autopsy the heart showed interstitial edema and severe myofibrillar degeneration without cell infiltrate.

Mucocutaneous lymph node syndrome (Kawasaki disease) is an idiopathic inflammatory condition of childhood associated with coronary angiitis and subsequent coronary aneurysm formation and coronary occlusion. Typical ECG patterns of inferior or anterior infarctions are commonly reported. Focal myocarditis may also occur. However, the infarct patterns are caused by the non-atherosclerotic coronary artery obstruction.[25,26]

The Q waves seen occasionally with acute myocarditis probably reflect a loss of myocardial potentials caused by the acute inflammatory process. The Q waves may represent either a temporary loss of myocardial function or, in cases of severe myocarditis, irreversible myocardial necrosis and fibrosis (Fig. 6-1). (Conduction abnormalities also contribute to Q wave pathogenesis in selected cases.) Similarly the ST-T changes, which may be indistinguishable from those of primary ischemia, reflect a true current of injury produced by the epicardial inflammation.

Differential diagnosis. The electrocardiographic pseudoinfarct patterns seen with acute myocarditis may be indistinguishable from the patterns of true infarction. In such cases the differential diagnosis is made clinically on the basis of serial virus titers and by means of cardiac catheterization and cardiac biopsy if indicated. Acute myocarditis should be considered in adults[51] as well as children and infants[22] with infarct patterns.

ACUTE METABOLIC INJURY
Transient Q Waves Caused by Reversible Ischemia and Other Metabolic Insults

There is a tendency in clinical practice to equate Q waves with *irreversible ischemic* injury, However, as illustrated by amyloidosis, tumor, and fibrosis, Q waves can also be caused by *nonischemic* injury as well as by infarction. Furthermore, Q waves caused by myocardial injury, ischemic or nonischemic, can appear *transiently* and do not necessarily signify irreversible damage to the heart muscle.[3,4,19,21,66,67,72]

Transient Q waves caused by ischemia have been documented in a number of clinical and experimental settings. Wilson et al.[75] described them in one patient, and Roesler and Dressler[62] reported their occurrence during otherwise typical attacks of angina. Evanescent Q waves may also occur with Prinzmetal's angina.[16,50] Mamlin, Weber, and Fisch[48] reported the case of a 64-year-old woman with pneumonia and septic shock in whom typical Q waves and ST-T changes of acute infarction developed but whose heart was completely normal at autopsy 2 days after the initial ECG changes appeared. Thomas et al.[71] described a similar case of septic shock in which transient Q waves and ST-T changes with acute infarction were observed. Shugoll[69] presented two cases of transient Q waves and ST-T changes in patients with shock. In neither case were there cardiac enzyme changes or symptoms of ischemic chest pain; R waves reappeared after a few days. Transient Q waves (and ischemic ST-T changes) may also occur in conjunction with anaphylactic shock,[64] during and after episodes of tachyarrhythmias,[65] following open heart surgery,[44] and in patients with acute pancreatitis and shock.[28] Experimentally, short periods of coronary occlusion have produced transient Q waves in dogs without subsequent evidence of myocardial damage at autopsy.[9,35]

In most of these examples transient Q waves (sometimes with typical ischemic ST-T changes) appear to be attributable to a temporary loss of electromotive potential. The precise pathophysiology of this dysfunction, however, is unclear. The appearance of new Q waves is consistent with this loss of myocardial forces, but it is impossible on the basis of one tracing to ascertain whether the myocardial cells are actually necrotic or have only been temporarily inactivated by a severe ischemic or other metabolic insult. DePasquale, Burch, and Phillips[19] referred to areas of myocardium that have lost their capacity to depolarize and repolarize but that are not necrotic as zones of "electrical silence." Such inactivated regions may still retain their capacity to recover electrical function, which accounts for the regeneration of R waves sometimes seen. Spontaneous R wave regeneration may occur during myocardial infarction. R wave regeneration may also occur after successful thrombolytic therapy[30] (see also p. 27) or balloon angioplasty[41] in patients with acute infarction.

The phenomenon of temporary ischemic inactivation followed by complete or partial restoration of normal potentials was initially called the *myocardial concussion syndrome*.[19] It is now referred to as *electrical stunning,* and may be accompanied by evidence of sometimes profound ventricular mechanical dysfunction (*myocardial stunning*).[3,4,11]

There are several possible explanations for transient Q waves in the context of myocardial ischemia without infarction. Severe ischemia affects the cell membrane and can cause a loss of electromotive potential without actual cell death. Transient conduction disturbances may cause alterations in ventricular activation sequence with noninfarctional Q waves[38] (Chapter 5). Finally, some transient Q waves represent an unmasking of a prior infarction; transient ischemia of the periinfarct zone may then allow for expression of these "anamnestic" Q waves.[40]

The examples of evanescent Q waves just cited all involve cases in which transient ischemia occurred in the context of anginal attacks, shock, tachyarrhythmias, etc. Not surprisingly, similar transient Q waves have also been described involving *nonischemic* metabolic or toxic insults[31] that produced temporary cardiac dysfunction. For example, Goldman, Gross, and Rubin[31] reported transient Q waves (lasting 5 days) after an episode of hypoglycemic coma in a 70-year-old woman. The heart was essentially normal at autopsy. Pietras et al.[55] reported on a man 30 years of age in whom the pattern of acute extensive infarction developed following ingestion of a phosphorous-containing poison. The Q waves disappeared after 9 days, and the authors suggested that the phosphorus might have produced direct derangements in myocardial function, resulting in a transient infarct pattern; however, the patient had also been markedly hypotensive, and this alone could have accounted for the ECG changes. Acute infarct patterns (ST elevations *without* Q waves) and myocardial failure have been observed following scorpion stings.[37] Scorpion venom exerts a direct toxic myocardial effect and may also evoke a sympathetic reaction, resulting in catecholamine-induced myocardial injury.[37]

Transient Q waves following acute pulmonary embolism probably do not reflect myocardial injury. (They are discussed separately in Chapter 4; those associated with intracranial bleeding are considered in greater detail on p. 295.) Transient Q waves have also been reported during exercise testing.[5,34] Although in some patients they may be due to ischemia,[5,61] they are neither a sensitive nor a specific marker of coronary disease. They have been reported in normal subjects[34,59] and in patients with hypertrophic cardiomyopathy.[76] In patients without ischemia, such exercise-induced Q waves could be due to positional factors or conduction alterations.

Two other conditions, severe hyperkalemia and acute pancreatitis, have been cited as causes of transient noninfarctional Q waves and are discussed next.

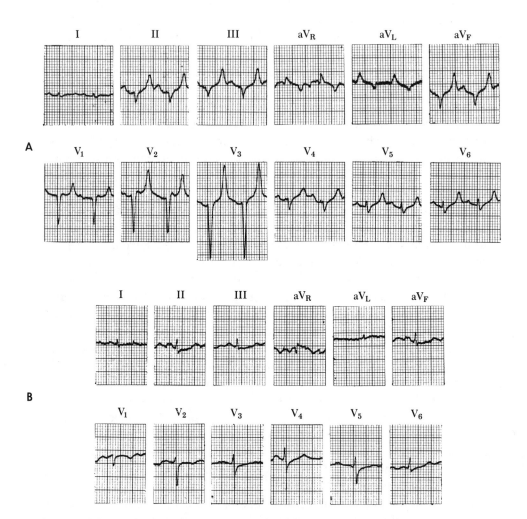

FIG. 6-3. Hyperkalemia simulating acute transmural anterior and inferior wall infarctions in a 51-year-old woman with renal disease. She was not hypotensive at admission, but her potassium level was 8.5 mEq/L with metabolic acidosis (arterial blood pH 7.15). **A,** Abnormal Q waves in II, III, and aV_F, with poor R wave progression in the anterior precordial leads consistent with an extensive infarct. The T waves are markedly peaked, especially in V_3. Note also the first-degree AV block and low voltage in the extremity leads. The QRS axis is −90 degrees. **B,** Several hours later. The serum K^+ has been lowered to 3.5 mEq/L, and the acidosis and dehydration are corrected. Notice the striking "regeneration" of depolarization forces in the anterior and inferior leads. Nonspecific ST-T abnormalities now replace the tall tented T waves, the PR interval is within normal range, and the QRS axis has shifted to about +80 degrees.

Transient Q Waves Associated with Hyperkalemia

Marked hyperkalemia may produce the following pseudoinfarct patterns, singly or in combination: (1) tall positive T waves simulating hyperacute infarction, (2) ST segment elevations simulating acute infarction, (3) transient Q waves simulating "transmural" infarction (Fig. 6-3). The pseudoinfarctional ST-T changes seen are discussed in detail in Chapters 10 and 19.

Noninfarctional Q waves are a well-documented finding with severe hyperkalemia.[2,19,27,53,73] Fig. 6-3 shows the pattern of transient anterior and inferior wall infarcts in a patient whose serum potassium level was 8.5 mEq/L.

Etiology. The Q waves associated with marked hyperkalemia are probably caused by the direct effect of increases in serum potassium concentration on the resting potential of myocardial cells.[19] Normally the ratio of intracellular to extracellular potassium is about 30:1, and this ratio is the primary determinant of the negative resting potential of normal cardiac fibers. Increasing extracellular potassium ion concentration will decrease this critical ratio and result in a lower resting potential. Decreasing the resting potential of cardiac cells in turn tends to lessen the amplitude of the action potentials generated by these cells due to inactivation of sodium channels.[2a] Experimentally, placing cardiac muscle in a solution of high potassium concentration can actually produce a complete loss of electrical activity, which reappears as soon as the muscle is restored to a physiologic milieu with a normal potassium concentration.[19]

The transient Q waves encountered clinically in some cases of marked hyperkalemia may be caused by a similar process of electrical dysfunction secondary to depolarization of cell membranes. In some cases transient Q waves may be related to slowing of conduction in the His-Purkinje system.[2]

DePasquale, Burch, and Phillips[19] initially suggested that local autolysis of necrotic cells following acute myocardial infarction produces local hyperkalemia, which in turn can lead to a transient inactivation of noninfarcted cells. These still viable cells may regain their normal electrical function when the potassium "flood" clears, possibly accounting (in at least some patients) for the partial regeneration of R waves sometimes seen after the acute phase of infarction (p. 26).

Transient Q Waves Associated with Acute Pancreatitis

There are a number of reports* (Table 6-1) of infarction patterns associated with acute pancreatitis. However, none of these cases convincingly fulfills the strict criteria for establishing a pseudoinfarct pattern (p. 10). For example, a number of the patients manifested hypotension and shock,[7,10,28,33] which alone can produce transient Q waves and ST-T changes without actual infarction (p. 130).

---

*References 7, 10, 13, 21, 28, 33, 45, 68, 69.

TABLE 6-1. Acute pancreatitis with ECG pattern of myocardial infarction: summary of published cases

Case	Clinical summary	ECG pattern
Dittler and McGavack[21]	Man 53 years of age with pancreatitis and chest pains; no myocardial necrosis at autopsy	ECG showed only atrial flutter and fibrillation with no evidence of "posterior infarction" described by authors
Gottesman, Casten, and Beller[33]*	Woman 68 years of age admitted in shock; died 5 hr after admission; heart was normal at autopsy	Q waves in II and III with ST segment elevations
Bockus and Raffensperger[10]†	Patient with massive pancreatic necrosis and in shock; patient survived	Q wave infarction pattern with persistent ECG abnormalities
Bauerlein and Stobbe[7]	Woman 51 years of age; shock(?); no myocardial necrosis at autopsy	Marked precordial ST elevations without Q waves
Caini and Modigliana[13]	Patient with pancreatitis who was in shock	ECG pattern consistent with "myocardial lesion"
Shamma'a and Rubeiz[68]	Man 43 years of age with history of atrial fibrillation; acute pancreatitis without apparent hypotension or electrolyte imbalance; patient survived, no follow-up data available	Inferolateral infarct pattern with Q waves persisting for 2 weeks
Fulton and Marriott[28]	Man 61 years of age with severe hypotensive episode	Precordial Q waves with ST elevations; Q waves disappeared after 2 days, but T wave inversions persisted
Lambert[45]	Man 43 years of age whose clinical course was not described; normal myocardium at autopsy	Precordial Q waves with T wave inversions
Spritzer et al.[70]	Man 47 years of age with pancreatitis and severe chest pain without hypotension; subsequent coronary arteriogram and exercise test were normal; patient healthy 1 year later	Q waves and ST elevations in inferior leads resolving in 36 hr
	Man 53 years of age with blood pressure drop to 99 mm Hg systolic; coronary arteriogram subsequently showed narrowing of left anterior descending coronary artery	Transient T wave inversions in V_1 to V_2 without Q waves
Cohen et al.[18]	Man 41 years of age without cardiac symptoms or hypotension; normal coronary arteriogram; patient survived	Anterior wall Q wave infarct pattern with T wave inversions; R waves returned after 2 days, but some ST-T changes persisted

*The authors also describe four other patients with pancreatitis and ST-T changes but no Q waves.
†The authors also mention two other patients with pancreatitis whose ST-T changes were consistent with ischemia.

In other cases without apparent hypotension, myocardial ischemia could not be definitely excluded. In three of the reported cases with alleged pseudoinfarct patterns, coronary arteriography was performed. One of these patients, described by Spritzer et al.[70] was a 47-year-old man with transient inferior ST segment elevations and Q waves in II, III, and aV_F associated with severe chest pain. In retrospect, the case is highly suggestive of coronary vasospasm, a well-documented case of transient ST segment elevations and sometimes transient Q waves.[50] The other patient reported by the same authors showed transient anterior T wave inversions without Q waves. A 50% stenosis of the left anterior descending coronary was noted. Subsequently, Cohen et al.[18] reported a 41-year-old man with pancreatitis and transient anterior Q waves and T wave inversions. It is noteworthy that in none of these three cases were cardiac enzyme studies available, nor were ventriculograms reported to exclude wall motion abnormalities.

For these reasons the significance of reported infarction patterns with acute pancreatitis remains uncertain.[58] Some authors[18,68,70] have suggested that proteolytic enzymes released by the injured pancreas might produce nonischemic myocardial injury. Intravenous infusion of trypsin in rabbits caused myocardial necrosis and ECG changes consistent with "cardiac injury."[43,46] However, Pollock and Bertrand[56] found no evidence of myocardial necrosis or abnormal Q waves in dogs following intravenous administration of trypsin or pancreatic juice, and there has been no documentation of proteolytic myocardial damage.

In summary: Although acute pancreatitis is a very common entity, infarction patterns have been reported only in exceptional cases. Furthermore, actual ischemia, including possible coronary artery vasospasm, was not convincingly excluded in any of these reports. In a retrospective survey of 50 patients with acute pancreatitis, Mautner et al.[49] observed a new infarct pattern in only one case, a patient with confirmed coronary occlusion. Therefore until more conclusive data are available, the appearance of Q waves or profound ST-T changes should not be ascribed to acute pancreatitis alone. Similarly, as noted in Chapter 1, there is no documentation that acute or chronic biliary disease can produce actual pseudoinfarct patterns.[24]

TRAUMATIC NONCORONARY MYOCARDIAL INJURY

Severe traumatic injury to the heart can produce classic infarct patterns (Q waves with ST-T changes).[39] Infarct patterns may appear following direct penetrating wounds of the myocardium (by bullet or knife) or following severe myocardial contusion caused by closed chest trauma (Fig. 6-4). The infarct patterns in such cases reflect actual myocardial damage but do not necessarily indicate direct injury of a coronary artery. Following cardiac trauma the abnormal Q waves and ST-T changes may persist, resolve completely, or leave nonspecific changes. Chest contusion may also be associated with intraventricular or AV conduction disturbances, as well as a positive technetium-99m-pyrophosphate scintigram.

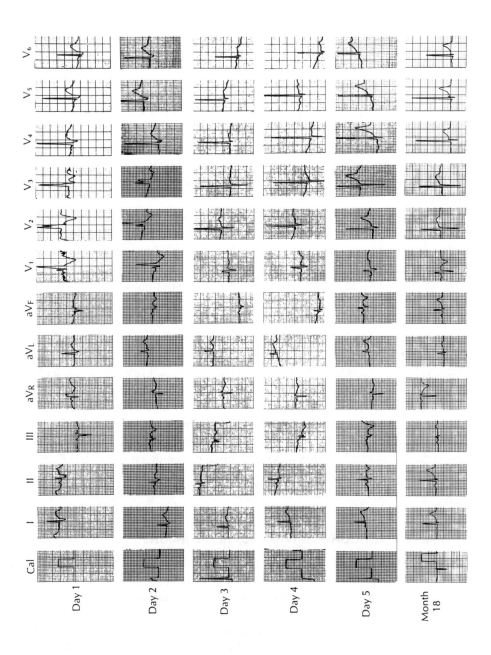

FIG. 6–4. Serial electrocardiograms of a 17-year-old boy who suffered blunt chest trauma, causing transient bifascicular block and an inferior wall myocardial contusion. **Day 1,** Note the pattern of right bundle branch block and left axis deviation, suggesting a bifascicular block. **Day 2,** Terminal QRS forces are slightly less superior, but evidence of the bifascicular block persists. The T waves in II, III, and aV_F have become inverted. **Day 3,** The right bundle branch block pattern has resolved, and the QRS axis is now about −30 degrees. T wave inversions persist in III and aV_F, and there is early precordial transition suggestive of posteroinferior wall injury. **Day 4,** Progression of the same pattern. **Day 5,** Deepening of the T wave inversions in II, III, and aV_F. **Month 18,** Follow-up tracing. The patient had no symptoms. Notice the early repolarization pattern, a normal variant, in I, II, aV_L, and V_2 to V_6. There is no evidence of the residual conduction defect or myocardial contusion. Calibration (*Cal*) is 1 mV. (From Carr KW, et al: West J Med 137:245, 1982. Reprinted with permission.)

Myocardial damage caused by lightning stroke has also been reported as a rare cause of Q waves and marked ST-T changes. The ECG pattern of transmural injury in these cases probably reflects a direct myocardial burn. Deep T wave inversions may appear and may have an unusual, widely splayed, shape suggestive of the pattern seen in conjunction with cerebrovascular accidents (p. 291). The T wave inversions seen with cerebrovascular accident have been attributed to excessive sympathetic stimulation, and Burda[12] has suggested that a similar "sympathetic storm" may be triggered following lightning stroke.

REFERENCES

1. Ainger LE, et al: Neonatal rubella myocarditis, Br Heart J 28:691, 1966.
2. Arnsdorf MF: Electrocardiogram in hyperkalemia: electrocardiographic pattern of anteroseptal myocardial infarction mimicked by hyperkalemia-induced disturbance of impulse conduction, Arch Intern Med 136:1161, 1976.
2a. Arnsdorf MF, Wasserstrom JA: Mechanisms of action of antiarrhythmic drugs: a matrical approach. In Fozzard HA, et al. (editors): The heart and cardiovascular system, New York, 1986, Raven Press.
3. Barold SS, et al: Significance of transient electrocardiographic Q waves in coronary artery disease, Cardiol Clin 5:367, 1987.
4. Bashour TT, et al: Transient Q waves and reversible cardiac failure during myocardial ischemia. Electrical and mechanical stunning of the heart, Am Heart J 106:780, 1983.
5. Bateman T, et al: Transient appearance of Q waves in coronary disease during exercise electrocardiography: consideration of mechanisms and clinical importance, Am Heart J 104:182, 1982.
6. Bateman TM, et al: Transient, pathologic Q waves during acute ischemic events. An electrocardiographic correlate of stunned but viable myocardium, Am Heart J 106:1421, 1983.
7. Bauerlein TC, Stobbe LHO: Acute pancreatitis simulating myocardial infarction with characteristic electrocardiographic changes, Gastroenterology 27:861, 1954.
8. Baumann BB, Morita ET: Systemic melioidosis presenting as myocardial infarction, Ann Intern Med 67:836, 1967.
9. Bayley RH, LaDue JS: Differentiation of the electrocardiographic changes produced in the dog by prolonged temporary occlusion of a coronary artery from those produced by postoperative pericarditis, Am Heart J 28:233, 1944.
10. Bockus HL, Raffensperger EC: Acute pancreatitis, NY J Med 48:2252, 1948.
11. Braunwald EB, Kloner RA: The stunned myocardium: prolonged postischemic ventricular dysfunction, Circulation 66:1146, 1982.
12. Burda CD: Electrocardiographic changes in lightning stroke, Am Heart J 72:521, 1966.
13. Caini B, Modigliana V: Cardiovascular syndrome of acute pancreatitis, Sett Med 44:349, 1956.
14. Case records of the Massachusetts General Hospital (case 20-1972), N Engl J Med 286:1100, 1972.
15. Case records of the Massachusetts General Hospital (case 32-1972), N Engl J Med 287:296, 1972.
16. Chava NR: Transient QRS changes in variant angina simulating acute myocardial infarction, Am Heart J 105:695, 1983.
17. Class RN, et al: Diphtheritic myocarditis simulating myocardial infarction, Am J Cardiol 16:580, 1965.
18. Cohen MH, et al: Electrocardiographic changes in acute pancreatitis resembling acute myocardial infarction, Am Heart J 82:672, 1971.
19. DePasquale NP, et al: Electrocardiographic alterations associated with electrically "silent" areas of myocardium, Am Heart J 68:697, 1964.
20. Desa'neto A, et al: Coxsackie B5 heart disease: demonstration of inferolateral wall myocardial necrosis, Am J Med 68:295, 1980.
21. Dittler EL, McGavack TH: Pancreatic necrosis associated with auricular fibrillation and flutter: report of a case simulating coronary thrombosis (autopsy findings), Am Heart J 16:354, 1938.

22. Dominguez P, et al: False "coronary patterns" in the infant electrocardiogram, Circulation 19:409, 1959.
23. Faruque AA: Acute fulminating puerperal myocarditis, Br Heart J 27:139, 1965.
24. Friedman GD: The relationship between heart disease and gallbladder disease: a critical review, Ann Intern Med 68:222, 1968.
25. Fujiwara H, et al: Clinicopathologic study of abnormal Q waves in Kawasaki disease (mucocutaneous lymph node syndrome), Am J Cardiol 45:797, 1980.
26. Fukushige J, et al: Spectrum of cardiovascular lesions in mucocutaneous lymph node syndrome: analysis of eight cases, Am J Cardiol 45:98, 1980.
27. Fuller PJ, et al: Transient anterior electrocardiographic changes simulating acute anterior myocardial infarction in diabetic ketoacidosis, Diabetes Care 5:118, 1982.
28. Fulton MC, Marriott HJL: Acute pancreatitis simulating myocardial infarction in the electrocardiogram, Ann Intern Med 59:730, 1963.
29. Gillis JG, Walters MB: Acute isolated myocarditis simulating coronary occlusion, Am Heart J 47:117, 1954.
30. Goldberg S, et al: Limitation of infarct size with thrombolytic agents—electrocardiographic indexes, Circulation 68(suppl I): I-77, 1983.
31. Goldman AG, et al: Transitory Q waves simulating the Q wave of myocardial infarction, Am Heart J 60:61, 1960.
32. Goldman AM: Acute myocarditis simulating myocardial infarction, Dis Chest 41:61, 1962.
33. Gottesman J, et al: Changes in the electrocardiogram induced by acute pancreatitis: a clinical and experimental study, JAMA 123:892, 1943.
34. Greenspan M, Anderson GJ: The significance of exercise-induced Q waves, Am J Med 67:454, 1979.
35. Gross H, et al: Transient abnormal Q waves in the dog without myocardial infarction, Am J Cardiol 14:669, 1964.
36. Gross H, et al: Abnormal Q waves in a child with myocarditis, NY J Med 67:283, 1967.
37. Gueron M, et al: Severe myocardial damage and heart failure in scorpion sting, Am J Cardiol 19:719, 1967.
38. Haiat R, Chiche P: Transient abnormal Q waves in the course of ischemic heart disease, Chest 65:140, 1974.

39. Harthorne JW, et al: Traumatic myocardial infarction: report of a case with normal coronary angiogram, Ann Intern Med 66:341, 1967.
40. Hassett MA, et al: Transient QRS changes simulating acute myocardial infarction, Circulation 62:975, 1980.
41. Ibba GV, et al: Disappearance of pathologic Q wave after PTCA in evolving myocardial infarction, Am Heart J 108:1538, 1989.
42. Judge KW, Ward NE: Fatal azide-induced cardiomyopathy presenting as acute myocardial infarction, Am J Cardiol 64:830, 1989.
43. Kellner A, Robertson T: Selective necrosis of cardiac and skeletal muscle induced experimentally by means of proteolytic enzyme solutions given intravenously J Exp Med 99:387, 1954.
44. Klein HO, et al: Transient electrocardiographic changes simulating myocardial infarction during open-heart surgery, Am Heart J 79:463, 1970.
45. Lambert H: Les altérations de l'électrocardiogramme dans la crise douloureuse de la pancréatite, Cardiologia 48:387, 1966.
46. Lieberman JS, et al: The effect of intravenous trypsin administration on the electrocardiogram of the rabbit, Circulation 10:338, 1954.
47. Limas CJ: Acute myocarditis simulating myocardial infarction, South Med J 64:1534, 1971.
48. Mamlin JJ, et al: Electrocardiographic pattern of massive myocardial infarction without pathologic confirmation, Circulation 30:539, 1964.
49. Mautner RK, et al: Electrocardiographic changes in acute pancreatitis, South Med J 75:317, 1982.
50. Meller J, et al: Transient Q waves in Prinzmetal's angina, Am J Cardiol 35:691, 1975.
51. Miklozek CL, et al: Myocarditis presenting as acute myocardial infarction, Am Heart J 115:768, 1988.
52. Miller R, et al: Focal mononucleosis myocarditis simulating myocardial infarction, Chest 63:102, 1973.
53. Nora TR, Pilz CG: Pseudoinfarction pattern associated with electrolyte disturbance, Arch Intern Med 104:300, 1959.
54. Palank EA, et al: Fatal acute bacterial myocarditis after dentoalveolar abscess, Am J Cardiol 43:1238, 1979.

55. Pietras RJ, et al: Phosphorus poisoning simulating acute myocardial infarction, Arch Intern Med 122:430, 1968.

56. Pollock AV, Bertrand CA: Electrocardiographic changes in acute pancreatitis, Surgery 40:951, 1956.

57. Potkin RT, et al: Evaluation of noninvasive tests of cardiac damage in suspected cardiac contusion, Circulation 66:627, 1982.

58. Pruitt RD, et al: The difficult electrocardiographic diagnosis of myocardial infarction, Prog Cardiovasc Dis 6:85, 1983.

59. Przybojewski JZ, Thorpe L: Transient "pathological" Q waves occurring during exercise testing: assessment of their direct significance in a presentation of a series of patients, J Electrocardiol 20:121, 1987.

60. Rafenstein EC: Acute gummatous myocarditis simulating acute myocardial infarction, Ann Intern Med 10:241, 1936.

61. Rebuzzi AG, et al: Transient Q waves followed by left anterior fascicular block during exercise, Br Heart J 54:107, 1985.

62. Roesler H, Dressler W: Transient electrocardiographic changes identical with those of acute myocardial infarction accompanying attacks of angina pectoris, Am Heart J 47:520, 1954.

63. Rosenbaum MB: Chagasic myocardiopathy, Prog Cardiovasc Dis 7:199, 1964.

64. Rosenfeld I, et al: Allergic shock in humans: report of two cases with electrocardiographic findings, Am Heart J 53:463, 1957.

65. Rubin IL, et al: Transitory abnormal Q waves during bouts of tachycardia, Am J Cardiol 11:659, 1963.

66. Rubin IL, et al: Transient abnormal Q waves during bouts of coronary insufficiency, Am Heart J 71:254, 1966.

67. Segers M, et al: Altérations électrocardiographiques transitoires simulant les images coronariennes, Acta Cardiol 6:39, 1951.

68. Shamma'a MH, Rubeiz GA: Acute pancreatitis with electrocardiographic findings of myocardial infarction, Am J Med 32:827, 1962.

69. Shugoll GI: Transient QRS changes dimulating myocardial infarction associated with shock and severe metabolic stress, Am Heart J 74:402, 1967.

70. Spritzer HW, et al: Electrocardiographic abnormalities in acute pancreatitis: two patients studied by selective coronary arteriography, Milit Med 134:687, 1969.

71. Thomas I, et al: Electrocardiographic changes in catastrophic illness mimicking acute myocardial infarction, Am J Cardiol 59:1224, 1987.

72. Uhley H: Transient abnormal Q waves [Editorial], Chest 65:123, 1974.

73. Weintraub LR, Reynolds EW: Electrocardiographic change simulating myocardial infarction in potassium intoxication, Univ Mich Med Bull 26:348, 1960.

74. Wenger NK, et al: Myocarditis. In Hurst JW (editor): The heart, ed 7, New York, 1989, McGraw-Hill Book Co, p 1256.

75. Wilson FN, et al: The precordial electrocardiogram, Am Heart J 27:19, 1944.

76. Zalman F, et al: Transient Q waves with exercise in hypertrophic cardiomyopathy, Am J Cardiol 56:491, 1985.

Noninfarctional myocardial injury: chronic myocardial injury patterns

A variety of chronic conditions discussed in this chapter can produce Q waves related to myocardial replacement or infiltration in the absence of coronary artery disease.

CARDIAC AMYLOIDOSIS

Prominent Q waves are relatively common with extensive cardiac amyloidosis. Buja, Khoi, and Roberts[12] reviewed 124 previously published cases of cardiac amyloidosis and found a 64% incidence of infarction patterns. Underlying coronary artery disease could not be excluded in some of these reported cases.

Fig. 7-1 shows an example of pseudoinfarctional QS waves in V_1 to V_3 in a patient with cardiac amyloidosis and no evidence of coronary disease at autopsy. This pattern of abnormal Q waves in the right to middle precordial leads that simulates anteroseptal infarction is particularly common with cardiac amyloidosis.[11,31] Noninfarctional Q waves extending from V_1 to V_6 have been reported.[7] Inferior wall infarct patterns also may occur.

Other common ECG abnormalities associated with amyloid heart disease[12] include low voltage, conduction disturbances (bundle branch block and AV block), arrhythmias (especially atrial fibrillation), and left axis deviation. Nonspecific ST-T alterations (Fig. 7-1) are also common findings. Deep T wave inversions or marked ST segment deviations, however, are not features of cardiac amyloidosis, and these findings suggest underlying ischemia.

Low voltage QRS complexes are especially common with amyloid heart disease. The presence of abnormal Q waves and low voltage together with the clinical manifestations of congestive heart failure should suggest the possibility of amyloid cardiomyopathy. However, this combination is nonspecific and may be seen with ischemic heart disease, myocarditis, or other types of chronic cardiomyopathy (see Fig. 7-11). With cardiac amyloid, the voltage is typically low in both the limb and the precordial leads. By contrast, dilated cardiomyopathy may be associated with *increased* precordial but *low* limb voltage (compare Figs. 7-1 and 7-13).

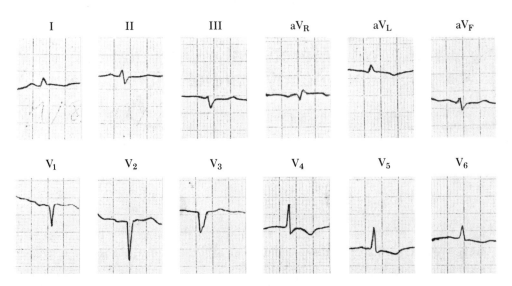

FIG. 7-1. Cardiac amyloidosis simulating anteroseptal infarction. This patient, a 44-year-old man, had systemic amyloidosis and congestive heart failure. Note the abnormal QS waves in V_1 to V_3 and the low voltage with borderline left axis deviation and nonspecific ST-T changes. At autopsy the heart was infiltrated with amyloid but there were no signs of coronary artery disease. Infarct patterns (anterior or inferior wall) are relatively common with cardiac amyloidosis. The noninfarctional Q waves are due to replacement of the myocardium by this electrically inert substance.

Other noninvasive tests may provide important diagnostic clues to the presence of cardiac amyloidosis. The echocardiogram typically reveals thickening of the right and left ventricular free walls as well as of the ventricular septum.[101] Thus the paradoxical presence of relatively low QRS voltage despite increased ventricular wall thickness should suggest cardiac amyloidosis.[18] (Myxedema may also produce this echocardiographic-ECG combination.)

Technetium-99m-pyrophosphate scintigraphy typically shows persistent, intense, diffuse uptake, in contrast to the more localized and transient pattern seen with acute infarction[30,117] (Chapter 22).

Definitive diagnosis of cardiac amyloidosis can be made in most cases by transvenous endocardial biopsy of the right ventricle; it is strongly suggested by amyloid in other sites (tongue, rectum, skin). However, cardiac amyloidosis with heart failure may occur as a relatively isolated finding in some patients.

At autopsy the hearts of such patients generally show extensive deposition of amyloid between the myocardial fibers, along with areas in which the myocardium has been totally replaced by the amyloid.[12] This replacement of myocardium with electrically inert material may account for the pathologic Q waves often seen in this condition. Amyloid typically spares the larger extramural coronary artery branches. However, involvement of the smaller intramural arteries and arterioles has been noted.[12,104] Occlusion of these distal vessels may cause secondary ischemia and possibly actual infarction. Finally, some patients with cardiac amyloid will have concomitant atherosclerosis.[88]

MUSCULAR DYSTROPHIES
Duchenne Muscular Dystrophy

An ECG pattern suggestive of posteroinferior or posterolateral wall infarction is a common finding in patients with Duchenne muscular dystrophy (Figs. 7-2 to 7-4). The specific features of the pseudoinfarct patterns seen with Duchenne muscular dystrophy include the following*:

1. Tall narrow R waves are seen in the right precordial leads, with an increased R/S ratio suggesting either posterior wall infarction or right ventricular hypertrophy (Fig. 7-4). An RSr' or polyphasic type of complex in V_1 may also be seen.

2. Deep, usually narrow, Q waves in the lateral precordial leads (e.g., V_5 and V_6) or in one or more of the limb leads (I, II, III, aV_L, and aV_F) suggest lateral or inferior wall infarction (Fig. 7-2). These Q waves may exceed 25% of the amplitude of the succeeding R wave; however, they are usually sharply inscribed and narrow (less than 0.04 sec duration). Rarely, wide Q waves like those shown in Figs. 7-3 and 7-4 will be present.

These pseudoinfarct patterns are very common with Duchenne muscular dystrophy. One series of 25 unselected cases included 20 patients (80%) with prominent R waves in the right precordial leads and 23 instances (92%) of deep Q waves.[12] Sanyal et al.[98] in a series of 75 patients noted a tall R wave in V_1 (R/S ratio >1) in 64% of patients and a narrow deep Q wave (>4 mm) in the lateral leads in 44% of patients.

Etiology. The cause of the typical ECG pattern seen with Duchenne muscular dystrophy has not been definitely established but most likely relates to the underlying cardiomyopathy with predominant posterobasal or lateral (apical) involvement. Right ventricular hypertrophy or right ventricular conduction defects were initially suggested as possible causes of the tall right precordial R waves[112] but could not be documented.[83] Other investigators attributed these findings to a persistence of the childhood ECG pattern, which also features tall right precordial R waves and sometimes deep narrow Q waves in the lateral leads.[74] Slucka[102] observed similar ECG patterns in the mothers of affected sons and suggested that the persistence of the childhood pattern might be genetically determined. However, De Leon et al.[26] presented serial tracings from a patient with Duchenne muscular dystrophy that showed an increase in the depth of the lateral lead Q waves over time, suggesting that additional factors were responsible for these ECG changes.

Autopsy examination of the hearts of patients with Duchenne muscular dystrophy reveals degenerative changes similar to those found in the skeletal mus-

---

*References 26, 35, 74, 83, 89, 99, 102.

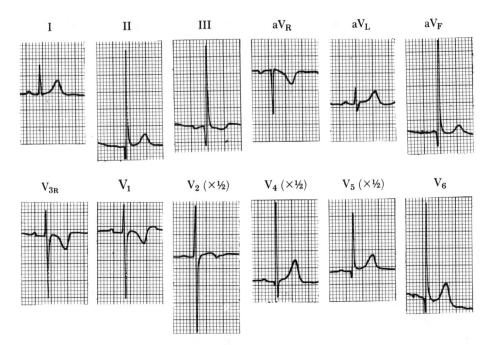

FIG. 7-2. Duchenne muscular dystrophy in a 7-year-old boy with no apparent cardiac disability. Prominent but narrow Q waves in the inferior and lateral leads are typical in these patients. Tall right precordial R waves also sometimes are seen (Fig. 7-4). T wave inversions in the right precordial leads, a normal finding in juveniles, may occasionally persist into adulthood.

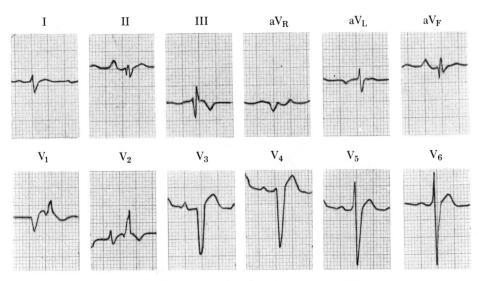

FIG. 7-3. Unusual Duchenne muscular dystrophy pattern in a 14-year-old boy with heart failure. Note the deep Q waves in the inferior leads. The QR complexes in V_1 and V_2 are consistent with right ventricular hypertrophy and dilation, and the giant P wave in V_1 is suggestive of bilateral atrial enlargement. The patient died 1 month after this tracing was taken. At autopsy the heart was massively hypertrophied (particularly the left ventricle) and weighed 860 g. Although there was biventricular dilation, the coronary arteries were entirely normal. Fibrosis was present throughout, most notably in the septum and left ventricular apex, and appeared at microscopic examination to have replaced the myocardium. This pattern represents terminal cardiomyopathy, reflecting ventricular fibrosis and hypertrophy, but it differs from the typical Duchenne pattern (which is characterized by deep narrow Q waves in the lateral or inferior leads and RS complexes in the right precordial leads).

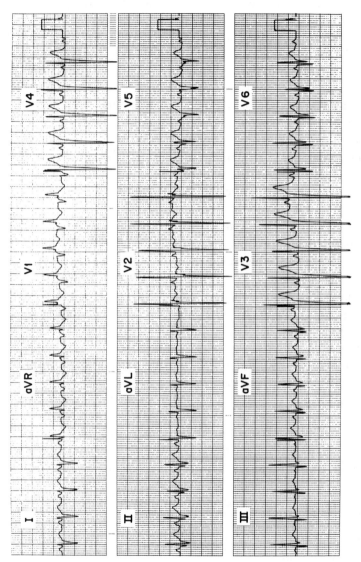

FIG. 7-4. Duchenne muscular dystrophy simulating an inferoposterolateral infarct. Note the characteristically narrow but prominent Q waves on this tracing from a 21-year-old male (in II, III, aV_F, and V_6) as well as the tall R wave (in V_1). In addition, there is sinus tachycardia with right axis deviation and marked left atrial abnormality.

cle of these children. Weisenfeld and Messinger[111] noted an increase in cardiac connective tissue with atrophy of the muscle cells and fatty replacement. Hypertrophy of remaining myocardial fibers was also seen. Rubin and Buchberg[95] attributed the deep Q waves seen with Duchenne muscular dystrophy to this dystrophic myocardial degeneration. De Leon et al.[26] subsequently reported a detailed ECG and pathologic correlative study of two patients with Duchenne muscular dystrophy. In both cases the ECGs showed the classic pattern of tall right precordial R waves with deep Q waves in the lateral leads. At autopsy, selective myocardial scarring involving primarily the posterobasal aspect of the left ventricle was noted in both patients. Similarly, Sanyal et al.[98] also observed multifocal degenerative changes predominantly involving the posterobasal portion of the left ventricle. These studies formed the basis of the hypothesis that loss of posterior depolarization forces secondary to dystrophic myocardial damage could account for a reciprocal increase in anterior forces (tall precordial R waves), analogous to the changes seen with posterior infarction (p. 50). The deep Q waves in the lateral or inferior leads might reflect extension of this process of primary myocardial injury.

This hypothesis is further supported by evidence of defects (particularly posteroapical) on resting thallium-201 perfusion scans.[118] However, Perloff et al.[84] reported that the apparent reduction or loss of posterolateral left ventricular electrical forces may not actually require transmural myocardial damage or replacement by connective tissue. Their studies of myocardial metabolism using positron emission tomography in 15 Duchenne patients with characteristic ECG abnormalities demonstrated viable though abnormal myofibers in the affected posterobasal or lateral segments.

Figs. 7-3 and 7-4 show two striking ECG patterns from children with Duchenne muscular dystrophy; these patterns are highly suggestive of dystrophic myocardial injury. In Fig. 7-3 a bizarre pattern with tall right precordial R waves and W-shaped complexes in the inferior leads suggests inferior wall injury. At autopsy marked ventricular fibrosis was noted. In Fig. 7-4 the more typical pattern, consistent with extensive posterolateral infarction and complete loss of lateral wall R waves and tall R waves in the right precordial leads, appears.

Clinically patients with Duchenne muscular dystrophy often have evidence of an underlying cardiomyopathy.[82,83] Persistent sinus tachycardia is common, although high-grade ventricular arrhythmias are surprisingly rare. A relatively short PR interval may be present without other evidence of preexcitation.[83] Patients may complain of palpitation and dyspnea. Chest pain is usually musculoskeletal in origin.[83] On physical examination, S_3 and S_4 gallops may be heard. Heart failure, caused by the underlying cardiomyopathy, occurs in the terminal stages.

Differential diagnosis. Exclusion of infarction in these patients is usually not difficult in light of the general clinical findings.[82,83] The Q waves seen with Duchenne muscular dystrophy are usually narrow and sharply inscribed, in contrast to the wide Q waves often seen with true infarction. However, wide Q waves may occur in rare cases of Duchenne muscular dystrophy, and these are indistinguishable from the Q waves of infarction. In such cases the youth of the patient should suggest an underlying cardiomyopathy. The MB isoenzyme fraction of the creatine kinase (CK) may also be elevated in Duchenne muscular dystrophy in the absence of myocardial infarction[38] (Chapter 22).

This ECG pattern also resembles the pattern sometimes seen with hypertrophic cardiomyopathy (Chapter 4), which often features tall right precordial R waves and deep lateral Q waves. However, the Q waves of idiopathic hypertrophic cardiomyopathy are usually broader than those of Duchenne muscular dystrophy.

The typical Duchenne pattern (tall right precordial R waves with deep narrow left precordial Q waves) has also been reported in asymptomatic female carriers of this X-linked recessive disorder. Mann et al.[73] noted this ECG pattern in three of 18 female carriers studied. The significance of their observation is not clear, but it suggests the possibility of underlying occult cardiomyopathy in these women.[73] A high percentage of female carriers, including all the subjects tested in the series of Mann et al.,[73] also have elevated levels of CK, a finding consistent with subclinical myopathy.

Other Hereditary Muscular Dystrophies

Abnormal Q waves similar to the pattern seen with Duchenne muscular dystrophy were also noted in three of 13 patients with Erb's limb girdle dystrophy studied by Perloff et al.[83]

There is also a case report of a Q wave inferior wall pseudoinfarct pattern (without pathologic confirmation) in a patient with fascioscapulohumeral dystrophy (Landouzy-Dejerine dystrophy).[116] Perloff, De Leon, and O'Doherty[83] however, did not note significant ECG abnormalities in the patients they studied with this syndrome.

MYOTONIA ATROPHICA

Myotonia atrophica (myotonia dystrophica, myotonic dystrophy, Steinert's disease) is a hereditary neuromuscular condition that occasionally simulates the ECG pattern of myocardial infarction (Fig. 7-5). It is characterized by the autosomal dominant inheritance of myotonia (slow muscle relaxation) and muscle atrophy in addition to cataracts, frontal baldness, testicular atrophy, mental retardation and cardiac involvement.

The cardiac and ECG features of this condition have been described by numerous authors.* The majority of patients in these series had abnormal ECGs. The most common findings were prolongation of the PR interval, intraventricu-

---

*References 17, 23, 31, 32, 34, 58, 77, 81, 82, 85, 113.

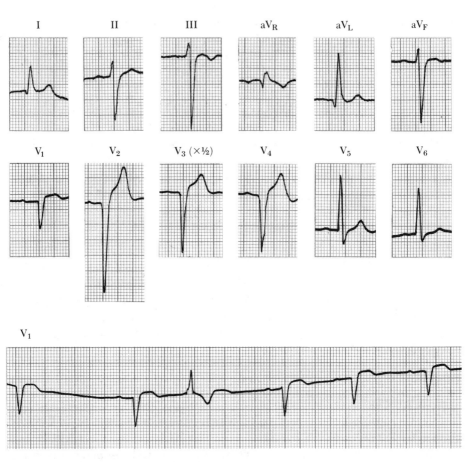

FIG. 7-5. Myotonia atrophica simulating anterior infarction in a 22-year-old black man. Note the Q waves in I, aV_L, and V_1 to V_4 as well as the left ventricular conduction disturbance (marked left axis deviation, borderline first-degree block, and sinus arrhythmia with ectopic beats). The ST in V_2 is also elevated (4 mm at the J point), suggesting acute anterior ischemia. However, prominent T waves with a high ST takeoff are frequently seen with uncomplicated left bundle branch block and the QS complexes in V_1 to V_4 can, likewise, be seen with LBBB. The distinguishing feature of this tracing that suggests underlying myocardial injury is the appearance of QR complexes in I and aV_L (p. 106).

lar conduction disturbances, left axis deviation, and sinus bradycardia. Other electrophysiologic abnormalities, including atrial flutter, atrial fibrillation, AV heart block, and ventricular arrhythmias, have been reported. Nonspecific ST-T changes also occur frequently.

Definitive pseudoinfarct patterns were seen in only a few cases. Fearrington, Gibson, and Churchill,[32] in their series of 17 cases, showed two examples of anterior wall infarct patterns and a third case with deep diffuse T wave inversions without Q waves. In none of these patients was there a history of cardiac abnormality. Wenger[113] presented an example of an anteroseptal pseudoinfarct pattern in a myotonic patient with no history of cardiac disease. Perloff et al.[85] prospectively studied 25 adult myotonic patients (ages 21 to 46 yr); one, a 38-year-old man, had an anteroseptal pseudoinfarct pattern with QS waves in V_1 to V_3; another had prominent Q waves in I and aV_L.

Fig. 7-5, obtained from a 22-year-old black man with myotonia atrophica, shows a pattern consistent with anterior wall infarction. Note also the intraventricular conduction disturbance, left axis deviation, sinus bradycardia, and premature beats.

ECG abnormalities are equally common in younger and older patients with myotonia, a finding consistent with a noncoronary cause.[86] Examination of the myocardium at autopsy may reveal diffuse fibrosis and fatty change; in addition, myocardial degeneration without significant coronary involvement may be present.[17,32,34] Mitochondrial damage and sarcoplasmic reticulum vacuolation were noted in one electron microscopy study,[14] but their cause was not known. Presumably the pseudoinfarct pattern occasionally seen in these patients reflects extensive replacement of myocardial fibers with electrically inert fibrous and fatty tissue or possibly regional dysfunction of viable myocardial fibers.

Clinically there is no direct correlation between skeletal muscle and cardiac involvement. Despite the high incidence of ECG abnormalities, major symptoms are surprisingly uncommon in patients with myotonia atrophica.[59] Mitral valve prolapse has been reported[58] but is not a consistent finding.[85] Cardiomegaly and heart failure may occur, in addition to AV heart block requiring a permanent pacemaker.[14] Syncope or sudden death due to sustained ventricular tachycardia has also occurred.[50] Although neuromuscular symptoms usually precede the cardiac symptoms, an abnormal ECG with any of the patterns just mentioned may be the first clue to the diagnosis of myotonia atrophica.[86]

FRIEDREICH'S ATAXIA

Friedreich's ataxia (Fig. 7-6) is a hereditary (usually recessive) neurodegenerative disease with associated cardiomyopathy. The neurologic deficits, which characteristically begin to appear in preadolescence, include ataxia, dysarthria, nystagmus, sensory impairments, loss of deep-tendon reflexes, abnormal Babinski responses, and skeletal deformities (scoliosis, pes cavus, hammer toe).[82,110]

ECG abnormalities are noted in over 90% of cases.[21,56,110] Prominent T wave inversions in the lateral precordial or limb leads are particularly common.* These may be deep with a coved appearance indistinguishable from the pattern seen with an evolving infarct (Fig. 7-6). Thoren[110] noted that such inversions transiently reverted to normal in over two thirds of patients following exercise. In about half of his cases the reversion occurred after administration of a ganglionic blocking agent. Although in some patients spontaneous reversion to normal was noted, generally the T wave inversions persisted.[110]

---

*10, 55, 65, 110.

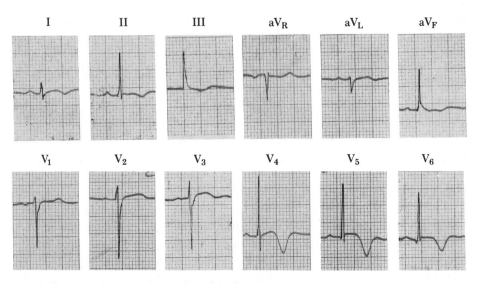

FIG. 7-6. Friedreich's ataxia simulating evolving infarction in a 14-year-old boy. Note the marked T wave inversions with a coved morphology in V_4 to V_6 and the nonspecific ST-T changes in II, III, and aV_F. Abnormal T wave inversions simulating an infarct are relatively common with Friedreich's and reflect the underlying cardiomyopathy. Occasionally noninfarctional Q waves will be seen in the lateral precordial or inferior leads.

Pseudoinfarctional Q waves have also been reported in Friedreich's ataxia but are less common than the repolarization changes just described. In Thoren's series[110] abnormal Q waves (chiefly in the lateral precordial or inferior limb leads) were observed in 20% of cases. Child et al.[21] reported abnormally broad inferolateral Q waves in 13% of the patients they studied. Of interest, 20% of their patients had prominent right precordial R waves simulating those seen with a posterior wall infarction (Fig. 7-7). The cause of this pattern remains obscure. Only 1 of the 15 patients with tall right-sided R waves had echocardiographic evidence of right ventricular hypertrophy.

Other frequently reported ECG findings include inappropriate sinus tachycardia, extrasystoles, other arrhythmias, and left and right ventricular hypertrophy.

There is no consensus regarding the nature of the cardiomyopathy of Friedreich's ataxia or the genesis of the pseudoinfarct patterns. Pathologic studies have revealed evidence of a diffuse chronic myocarditis with extensive interstitial fibrosis and focal muscle degeneration.[56] Other reports[63,110] have noted significant degenerative involvement of the smaller intramural branches of the coronary arteries. James and Fisch,[63] for example, described the case of a patient with extensive disease of the smaller coronary and pulmonary arteries characterized by intimal hyperplasia, degeneration of the tunica media, and endothelial deposits. There is some debate as to whether this arteriopathy is the

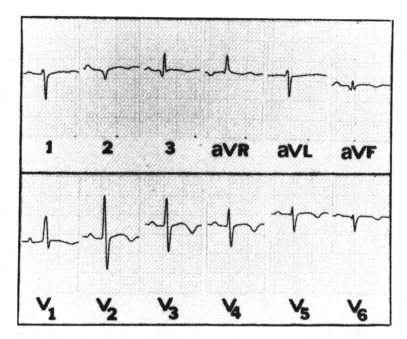

FIG. 7-7. Friedreich's ataxia simulating an inferoposterolateral infarct in a 28-year-old man. The echocardiogram did not show ventricular hypertrophy or a regional wall motion abnormality. (From Child CS, et al: J Am Coll Cardiol 7:1370, 1986.)

underlying cause of the myocardial degeneration[63] or only a secondary consequence of some primary myocardial process.[56] In either case the pseudoinfarct ECG patterns may reflect the resulting myocardial injury.

An alternative explanation for the noninfarctional Q waves comes from a number of reports[25,37,47,103] suggesting a correlation between Friedreich's ataxia and hypertrophic cardiomyopathy, a well-known cause of pseudoinfarct patterns (Chapter 4). For example, in the case of Friedreich's ataxia with hypertrophic cardiomyopathy described by Gach, Andriange, and Franck,[37] the ECG showed prominent inferolateral Q waves. However, the association of Friedreich's ataxia and hypertrophic cardiomyopathy has been challenged by other authors,[48,105] who noted a primarily concentric rather than asymmetric type of ventricular hypertrophy in their patients.

Child et al.,[21] in a more recent study, proposed that there are two distinct manifestations of heart disease in Friedreich's ataxia: *hypertrophic* and *dystrophic*. The hypertrophic form may be either concentric or asymmetric. The dystrophic form is usually segmental, but may become global, and is associated with a dilated type of cardiomyopathy. However, the relationship between these two forms of heart disease and the typical neurodegenerative process of Fried-reich's remains to be defined.

Clinically patients with Friedreich's ataxia may complain of exertional dysp-nea and palpitation and less frequently of angina-like pain. Physical examina-tion often reveals a systolic murmur, and signs of congestive failure may appear late in the course of the disease. Cardiac symptoms will rarely precede neuro-logic manifestations.[110]

SCLERODERMA

Progressive systemic sclerosis (scleroderma) occasionally produces pseudo-infarctional ECG patterns. The Q waves in such cases reflect myocardial atro-phy and fibrosis in the absence of atherosclerotic coronary artery disease.

Beigelman, Goldner, and Bayles[6] described a patient with cardiac sclero-derma characterized by diffuse myocardial fibrosis without coronary disease. The ECG in this patient was compatible with extensive anterior wall infarction. Windesheim and Parkin[115] reported a variety of ECG abnormalities in 8 of 90 patients with scleroderma, including two probable anterior wall pseudoinfarct patterns (without pathologic confirmation). Sackner, Heinz, and Steinberg[97] presented a case of apparent apicolateral wall infarction in a patient whose heart revealed marked myocardial degeneration and atrophy. Gupta et al.[51] described a 41-year-old woman with scleroderma and the ECG pattern of inferior wall in-farction. Cardiac catheterization revealed diffuse left ventricular hypokinesis and patent coronary arteries. Slow runoff of the angiographic dye was observed, suggesting the possibility of small vessel disease. Fig. 7-8 shows a pattern con-sistent with inferior and anterior wall infarction; the patient was a 24-year-old woman with multisystem scleroderma and heart failure.

Although actual pseudoinfarct patterns are relatively rare in scleroderma, myocardial fibrosis is a common autopsy finding. In one large series of 52 post-mortem cases, 50% showed some areas of myocardial fibrosis. In 25% of cases the fibrotic changes were extensive with normal coronary arteries.[13]

The cause of the myocardial lesion in scleroderma has not been fully re-solved. The hypotheses that have been proposed implicate (1) primary myocar-dial degeneration caused by the collagen disease process,[97] (2) myocardial fi-brosis secondary to small vessel coronary disease, and (3) myocardial fibrosis caused by small vessel spasm.[13] In patients with sclerodermatous cardiomyopa-thy, the larger extramural coronary arteries are typically normal,[13,28,97] and the fibrotic changes are patchy in distribution. James[62] reported small vessel in-volvement with narrowing of the intramural coronary branches by intimal pro-liferation, fibrosis, and fibrinoid necrosis. On the other hand, Bulkley et al.[13] found no evidence of small vessel narrowing and postulated intermittent small vessel spasm as the cause of the contraction band necrosis and replacement fi-brosis frequently observed in their autopsy series.

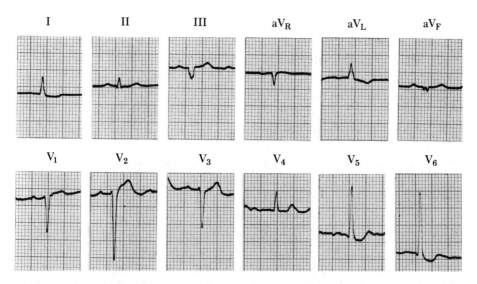

FIG. 7-8. Infarction pattern associated with scleroderma. This 24-year-old woman had multisystem involvement and heart failure. Poor R wave progression in the precordial leads suggests anterior wall injury. The prominent Q waves in III and aV$_F$ are consistent with inferior wall injury. In addition, note the low-voltage complexes in the extremity leads and the nonspecific ST-T changes in the lateral leads.

However, even patients with extensive pathologic evidence of cardiac involvement may have normal or only nonspecifically abnormal ECG patterns. ECG abnormalities in scleroderma* include nonspecific low-voltage ST-T alterations, left axis deviation, conduction disturbances (e.g., bundle branch block and varying degrees of AV block), ventricular and atrial arrhythmias, left ventricular hypertrophy patterns secondary to renal hypertension, and right ventricular hypertrophy patterns secondary to pulmonary sclerosis and cor pulmonale.

In some patients with scleroderma congestive heart failure may develop from primary myocardial fibrosis or pericardial disease (causing effusion or, rarely, constriction). In others heart failure may be secondarily related to hypertension from renal disease or cor pulmonale from pulmonary vascular disease. Angina-like pain occurs despite patent coronary arteries.[13] The cause of the chest pain in such cases is unclear but could be related to the small vessel ischemia just described. Death from arrhythmias and conduction disturbances may be sudden.

SARCOIDOSIS

Cardiac involvement with sarcoidosis may occur in as many as 25% of cases; however, extensive myocardial replacement with granulomatous or fibrous tis-

---

*References 24, 44, 79, 97, 115.

sue is relatively rare.[19,61,100] The most common ECG manifestations of cardiac sarcoidosis are AV conduction disturbances (including complete heart block), various arrhythmias, bundle branch block, and nonspecific ST-T changes.[4] Occasionally, extensive myocardial replacement by sarcoid granuloma or fibrosis has produced pseudoinfarctional Q waves.

Gold and Cantor[41] reported the first case of possible pseudoinfarct Q waves in sarcoidosis. Their patient had the typical pattern of an evolving anteroseptal infarct marked by a return of normal R wave progression 6 weeks after the initiation of steroid therapy. The authors suggested that the infarct pattern might have been caused either by granulomatous infiltration of the myocardium or possibly by direct involvement of a coronary artery. The patient survived, and direct ischemic injury could not be excluded.

Subsequent case reports have documented pseudoinfarct patterns with actual aneurysm formation caused by myocardial sarcoidosis.[4,22,72] Hines and Sancetta[57] described a patient whose ECG showed right bundle branch block and QS waves in V_5, V_6, and aV_L. The patient died suddenly, and postmortem examination revealed normal coronary arteries with dense fibrosis and aneurysm formation of the left ventricular free wall. There was no evidence of active sarcoid granuloma in the myocardium. The authors suggested that the cardiac fibrosis represented end-stage sarcoid disease. They also speculated that some cases of so-called idiopathic myocardial fibrosis might include patients with unrecognized "burnt-out" sarcoidosis.

Bashour et al.[4] described a similar case of a 43-year-old black woman with precordial Q waves (present for 6 yr) with persistent ST segment elevations suggestive of ventricular aneurysm, which was documented fluoroscopically. Although coronary involvement could not be excluded in this case, the ECG pattern was consistent with extensive myocardial sarcoidosis. Lull, Dunn, and Gregoratos[72] reported the dramatic case of a young black man with ventricular arrhythmias and congestive heart failure who was found to have a large apical aneurysm. The ECG showed deep Q waves and T wave inversions. Aneurysmectomy produced marked clinical improvement and disappearance of the Q waves. The coronary arteries were patent. Ishikawa et al.[61] described a 25-year-old woman with left ventricular dysfunction and QS waves in I and aV_L. Following steroid administration her ventricular function improved and the Q waves resolved.

Clinically patients with sarcoidosis may have a wide range of cardiac problems, including congestive failure, pericarditis (sometimes with effusion), papillary muscle dysfunction, and syncope or even sudden death caused by ventricular arrhythmias or complete AV block.[89,100] In some cases cardiac problems will be the initial feature of the disease.[72,89]

By way of summary: The occurrence of pseudoinfarctional Q waves in sarcoidosis is relatively rare and reflects extensive myocardial replacement by granuloma or fibrosis. In such cases actual aneurysm formation may be present.

CARDIAC TUMORS

The most common ECG abnormalities seen in association with primary or metastatic cardiac tumors are nonspecific ST-T changes, arrhythmias (often refractory to management), AV conduction disturbances, bundle branch block, and low voltage secondary to pericardial effusion.[1,60,119] In rare cases abnormal Q waves and even ST-T changes simulating infarction (Fig. 7-9) have been reported.

Theoretically, extensive myocardial infiltration with neoplastic tissue could produce Q waves secondary to the replacement of myocardium by electrically inert tissue. Pilcher[87] described a case of cardiac lymphosarcoma in which the ECG (not published) was said to be suggestive of anterior infarction. Bisel, Wroblewski, and LaDue[9] reported their ECG findings in a large series of patients with cardiac metastases. Of 59 ECGs available, only two showed Q waves that could be attributed to tumor involvement. In one case[76] pathologic inferior and anterior lead Q waves with evolving ST-T changes were reported in a patient with reticulum cell sarcoma and myocardial infiltration. Metastatic bronchogenic carcinoma has also been reported as a cause of documented pseudoinfarctional Q waves.[45,91]

Several reports describe persistent ST elevations mimicking the pattern of ventricular aneurysm in patients with metastatic tumor of the heart. Rosenbaum, Johnston, and Alzamora[91] reported the first case, that of a patient with extensive esophageal carcinoma involving the pericardium and myocardium. The authors suggested that the persistent ST elevations might have been caused by a number of factors including actual coronary occlusion not evident at autopsy, pericardial inflammation, or continuous myocardial injury secondary

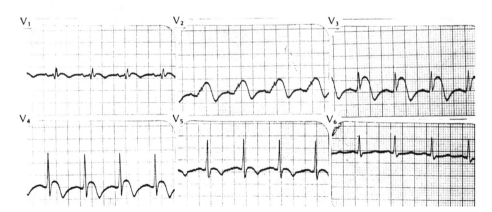

FIG. 7-9. Metastatic epidermoid carcinoma of the tongue involving the myocardium in a 61-year-old man. This ECG shows an intraventricular conduction delay and prominent ST elevations simulating acute anteroseptal infarction. The serial tracings were unchanged, cardiac enzymes were normal, and at autopsy the coronary arteries were patent without evidence of myocardial infarction. (From Zatuchni J, et al: Am Heart J 101:674, 1981.)

to mechanical pressure, chemical contact, or local ischemia from neoplastic encroachment.

Harris, Copeland, and Brody[54] described a similar case of cardiac tumor with ST elevations that persisted for 2½ months. Q waves also were present. At autopsy the myocardium was extensively infiltrated by bronchogenic carcinoma; areas of myocardial necrosis surrounded the tumor. The authors speculated that the neoplastic process might have produced local cardiac injury and leakage of potassium ions from the necrotic tissue; the resultant increase in extracellular K^+ concentration might in turn have depolarized the surrounding myocardial fibers, producing a current of injury pattern similar to that seen with ischemic damage. Subsequently another case of metastatic bronchogenic carcinoma causing localized ST elevations in the lateral leads without Q waves was described.[108] Zatuchni et al.[120] reported two patients with persistent ST elevations, simulating anterior infarction in one case and inferior infarction in the other, associated with metastatic epidermoid carcinoma of the tongue. Fig. 7-10 shows a dramatic example of Q waves simulating anterior and inferior wall infarctions in a patient with metastatic breast carcinoma.

Pseudoinfarctional Q waves have also been reported in children with benign intramural fibromas of the left ventricle.[40] Two-dimensional echocardiography may provide preoperative delineation of the tumor in such cases.[8] Clinically these children may have congestive failure, arrhythmias, unusual murmurs,

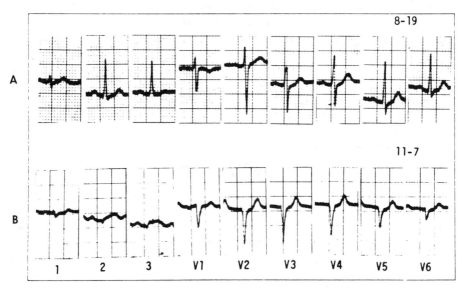

FIG. 7-10. Metastatic breast carcinoma with extensive cardiac involvement causing anterior and inferior wall pseudoinfarct patterns. **A,** Normal baseline ECG. **B,** Three months later. There is extensive loss of inferior and anterior R waves, with reduction of the QRS voltage and subtle elevation of the ST segments in the inferior leads. (From Fisch C: In Likoff W, et al [editors]: Atherosclerosis and coronary artery disease, New York, 1972, Grune & Stratton Inc.)

and an irregular cardiac x-ray silhouette. Deep T wave inversions without Q waves were reported with a coronary hemangiomatous tumor in a 15-year-old girl.[107]

Metastatic cardiac tumors may also simulate the pattern of atrial infarction. ECG signs of atrial infarction include PR deviation (caused by an atrial injury current), changes in P wave morphology, and atrial arrhythmias. In one case[94] metastatic tumor to the left atrium was found to cause P wave alteration and PR elevation in aV_L along with atrial ectopy. Subsequently another case of metastatic right atrial tumor has been reported,[43] with the premortem diagnosis suggested by PR segment elevations in aV_R and atrial ectopy.

These pseudoinfarct patterns caused by the primary replacement or infiltration of myocardial fibers by neoplastic tissue must be distinguished from the rare but documented occurrence of actual infarction caused by direct coronary occlusion by metastatic tumor.[36] Metastatic cardiac tumor has also been reported as a possible cause of positive results with technetium-99m-pyrophosphate cardiac scans in the absence of typical myocardial infarction.[53]

CHRONIC CHAGASIC MYOCARDITIS

Chagas' disease, caused by the protozoan parasite *Trypanosoma cruzi*, is endemic in certain areas of Central and South America, particularly in Argentina. In rare instances it produces a fulminant acute myocarditis associated with progressive heart failure and sometimes marked ST elevations simulating acute infarction.[92,93]

More commonly Chagas' disease causes a chronic slowly developing cardiomyopathy that may produce ECG abnormalities and heart failure years after the initial infection. Pathologically the disease is marked by widespread myocardial degeneration with fibrotic replacement. Occasionally the fibrosis is extensive enough to produce abnormal Q waves in the absence of coronary disease. Coved T wave inversions may also be present. Right bundle branch block with left axis deviation (bifascicular block) and arrhythmias are common manifestations of chagasic myocarditis.

The ECG appearance of right bundle branch block, left axis deviation, or Q waves and T wave inversions in a patient who has previously lived in an endemic area should suggest the possibility of chronic chagasic myocarditis.

CARDIAC ECHINOCOCCOSIS

A large echinococcal cyst in the left ventricular free wall is a rare cause of pathologic Q waves.[67] Deep coved plane or symmetric T wave inversions may also be present.[16,67] One case in which a cardiac hydatid cyst produced an ECG pattern suggesting ventricular aneurysm has been reported.[90] Hydatid cysts can be visualized with two-dimensional echocardiography.[78]

The abnormal Q waves in such cases are caused by replacement of functional myocardium by the electrically inert cyst.[67] The T wave inversions probably reflect local injury produced by the cyst.[90] The chest x-ray may show a left ventricular bulge.[67]

ENDOCARDIAL FIBROELASTOSIS

Endocardial fibroelastosis, a cardiomyopathy of unknown cause, is characterized by proliferation of elastic and collagen tissue primarily in the inner layers of the left ventricle. Endocardial fibroelastosis is a relatively important cause of acyanotic heart failure in the first year of life. The ECG generally shows signs of left ventricular hypertrophy. Pseudoinfarct patterns have been reported rarely.

Auld and Watson[2] described an unusual case of endocardial fibroelastosis in a 15-year-old boy with progressive heart failure. The ECG showed the pattern of extensive anterior wall infarction. At autopsy examination of the heart revealed diffuse myocardial fibrosis in addition to the classic findings of endocardial fibroelastosis.

Linde and Adams,[70] reporting on a series of 17 cases of endocardial fibroelastosis, described one infant with prominent Q waves in the lateral precordial leads. A follow-up ECG 4 years later showed only signs of left ventricular hypertrophy, with complete regression of the abnormal Q waves.

Graham[49] presented the case of an infant 16 months of age with endocardial fibroelastosis and a pattern of extensive anterior and inferior transmural infarction. At autopsy there was no infarct, but examination of the myocardium revealed large strands of hyaline fibrous tissue deep within the muscle and areas of early calcification.

Lintermans et al.[71] described three cases of endocardial fibroelastosis with vectorcardiographic patterns suggestive of anterior infarction. However, in none of these cases did the conventional ECGs show pathologic Q waves.

By way of summary: Pathologic Q waves are a relatively rare finding with endocardial fibroelastosis. Their presence in pediatric patients should always raise the possibility of other diagnoses, including myocarditis, anomalous origin to the left coronary artery, and myocardial fibroma (p. 156). An anomalous left coronary artery produces true left ventricular ischemia, sometimes with the pattern of lateral wall Q wave infarction. Lintermans et al.[71] concluded that the pseudoinfarct patterns caused by anomalous origin of the left coronary artery and those produced by endocardial fibroelastosis could not be distinguished on the basis of the ECG or vectorcardiogram alone.

MYOCARDIAL FIBROSIS ASSOCIATED WITH CHRONIC CONSTRICTIVE PERICARDITIS

The electrocardiogram with acute pericarditis (Chapter 10) is characterized by diffuse ST segment elevations that simulate acute infarction (Fig. 10-2). With subacute (evolving) pericarditis the T waves become inverted, mimicking ischemic T waves in some cases (Fig. 10-4). In patients with chronic constrictive pericarditis the ECG commonly shows low-voltage complexes, nonspecific ST-T alterations (including T wave inversions), and occasionally wide P waves that simulate the P mitrale pattern.[69] (These are the broad often notched P waves seen with left atrial enlargement.)

In general, pathologic Q waves are conspicuously absent with acute or subacute pericarditis. The absence of depolarization abnormalities is often a useful differential point in the diagnosis of infarction versus pericarditis. However, Levine[69] reported a small group of patients with chronic constrictive pericarditis and Q wave patterns without significant coronary artery disease. Sixty-seven patients with constrictive pericarditis of varying cause were studied. In seven the ECG was considered diagnostic of infarction. Eleven other patients had ECG findings compatible with though not necessarily diagnostic of infarction.

The hearts of three of the patients with definite infarct patterns were examined at autopsy. In one case there was aneurysmal thinning of the left ventricular wall without significant coronary disease. Autopsy of the second case revealed marked myocardial fibrosis without apparent coronary obstruction. The third patient with Q waves had sustained a perioperative infarct, confirmed at postmortem examination. Two other patients had ECG findings compatible with infarction. They also showed evidence of marked myocardial fibrosis without coexistent coronary disease. Levine[69] concluded that, contrary to prevailing concepts, Q waves do appear in association with chronic constrictive pericarditis and may reflect myocardial fibrosis in the absence of significant coronary artery disease. The myocardial fibrosis in these cases was thought to be caused by subepicardial extension of the primary pericardial inflammatory process. Fig. 7-11 shows an example of the anterior wall pseudoinfarct pattern associated with chronic constrictive pericarditis.

Tall right precordial R waves simulating right ventricular hypertrophy or posterior infarction have also been reported in rare cases of chronic constrictive pericarditis. In one series of 122 patients with pericardial constriction,[20] they were noted in six cases. One patient with this pattern had ECG findings attributable to subpulmonic constriction with secondary right ventricular hypertrophy, but in the other five patients the cause of the abnormal right precordial R waves was not apparent.

DILATED (CONGESTIVE) CARDIOMYOPATHY

The term *cardiomyopathy* is generally used to refer to primary myocardial disease in the absence of extrinsic factors such as coronary disease, hypertension, or valvular disease. Clinically patients with cardiomyopathy can be subdivided into three relatively distinct hemodynamic subsets[46]: (1) dilated (congestive) cardiomyopathy, (2) hypertrophic cardiomyopathy, and (3) restrictive cardiomyopathy.

Patients with dilated cardiomyopathy, as the name implies, have impairment of left ventricular systolic function, with left (and often right) ventricular dila-

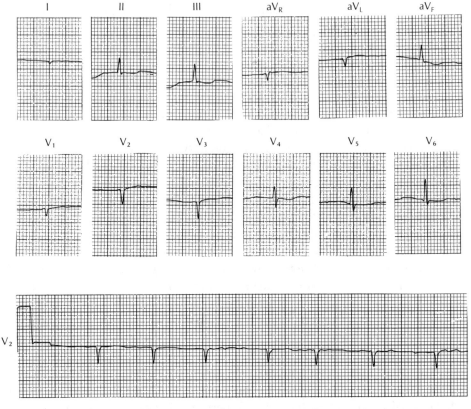

FIG. 7-11. Chronic constrictive pericarditis simulating anteroseptal infraction in a 67-year-old man. Note the presence of atrial fibrillation, low voltage, and right axis deviation. No significant coronary disease was detected at angiography.

tion and failure. The left ventricular ejection fraction is typically less than 40% (normal >55%).[65] Hypertrophic cardiomyopathy has been previously discussed (Chapter 4). Restrictive cardiomyopathy, which may be idiopathic or caused by specific factors such as amyloidosis (p. 141), is characterized by a stiff poorly compliant myocardium, resulting in elevated diastolic filling pressures. Systolic function may be normal or only moderately impaired. Restrictive cardiomyopathy sometimes mimics the clinical picture of constrictive pericarditis.

Pathologic but noncoronary Q waves are a relatively common finding with all three types of cardiomyopathy. Q waves due to replacement of myocardial fibers by amyloid were described earlier in this chapter. Pseudoinfarct patterns associated with hypertrophic cardiomyopathy may be caused either by augmentation of septal depolarization forces or by altered septal activation (p. 93).

Pathologic Q waves are also well described in patients with dilated cardiomyopathy[3,39,75] and may simulate anterior or inferior wall infarction. Two examples are shown in Figs. 7-12 and 7-13.

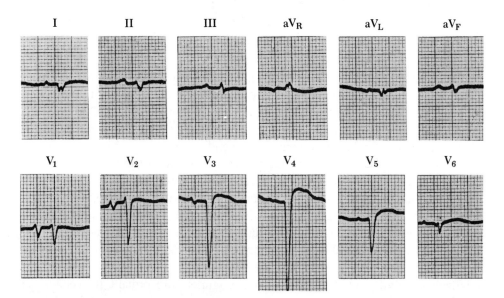

FIG. 7-12. Idiopathic dilated cardiomyopathy simulating extensive anterior wall infarction in a 49-year-old white man with severe idiopathic cardiomyopathy, congestive heart failure, chronic obstructive pulmonary disease, and a history of pulmonary embolism. Cardiac catheterization 3 months earlier had shown a markedly dilated, poorly contractile left ventricle with normal coronary arteries. Note on this tracing the sinus rhythm with borderline first-degree AV block, the left atrial enlargement and low-voltage complexes in the limb leads, the striking loss of R wave progression across the entire precordium, and the persistent ST elevations (compatible with widespread anterior wall injury). The electrical axis is shifted to the extreme right (+180 degrees). Pseudoinfarct patterns are not uncommon with cardiomyopathies and are caused by extensive replacement of or damage to the myocardial fibers. This combination of low voltage in the limb leads and poor R wave progression is characteristic but nondiagnostic in such cases. Here the underlying chronic obstructive pulmonary disease probably contributed to the low voltage and delayed R wave progression.

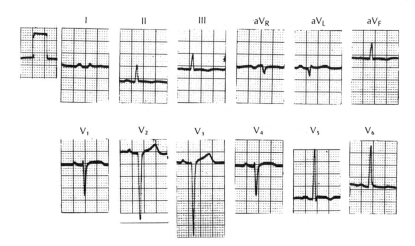

FIG. 7-13. Severe idiopathic dilated cardiomyopathy in a 29-year-old man. Note the poor precordial R wave progression simulating anterior infarction. The combination of low limb lead QRS voltage, prominent precordial QRS voltage, and poor R wave progression is highly specific for dilated cardiomyopathy.[42]

The pathologic Q waves of dilated cardiomyopathy result from a number of different mechanisms, including myocardial fibrosis,[39] left or right ventricular hypertrophy and dilation (Chapter 4), and ventricular conduction disturbances (Chapter 5). In some cases a number of factors will contribute simultaneously to a pseudoinfarct pattern. For example, loss of normal R wave progression, common in these patients, may reflect anterior wall fibrosis, left or right ventricular enlargement, and an intraventricular conduction delay.

Several other ECG abnormalities commonly occur in the setting of dilated cardiomyopathy, including atrial and ventricular arrhythmias, AV conduction disturbances, left atrial abnormality, and left ventricular hypertrophy patterns. Repolarization abnormalities are usually nonspecific, although prominent T wave inversions simulating coronary disease may be observed. Precordial QRS voltage in patients with dilated cardiomyopathy tends to be increased, whereas limb lead voltage may be relatively low. The triad of poor R wave progression, relatively low limb lead QRS voltage, and prominent precordial QRS voltage is a highly specific but insensitive sign in congestive cardiomopathy[42] (Fig. 7-13).

Patients with dilated cardiomyopathy may also complain of chest pain suggesting angina, adding to diagnostic confusion. Evidence of subendocardial ischemia has been noted in some cases of dilated cardiomyopathy, during both rest and atrial pacing.[80] Myocardial ischemia occurs in such cases, despite patent coronary arteries, probably because of the increased myocardial oxygen demands related to tachycardia and left ventricular dilation.

Noninfarctional Q waves have also been reported in a number of specific diseases that produce the clinical picture of a dilated cardiomyopathy, including "alcoholic" cardiomyopathy and several other conditions.

Alcoholic Cardiomyopathy

Excessive consumption of alcohol has been associated with a dilated type of cardiomyopathy characterized by left and right ventricular failure, often with conduction disturbances and atrial and ventricular arrhythmias.[27] Although the precise etiologic role of alcohol in such cases remains to be defined, the term *alcoholic cardiomyopathy* is widely applied in clinical practice.

Whereas nonspecific ST-T changes are commonly reported with alcoholic cardiomyopathy, pathologic Q waves are relatively rare. Evans,[29] in an early study of ECG patterns associated with alcoholic cardiomyopathy, primarily reported T wave alterations and made no mention of pathologic Q waves in any of his cases. Hamby and Raia,[52] in a subsequent study of 60 patients with primary myocardial disease, cited two cases of alcoholic cardiomyopathy with anterior infarction patterns.

Bashour, Fahdul, and Cheng[5] reported on 65 patients with presumed alcoholic cardiomyopathy. Pathologic Q waves were present in only 3 cases. In another series involving cardiomyopathy associated with alcohol abuse,[27] Q waves were seen in 4 of 57 cases. Additional cases with pseudoinfarct patterns in alcoholic cardiomyopathy have been reported.[96]

The significance of these noncoronary Q waves in alcoholic cardiomyopathy is not clear. Rubler et al.[96] suggested that the infarct patterns could reflect direct alcohol-induced myocardial damage. The toxic myocardial effects of the alcohol might be exerted on the oxidative enzyme system or on the cell membrane, leading to nonischemic myocardial necrosis with fibrotic replacement. Ferrans et al.[33] described cases of alcoholic cardiomyopathy with marked myocardial fibrosis in the absence of significant coronary disease. However, it is not certain whether the pathologic fibrosis in such cases is caused entirely or even partly by direct or indirect effects of alcohol.

Other Causes of Dilated Cardiomyopathy

Pseudoinfarct patterns have been described with a number of other specific causes of dilated cardiomyopathy. For example, Adriamycin (doxorubicin) can induce congestive failure resulting from myocardial degeneration. Loss of precordial R wave progression in such cases may simulate anterior wall infarction.[68]

Pseudoinfarct patterns associated with myocarditis, muscular dystrophy and other neuromuscular diseases, scleroderma, sarcoidosis, and Chagas' disease are discussed in this chapter. Pseudoinfarct patterns have also been described in patients with myocardial fibrosis of obscure etiology[109] as well as in familial types of cardiomyopathy.[66,114]*

Finally, in some patients with coronary artery disease severe congestive failure may develop. Use of the term *ischemic cardiomyopathy* has been advocated by some authors[15] but discouraged by others,[65] who reserve "cardiomyopathy" for use in cases of primary heart muscle disease. Regardless of the terminology, clinicians should recognize that patients with heart failure caused by severe coronary artery disease do not fit into any discrete subset. For example, some individuals may have sustained one large infarct; others may have had multiple infarcts; still others, without anginal pain, may be suffering congestive failure, even though they have no history of infarction. In this last group heart failure is the result, presumably, of one or more silent infarcts. Furthermore, patients with severe heart failure associated with ischemic heart disease may not necessarily have pathologic Q waves.[64] Therefore, just as the presence of Q waves in a patient with dilated cardiomyopathy does not ensure the diagnosis of coronary artery disease, so the absence of Q waves does not exclude "ischemic cardiomyopathy."

---

*Some of the cases of "familial cardiomyopathy" reported earlier in the literature may have represented undiagnosed hypertrophic cardiomyopathy.

REFERENCES

1. Aronson SF, Leroy E: Electrocardiographic findings in leukemia, Blood 2:356, 1947.
2. Auld WHR, Watson H: Fibroelastosis of the heart in adolescence, Br Heart J 19:186, 1957.
3. Banta HD, Estes EH: Electrocardiographic and vectorcardiographic findings in patients with idiopathic myocardial hypertrophy, Am J Cardiol 14:218, 1964.
4. Bashour FA, et al: Myocardial sarcoidosis, Dis Chest 53:413, 1968.
5. Bashour TT, et al: Electrocardiographic abnormalities in alcoholic cardiomyopathy, Chest 68:24, 1975.
6. Beigelman PM, et al: Progressive systemic sclerosis (scleroderma), N Engl J Med 249:45, 1953.
7. Bernreiter M: Cardiac amyloidosis: electrocardiographic findings, Am J Cardiol 1:644, 1958.
8. Biancaniello TM, et al: Primary benign intramural ventricular tumors in children: pre- and postoperative electrocardiographic, echocardiographic, and angiographic evaluation, Am Heart J 103:852, 1982.
9. Bisel HF, et al: Incidence and clinical manifestations of cardiac metastases, JAMA 153:712, 1953.
10. Boyer SH, et al: Cardiac aspects of Friedreich's ataxia, Circulation 25:493, 1962.
11. Brandt K, et al: A clinical analysis of the course and prognosis of forty-two patients with amyloidosis, Am J Med 44:955, 1968.
12. Buja LM, et al: Clinically significant cardiac amyloidosis: clinicopathologic findings in 15 patients, Am J Cardiol 26:394, 1970.
13. Bulkley BH, et al: Myocardial lesions of progressive systemic sclerosis: a cause of cardiac dysfunction, Circulation 53:483, 1976.
14. Bulloch RT, et al: Dystrophia myotonica with heart block: a light and electron microscopic study, Arch Pathol 84:130, 1967.
15. Burch GE, et al: Ischemic cardiomyopathy, Am Heart J 79:291, 1970.
16. Canabal EJ, et al: Echinococcus disease of the left ventricle: a clinical, radiologic, and electrocardiographic study, Circulation 12:520, 1955.
17. Cannon PJ: The heart and lungs in myotonic muscular dystrophy, Am J Med 32:765, 1962.
18. Carroll JD, et al: Amyloid cardiomyopathy: characterization by a distinctive voltage/mass relation, Am J Cardiol 49:9, 1982.
19. Case records of the Massachusetts General Hospital (case 34-1985), N Engl J Med 313:498, 1985.
20. Chesler E, et al: The ECG of constrictive pericarditis: pattern resembling right ventricular hypertrophy, Am Heart J 91:420, 1976.
21. Child JS, et al: Cardiac involvement in Friedreich's ataxia: a clinical study of 75 patients, J Am Coll Cardiol 7:1370, 1986.
22. Chun SK, et al: Ventricular aneurysm in sarcoidosis [Letter to the editor], Chest 68:392, 1975.
23. Church SC: The heart in myotonia atrophica, Arch Intern Med 119:176, 1967.
24. Clements PJ, et al: The relationship of arrhythmias and conduction disturbances to other manifestations of cardiopulmonary disease in progressive systemic sclerosis (PSS), Am J Med 71:38, 1981.
25. Cote A, et al: Hemodynamic findings in Friedreich's ataxia, Can J Med Sci 3:333, 1976.
26. De Leon AC, et al: Distinctive electrocardiogram of Duchenne's progressive muscular dystrophy: an electrocardiographic-pathologic correlative study, Am J Med 42:179, 1967.
27. Demakis JG, et al: The natural course of alcoholic cardiomyopathy, Ann Intern Med 80:293, 1974.
28. Escudero J, McDevitt E: The electrocardiogram in scleroderma: analysis of 60 cases and review of the literature, Am Heart J 56:846, 1958.
29. Evans W: The electrocardiogram in alcoholic cardiomyopathy, Br Heart J 21:445, 1959.
30. Falk RH, et al: Sensitivity of technetium-99m-pyrophosphate scintigraphy in diagnosing cardiac amyloidosis, Am J Cardiol 51:826, 1983.
31. Farrokh A, et al: Amyloid heart disease, Am J Cardiol 13:750, 1964.
32. Fearrington EL, et al: Vectorcardiographic and electrocardiographic findings in myotonia atrophica: a study employing the Frank lead system, Am Heart J 67:599, 1964.

33. Ferrans VJ, et al: Alcoholic cardiomyopathy: a histochemical study, Am Heart J 69:748, 1965.

34. Fisch C: The heart in dystrophia myotonica, Am Heart J 41:525, 1951.

35. Fitch CW, Ainger LE: The Frank vectorcardiogram and the electrocardiogram in Duchenne progressive muscular dystrophy, Circulation 35:1124, 1967.

36. Franciosa JA, Lawrinson W: Coronary artery occlusion due to neoplasm, Arch Intern Med 128:797, 1971.

37. Gach JV, et al: Hypertrophic obstructive cardiomyopathy and Friedreich's ataxia: report of a case and review of literature, Am J Cardiol 27:436, 1971.

38. Galen RS, Gambino SR: Isoenzymes of CPK and LDH in myocardial infarction and certain other diseases, Pathobiol Annu 5:283, 1975.

39. Gau GT, et al: Q waves and coronary arteriography in cardiomyopathy, Br Heart J 34:1034, 1972.

40. Geha AS, et al: Intramural ventricular cardiac fibroma: successful removal in two cases and review of the literature, Circulation 36:427, 1967.

41. Gold JA, Cantor PJ: Sarcoid heart disease: a case with an unusual electrocardiogram, Arch Intern Med 104:101, 1959.

42. Goldberger AL: A specific ECG triad associated with congestive heart failure, PACE 5:593, 1982.

43. Goldberger AL, Ludwig M: Metastatic atrial tumor: case report with electrocardiographic-pathologic correlation, J Electrocardiol 11:297, 1978.

44. Goldman AP, Kotler MN: Heart disease in scleroderma, Am Heart J 110:1043, 1985.

45. Goldman MJ: Principles of clinical electrocardiography, ed 7, Los Altos Calif, 1970, Lange Medical Publications.

46. Goodwin JF: Congestive and hypertrophic cardiomyopathies: a decade of study, Lancet 1:732, 1970.

47. Gottdiener JS, et al: Characteristics of the cardiac hypertrophy in Friedreich's ataxia, Am Heart J 103:525, 1982.

48. Gottiker HF, et al: Echocardiographic findings in Friedreich's ataxia, Can J Neurol Sci 3:329, 1976.

49. Graham GR: Fibroelastosis. In Westenholme GEW, O'Connor M (editors): Cardiomyopathies, London, 1964, J&A Churchill Ltd.

50. Grigg LE, et al: Ventricular tachycardia and sudden death in myotonic dystrophy: clinical, electrophysiologic, and pathologic features, J Am Coll Cardiol 6:254, 1985.

51. Gupta MP, et al: Scleroderma heart disease with slow flow velocity in coronary arteries, Chest 67:116, 1975.

52. Hamby RI, Raia R: Electrocardiographic aspects of primary myocardial disease in 60 patients, Am Heart J 76:316, 1968.

53. Harford W, et al: Positive ^{99m}Tc–stannous pyrophosphate myocardial image in a patient with carcinoma of the lung, Radiology 122:747, 1977.

54. Harris TR, et al: Progressive injury current with metastatic tumor of the heart: case report and review of the literature, Am Heart J 69:392, 1965.

55. Heck AF: Heart disease in Friedreich's ataxia, Neurology 13:587, 1963.

56. Hewer RS: The heart in Friedreich's ataxia, Br Heart J 31:5, 1969.

57. Hines J, Sancetta S: Myocardial sarcoidosis simulating healed myocardial infarction, Ohio State Med J 59:689, 1963.

58. Hiromasa S, et al: Ventricular tachycardia and sudden death in myotonic dystrophy, Am Heart J 115:914, 1988.

59. Holt JM, Lambert EHN: Heart disease as the presenting feature in myotonia atrophica, Br Heart J 26:433, 1964.

60. Hurst JW, Cooper HR: Neoplastic disease of the heart, Am Heart J 50:782, 1955.

61. Ishikawa T, et al: Steroid therapy in cardiac sarcoidosis: increased left ventricular contractility concomitant with electrocardiographic improvement after prednisolone, Chest 85:445, 1984.

62. James TN: De subitaneis mortibus. VIII. Coronary arteries and conduction system in scleroderma heart disease, Circulation 50:844, 1974.

63. James TN, Fisch C: Observations on the cardiovascular involvement in Friedreich's ataxia, Am Heart J 66:164, 1963.

64. Johnson AD, et al: Non-invasive diagnosis of ischemic cardiomyopathy by fluorescent detection of coronary artery calcification, Am Heart J 96:521, 1978.

65. Johnson RA, Palacios I: Dilated cardiomyopathies of the adult. I, N Engl J Med 307:1051, 1982.

66. Kariv I, et al: Familial cardiomyopathy with special consideration of electrocardio-

graphic and vectorcardiographic findings, Am J Cardiol 13:734, 1964.

67. Langer L, et al: Onda Q patologica en el electrocardiograma de la equinococosis miocardica, El Torax 9:40, 1960.

68. Lefrak EA, et al: A clinicopathologic analysis of Adriamycin cardiotoxicity, Cancer 32:302, 1973.

69. Levine HD: Myocardial fibrosis in constrictive pericarditis: electrocardiographic and pathologic observations, Circulation 48:1268, 1973.

70. Linde LM, Adams FH: Prognosis in endocardial fibroelastosis, Am J Dis Child 105:329, 1963.

71. Lintermans JP, et al: Infarction patterns in endocardial fibroelastosis, Circulation 33: 202, 1966.

72. Lull RJ, et al: Ventricular aneurysm due to cardiac sarcoidosis with surgical cure of refractory ventricular tachycardia, Am J Cardiol 30:282, 1972.

73. Mann O, et al: Duchenne's muscular dystrophy: the electrocardiogram in female relatives, Am J Med Sci 255:376, 1968.

74. Manning GW, Cropp GJ: Electrocardiogram in progressive muscular dystrophy, Br Heart J 20:416, 1958.

75. Marriott HJL: Electrocardiographic abnormalities, conduction disturbances, and arrhythmias in primary myocardial disease, Prog Cardiovasc Dis 7:99, 1964.

76. Miwa K, et al: Abnormal electrocardiograms resembling infarction in a case of reticulum cell sarcoma, Jpn Circ J 45:329, 1981.

77. Nguyen HH, et al: Pathology of the cardiac conduction system in myotonic dystrophy: a study of 12 cases, J Am Coll Cardiol 11:662, 1988.

78. Oliver JM, et al: Two-dimensional echocardiographic features of echinococcosis of the heart and great blood vessels, Circulation 78:327, 1988.

79. Oram S, Stokes W: The heart in scleroderma, Br Heart J 23:243, 1961.

80. Pasternac A, et al: Pathophysiology of chest pain in patients with cardiomyopathy and normal coronary arteries, Circulation 65:778, 1982.

81. Payne CA, Greenfield JC Jr: Electrocardiographic abnormalities associated with myotonic dystrophy, Am Heart J 65:436, 1963.

82. Perloff JK: Neurologic disorders and heart disease. In Braunwald EB (editor): Heart disease: a textbook of cardiovascular medicine, ed 3, Philadelphia, 1988, WB Saunders Co, p 1782.

83. Perloff JK, et al: The cardiomyopathy of progressive muscular dystrophy, Circulation 33:625, 1966.

84. Perloff JK, et al: Alterations in regional myocardial metabolism, perfusion, and wall motion in Duchenne muscular dystrophy studied by radionuclide imaging, Circulation 69:33, 1984.

85. Perloff JK, et al: Cardiac involvement in myotonic dystrophy (Steinert's disease): a prospective study of 25 patients, Am J Cardiol 54:1074, 1984.

86. Petkovich NJ, et al: Myotonia dystrophica with A-V dissociation and Stokes-Adams attacks: a case report and review of the literature, Am Heart J 68:391, 1964.

87. Pilcher RB: Lymphosarcoma invading the heart: report of three cases with autopsy findings, Med J Aust 37:366, 1950.

88. Roberts WC, Barbour DJ: Frequency of acute and healed myocardial infarcts in fatal cardiac amyloidosis, Am J Cardiol 62:1134, 1988.

89. Roberts WC, et al: Sarcoidosis of the heart: a clinicopathologic study of 35 necropsy patients (group I) and review of 78 previously described necropsy patients (group II), Am J Med 63:86, 1977.

90. Robertson GH: Hydatid cyst of the heart simulating an aneurysm, NZ Med J 51:388, 1952.

91. Rosenbaum FF, et al: Persistent displacement of the RS-T segment in a case of metastatic tumor of the heart, Am Heart J 27:667, 1944.

92. Rosenbaum MB: Chagasic myocardiopathy, Prog Cardiovasc Dis 7:199, 1964.

93. Rosenbaum MB, Alvarez AJ: The electrocardiogram in chronic chagasic myocarditis, Am Heart J 50:492, 1955.

94. Rothfield EL, Zirkin RM: Unusual electrocardiographic evidence of metastatic cardiac tumor resembling atrial infarction, Am J Cardiol 10:882, 1962.

95. Rubin IL, Buchberg AS: Heart in progressive muscular dystrophy, Am Heart J 43:161, 1952.

96. Rubler S, et al: Cardiomyopathy simulating myocardial infarction: electrocardiographic and vectorcardiographic findings, NY J Med 73:1111, 1973.

97. Sackner MA, et al: The heart in scleroderma, Am J Cardiol 17:542, 1966.

98. Sanyal SK, et al: An ultrastructural basis for electrocardiographic alterations associated with Duchenne's progressive muscular dystrophy, Circulation 57:1122, 1978.

99. Schott J, et al: Electrocardiographic patterns in the differential diagnosis of progressive muscular dystrophy, Am J Med Sci 229:517, 1955.

100. Silverman KJ, et al: Cardiac sarcoid: a clinicopathologic study of 84 unselected patients with systemic sarcoidosis, Circulation 58:1204, 1978.

101. Siqueira-Filho AG, et al: M-mode and two-dimensional echocardiographic features in cardiac amyloidosis, Circulation 63:188, 1981.

102. Slucka C: The electrocardiogram in Duchenne progressive muscular dystrophy, Circulation 38:933, 1968.

103. Smith ER, et al: Hypertrophic cardiomyopathy: the heart disease of Friedreich's ataxia, Am Heart J 94:428, 1977.

104. Smith RRL, Hutchins GM: Ischemic heart disease secondary to amyloidosis of intramyocardial arteries, Am J Cardiol 44:413, 1979.

105. St John Sutton MG, et al: Left ventricular function in Friedreich's ataxia, Br Heart J 44:309, 1980.

106. Stumpf DA: Friedreich's ataxia: a metabolic cardiomyopathy, Am Heart J 104:887, 1982.

107. Sulayman R, Cassels DE: Myocardial coronary hemangiomatous tumors in children, Chest 68:113, 1975.

108. Swirsky MH, et al: Electrocardiographic diagnosis of a metastatic heart tumor, Conn Med 40:375, 1976.

109. Tavel ME, Fisch C: Abnormal Q waves simulating myocardial infarction in diffuse myocardial diseases, Am Heart J 68:534, 1964.

110. Thoren C: Cardiomyopathy in Friedreich's ataxia with studies of cardiovascular and respiratory function, Acta Paediatr Scand 53(suppl 153):1, 1964.

111. Weisenfeld S, Messinger WJ: Cardiac involvement in progressive muscular dystrophy, Am Heart J 43:170, 1952.

112. Welsh JD, et al: Cardiac findings in 73 patients with muscular dystrophy, Arch Intern Med 112:199, 1963.

113. Wenger NK: Myocardial involvement in systemic disease. In Hurst JW, Logue RB (editors): The heart, ed 2, New York, 1970, McGraw-Hill Book Co.

114. Whitfield AGW: Familial cardiomyopathy, Q J Med 30:119, 1961.

115. Windsheim JH, Parkin TW: Electrocardiograms of ninety patients with acrosclerosis and progressive diffuse sclerosis (scleroderma), Circulation 17:874, 1958.

116. Witchitz S, Diamant-Berger F: Les faux aspects d'infarctus du myocarde et les anomalies de l'onde P au cours des myopathies, Coeur Med Int 9:313, 1970.

117. Wizenberg TA, et al: Value of positive myocardial technetium-99m-pyrophosphate scintigraphy in the noninvasive diagnosis of cardiac amyloidosis, Am Heart J 103:468, 1982.

118. Yamamoto S, et al: A comparative study of thallium-201 single-photon emission computed tomography and electrocardiography in Duchenne and other types of muscular dystrophy, Am J Cardiol 61:836, 1988.

119. Young JM, Goldman IR: Tumor metastasis to the heart, Circulation 9:220, 1954.

120. Zatuchni J, et al: Metastatic epidermoid cardiac tumor manifested by persistent ST segment elevation, Am Heart J 101:674, 1981.

Review 1: Differential diagnosis of Q waves (Chapters 2 through 7)

Q waves are classified according to their pathophysiology into four major groups: (1) those caused by physiologic (positional) variants, (2) those associated with ventricular enlargement, (3) those associated with ventricular injury or replacement, and (4) those due to altered ventricular depolarization. In this brief review the data from the preceding six chapters are reassembled in terms of a more general clinical approach to Q waves.

Q waves with a widened QRS complex. The diagnosis of infarction should always be made with great caution in the presence of a prolonged QRS. All the major patterns of altered conduction (left or right bundle branch block, Wolff-Parkinson-White, and ventricular pacemaker) frequently produce pseudoinfarctional Q waves.

Q waves in young adults. Prominent Q waves in young patients are usually an unexpected finding. In subjects with no symptoms, normal variant patterns like a QS in V_1 and V_2, Q waves in III and aV_F, or a QS or Qr in aV_L should be considered. Dextrocardia can be readily diagnosed; however, even prominent pectus excavatum may be overlooked at first. Complete corrected transposition of the great vessels, an acyanotic anomaly, may be associated with loss of septal r waves and sometimes with the presence of inferior QS waves. Wide QR waves are seen in the anterior precordial leads, and sometimes in the inferior limb leads, with Ebstein's anomaly of the tricuspid valve. Left pneumothorax may lead to chest pain, dyspnea, and apparent loss of anterior forces. Hypertrophic cardiomyopathy is a particularly important cause of Q waves in this age group, and the diagnosis can usually be readily confirmed by means of two-dimensional echocardiography. Concentric left ventricular hypertrophy due, for example, to valvular aortic stenosis may also account for poor precordial R wave progression. In Friedreich's ataxia and myotonia atrophica, ECG abnormalities will occasionally precede gross neurologic manifestations. (Female carriers of Duchenne muscular dystrophy may have an ECG pattern similar to that of affected males.) Sarcoidosis and scleroderma sometimes cause pathologic Q waves, as does myocarditis from a variety of causes. Acute myocarditis may exactly simulate the ECG changes of infarction. Dilated (congestive) cardiomyopathy is suggested by global hypokinesis on echocardiographic study and may be confirmed by cardiac catheterization. Finally, in cases of unexplained Q waves a history of myocardial trauma or contusion should be sought.

Not all Q waves in younger patients reflect pesudoinfarct patterns. Actual myocardial infarction is well described in young adults and even rarely in children. It can result from a number of factors—premature atherosclerosis, coronary vasospasm (idiopathic or due to cocaine), Kawasaki's disease or other causes of coronary arteritis, congenital coronary artery anomaly (e.g., origin of the left coronary artery from the pulmonary artery).

Q waves with a low-voltage pattern. Although myocardial infarction commonly causes low voltage and Q waves, this pattern should also suggest the possibility of emphysema, amyloidosis, myocarditis, chronic constrictive pericarditis, or idiopathic cardiomyopathy.

Q waves in chronic cor pulmonale. Patients with pulmonary emphysema commonly have poor precordial R wave progression and occasionally noninfarctional Q waves in the inferior limb leads. Particular care must be taken to prevent misdiagnosing these cases as infarction.

Transient Q waves. Transient Q waves may appear with severe but reversible ischemia (hypotension, cardiac surgery, tachycardia) or with hyperkalemia.

Q waves with refractory cardiac failure. Cardiac tumor, amyloidosis, or other myocardial diseases (endocardial fibroelastosis, idiopathic dilated cardiomyopathy) should be considered in addition to ischemic heart disease.

Q waves with parasitic infections. Cardiac echinococcosis and chronic chagasic myocarditis both can produce pseudoinfarct Q waves patterns and should be considered in patients who have lived in endemic areas.

Q waves and the Bayes theorem. According to the Bayes theorem of conditional probability (p. 260), the likelihood that a patient has a disease process (e.g., a myocardial infarct) after a test is the product of the probability that he had the disease before the test and the diagnostic accuracy of the test itself. Clinicians should approach ECGs from a Bayesian point of view.[1,2] Thus the likelihood of a patient's having had a myocardial infarction, given the presence of Q waves, is related in part to the probability that the patient had an infarct *before* the ECG was obtained. For this reason the positive predictive value* of Q waves in diagnosing infarction will be higher in an elderly population, with a relatively high incidence of coronary disease, than in a younger population, with a low incidence of severe coronary artery disease. Conversely, Q waves are more likely to represent a pseudoinfarct pattern in the younger age groups.

However, such statistical considerations, though important in conditioning the clinician's index of suspicion, are not absolute guides. As noted, myocardial infarction may occur in young adults and normal-variant Q waves may be seen in the elderly. Electrocardiograms therefore must be interpreted in the widest clinical context, integrating data from multiple sources (Chapter 22).[1]

The lists that follow summarize the differential diagnosis of Q wave infarction patterns from a topographic viewpoint in terms of the traditional categories of anteroseptal, anterolateral, inferior, and posterior infarction.†

---

*The positive predictive value of Q waves equals the true-positive Q waves divided by the sum of true-positive and false-positive Q waves.

†However, precise localization of an infarction based on the distribution of QRS changes is of limited accuracy (Chapter 2).

Conditions simulating ANTEROSEPTAL myocardial infarction
(QS waves in one or more of V_1 to V_3)

A. Physiologic/positional factors
   1. Misplacement of chest leads
   2. Normal-variant QS in V_1 to V_2
   3. Left pneumothorax
   4. Congenital absence of left pericardium
   5. Complete corrected transposition of great vessels
   6. Pectus excavatum
B. Ventricular enlargement
   1. Left ventricular hypertrophy
   2. Right ventricular overload (right ventricular hypertrophy, acute or chronic cor pulmonale)
   3. Hypertrophic cardiomyopathy
C. Altered ventricular depolarization
   1. Left bundle branch block
   2. Left anterior hemiblock (qrS pattern in right precordial leads)
   3. Pacemaker patterns
   4. Right bundle branch block (qR in V_1 and V_2); QR waves may occur in V_1 to V_4 with Ebstein's anomaly of the tricuspid valve
   5. Wolff-Parkinson-White pattern (Type B)
D. Myocardial injury
   1. Acute: myocarditis, metabolic disturbances (transient ischemia, hyperkalemia), myocardial trauma
   2. Chronic: dilated cardiomyopathy, amyloidosis, sarcoidosis, scleroderma, chronic constrictive pericarditis, tumor, chagasic myocarditis, myotonia atrophica, endocardial fibroelastosis, echinococcus cyst

Conditions simulating ANTEROLATERAL myocardial infarction
(Q waves in one or more of I, aV_L, and V_4 to V_6)

A. Physiologic/positional factors
   1. Limb lead reversal
   2. Normal-variant QS or Qr in aV_L
   3. Normal-variant "septal" q waves
   4. Left pneumothorax
   5. Pectus excavatum (rare cause of deep narrow inferolateral q waves)
B. Ventricular enlargement
   1. Right ventricular overload (particularly right ventricular hypertrophy or chronic cor pulmonale)
   2. Hypertrophic cardiomyopathy
C. Altered ventricular depolarization
   1. Left bundle branch block
   2. Pacemaker patterns
   3. Wolff-Parkinson-White pattern
D. Myocardial injury
   1. Acute: myocarditis, metabolic disturbances (transient ischemia, hyperkalemia), myocardial trauma
   2. Chronic: dilated cardiomyopathy, amyloidosis, sarcoidosis, scleroderma, chronic constrictive pericarditis, Duchenne muscular dystrophy, tumor, chagasic myocarditis, myotonia atrophica, Friedreich's ataxia, endocardial fibroelastosis, echinococcus cyst

Conditions simulating INFERIOR myocardial infarction
(Q waves in one or more of II, III, and aV$_F$)

A. Physiologic/positional factors
   1. Limb lead reversal
   2. Normal variant
   3. Pectus excavatum (rare cause of deep narrow inferolateral q waves)
   4. Complete corrected transposition of great vessels
B. Ventricular enlargement
   1. Acute cor pulmonale (S$_I$Q$_{III}$ pattern)
   2. Chronic cor pulmonale
   3. Hypertrophic cardiomyopathy
C. Altered ventricular depolarization
   1. Left bundle branch block
   2. Right bundle branch block
   3. Wolff-Parkinson-White patterns
   4. Pacemaker patterns
D. Myocardial injury
   1. Acute: myocarditis, metabolic disturbances (transient ischemia, hyperkalemia), trauma
   2. Chronic: dilated cardiomyopathy, amyloidosis, scleroderma, sarcoidosis, Duchenne muscular dystrophy, chronic constrictive pericarditis, myotonia atrophica, Friedreich's ataxia, chagasic myocarditis, endocardial fibroelastosis, echinococcal cyst

Conditions simulating POSTERIOR myocardial infarction
(Relatively tall R wave in right precordial leads)

A. Physiologic/positional factors
   1. Misplacement of chest leads
   2. Normal variants
   3. Displacement of heart toward right chest (dextroversion): congenital or acquired
B. Ventricular enlargement
   1. Right ventricular hypertrophy
   2. Hypertrophic cardiomyopathy
C. Altered ventricular depolarization
   1. Right ventricular conduction abnormalities
   2. Wolff-Parkinson-White pattern (Type A)
D. Myocardial injury
   1. Duchenne muscular dystrophy
   2. Friedreich's ataxia*
   3. Chronic constrictive pericarditis (rarely)

---

*The prominent right precordial R waves may be associated with myocardial dystrophy, hypertrophic cardiomyopathy, or right ventricular hypertrophy (see p. 150).

REFERENCES

1. Goldberger AL: ECG simulators of infarction. II. Pathophysiology and differential diagnosis of pseudo-infarction ST-T patterns, PACE 5:414, 1982.

2. Selzer A: The Bayes theorem and clinical electrocardiography, Am Heart J 101:360, 1981.

PART

II

Repolarization (ST-T) Patterns Simulating Myocardial Infarction

Myocardial infarction often produces characteristic repolarization changes in the ST-T complex in addition to the Q waves as described in Part One. The differential diagnosis of these ischemic ST-T patterns is considered in the following chapters, which deal with (1) patterns associated with ST segment elevations, (2) patterns associated with ST segment depressions, (3) patterns associated with deep T wave inversions, and (4) patterns associated with tall positive T waves.

ST segment elevations: ischemic causes

ST segment elevation is a major electrocardiographic hallmark of ischemia. The first part of this chapter considers the clinical settings in which ST elevation may be seen on the resting ECG of patients with ischemic heart disease, including the effects of thrombolytic therapy. The significance of ST elevations during exercise testing is then reviewed. The final section discusses the pathophysiology of ischemic ST elevations ("current of injury" pattern).

ST ELEVATIONS ON THE RESTING ECG

ST elevations on the resting ECG may occur in three settings associated with ischemia or infarction: acute myocardial infarction, Prinzmetal's variant angina, and ventricular wall motion abnormalities (including ventricular aneurysm).

Acute myocardial infarction. ST segment elevations appear in the acute phase of infarction and are most often followed after a variable time (usually from hours to weeks) by characteristic T wave inversions. Reciprocal ST depressions may be seen in leads facing uninjured areas of the myocardium.

Thrombolytic therapy has been reported to cause more rapid resolution of ST elevations.[73] However, there is considerable intersubject variability, probably related to multiple factors, including the duration and extent of ischemia, the location of infarction, and the degree of reperfusion achieved.[1,4,11,34,60] Bar et al.[3] reported that intravenous thrombolytic therapy was most likely to limit significantly the size of anterior or inferior wall infarcts in patients with more marked degrees of initial ST elevation. (See also pp. 27 to 30.)

Unfortunately, the ECG is of limited value in predicting coronary artery patency within the first 90 minutes of intravenous thrombolytic therapy. In one large series including 386 patients treated with tissue plasminogen activator,[11] *complete* resolution of ST elevations was the only specific ECG marker of successful reperfusion detected by coronary angiography. However, this sign was of limited sensitivity, because reperfusion can occur despite unresolved or partially resolved ST elevation. Furthermore, cardiac arrhythmias (e.g., ventricular tachycardia, accelerated idioventricular rhythm, bradyarrhythmias) are not spe-

175

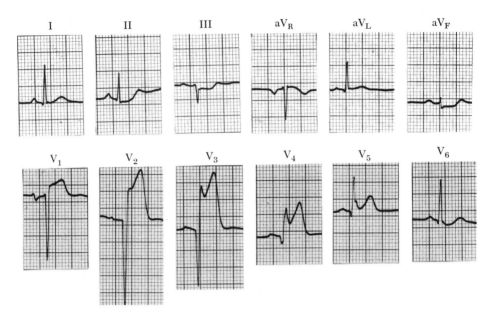

FIG. 8-1. Acute anterior wall infarction. Note the marked ST elevations (current of injury pattern) in V_1 to V_5, with prominent Q waves in these leads, as well as the slight reciprocal ST depressions in II, III, and aV_F with left atrial abnormality. This tracing was obtained after several hours of chest pain.

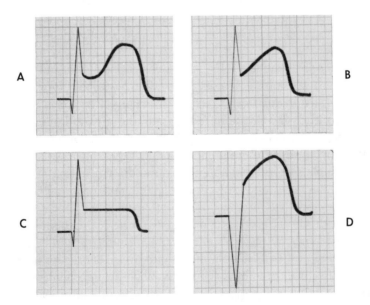

FIG. 8-2. Types of ST elevation seen with acute myocardial infarction (current of injury pattern). **A,** Upwardly concave. The ST segment appears to have been lifted evenly off the baseline. A similar pattern occurs with benign early repolarization variant (Fig. 9-6) and acute pericarditis. **B,** Obliquely straightened. **C,** Plateau shaped. **D,** Convex. (Similar elevations to this are sometimes seen in the right precordial leads with left bundle branch block and left ventricular hypertrophy in the absence of infarction.)

cific or sensitive predictors of successful reperfusion.[11,35]

Recurrent ST elevations following their resolution after thrombolytic therapy are not uncommon and strongly suggest re-thrombosis of the artery.[37]

ST elevations seen with acute (Q wave or non–Q wave) infarction may vary in amplitude from less than 1 to more than 10 mm (Fig. 8-1) above the baseline. Occasionally, as shown in Fig. 11-7, the reciprocal ST depressions seen during the acute phase of myocardial infarction will be more pronounced than the primary ST elevations.

The morphology of the ST complex during acute infarction is also variable. The ST segment may retain its normal upward concavity (scooped appearance), or it may become convex (dome shaped), rise obliquely in a straight line, or become plateau shaped.[25] These variations are shown diagrammatically in Fig. 8-2.

These ST elevations, as described later in the chapter, are attributable to a transmural (subepicardial) current of injury (see Fig. 8-10). However, it is important to recognize that ischemic ST elevations are not invariably the precursor of acute Q wave infarction; they also may be a marker of transient transmural ischemia without infarction (Prinzmetal's angina, described next) or may precede acute non–Q wave infarction, as summarized in the box below. Several studies[6,33,78] have shattered the myth that non–Q wave infarction is associated only with ST depressions, T wave inversions, or nonspecific repolarization changes. For example, Huey et al.[32] studied 150 consecutive patients with enzymatically confirmed acute infarction who had ST segment elevations (≥ 1 mm in at least two contiguous leads) on their admission electrocardiogram. Q wave infarcts developed in 115 of these patients (77%). However, an important subset (23%) had non–Q wave infarcts (Fig. 8-3). Similar observations have been made by Willich et al.[78] and Boden et al.[6]

From a pathophysiologic perspective, the association of early ST elevations with subsequent non–Q wave infarction is of considerable interest. This finding suggests that the infarct in at least some patients may be initiated by transient thrombotic or vasospastic occlusion of a coronary artery followed by spontaneous reperfusion.[6,32] Such a scenario would be consistent with the clinical observation that acute non–Q wave infarcts do indeed tend to be smaller than Q wave infarcts and to be associated with a higher patency rate of the infarct-related artery when coronary arteriography is performed shortly after the acute episode[6] (pp. 23 to 25).

FATE OF ISCHEMIC ST ELEVATIONS

1. Resolve without infarction (Prinzmetal's variant angina)
2. Be followed by Q wave infarction
3. Be followed by non–Q wave infarction

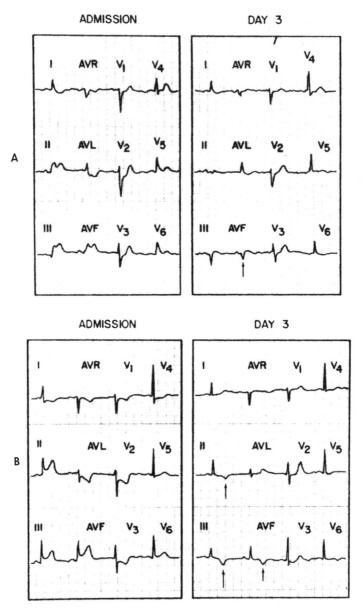

FIG. 8-3. Comparison of Q wave and non–Q wave myocardial infarctions. **A,** Admission and Day 3, from a patient with an inferior wall Q wave infarct. Note the ST elevations in II, III, and aV$_F$ at admission and the subsequent development of Q waves *(arrow)*. **B,** Admission and Day 3, from a patient with an inferior wall non–Q wave infarct. Despite significant ST elevations in II, III, and aV$_F$ at admission, no abnormal Q waves developed subsequently. Serial ECGs showed only T wave inversions *(arrows)*. (From Huey B, et al: J Am Coll Cardiol 9:18, 1987. Used by permission.) (See also Figs. 2-1 and 2-2.)

I	II	III	aV_R	aV_L	aV_F

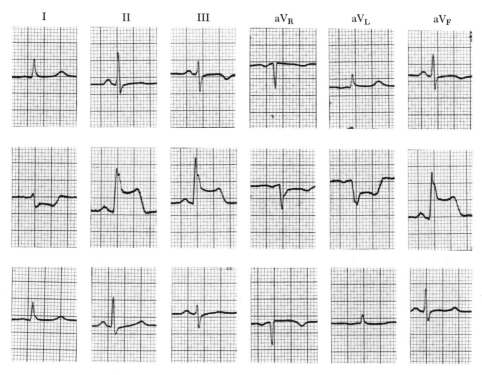

FIG. 8-4. Prinzmetal's (variant) angina with transient ST elevations. This 30-year-old man had a history of angina with both rest and exertion. **A,** The baseline resting ECG shows nonspecific inferior lead ST-T changes. **B,** With chest pain, note the marked ST elevations in II, III, and aV_F and the reciprocal ST depressions in I and aV_L. There is also shift of the axis to the right and slight widening of the QRS consistent with left posterior hemiblock. **C,** After nitroglycerin administration the ST segments return to baseline. Cardiac catheterization showed a 95% right coronary artery lesion with intermittent spasm producing total occlusion and transient elevation of the ST segments.

Prinzmetal's variant angina. The classic ECG pattern seen in some but not by any means in all cases of typical exertional angina (Chapter 20) is diffuse depression of the ST segment (except in aV_R, which may show ST elevation). This "coronary insufficiency" pattern (discussed in Chapter 11) is generally attributed to predominant subendocardial ischemia. Prinzmetal et al.[56] subsequently described a variant form of angina that was associated with ST elevations and simulated the pattern of acute infarction (Fig. 8-4). However, in Prinzmetal's angina syndrome the ST elevations characteristically return to baseline following the ischemic episode and further evolution of Q waves does not occur.* In addition, cardiac enzyme studies are negative.

The transient ST elevations that characterize Prinzmetal's angina appear to reflect reversible transmural ischemia.[42,47] Furthermore, elegant coronary arteriographic studies[47,53] have demonstrated that such ischemia is caused by coro-

---

*Transient Q waves have subsequently been reported with this type of angina (p. 130).[48]

nary vasospasm that may involve a single vessel or, occasionally, multiple vessels.

The ECG is of some value in predicting the coronary system involved.[43] Elevations of the ST segment in V_2 and V_3 are highly predictive of left anterior descending involvement. Elevations in II, III, and aV_F usually indicate right coronary or left circumflex involvement (Fig. 8-4). Elevations in V_5 or V_6 are nonspecific and may be seen with spasm of any of the three major coronary branches.

Current evidence shows that Prinzmetal's angina is not a monolithic syndrome. There are multiple subsets. For example, some patients will have coronary vasospasm superimposed on apparently normal coronary vessels without evidence of atherosclerosis.[53,67] Attacks in this subset occur spontaneously or may be secondary to drugs such as cocaine.[38*] Others will have vasospasm in the area of a fixed but subcritical stenosis. In still others vasospasm will occur in association with severe coronary atherosclerosis involving one or more vessels.[47]

Not all patients with coronary vasospasm will have ST segment elevations. Some with an abnormal baseline and ST depressions or T wave inversions will, during episodes of vasospasm, show transient normalization of the repolarization complex without ST elevations.[47] This pattern has been aptly termed "pseudo-" or "paradoxical" T wave normalization[51] and is discussed further in Chapter 18. An example is shown in Fig. 18-8. Paradoxical T wave normalization is well documented during Prinzmetal's angina[47] and also in some cases during the earliest phase of myocardial infarction. (Whether transient paradoxical normalization of T waves invariably denotes coronary vasospasm remains to be proved.)

In addition to paradoxical T wave normalization, several other ECG patterns may be seen with coronary vasospasm. Hyperacute T waves (Chapter 18) indicative of transmural ischemia may appear transiently. Surprisingly, some subjects will have ST depressions, the pattern classically associated with exertional angina and subendocardial ischemia.[5,47,79] Maseri et al.[47] clearly documented episodes of ST segment depression in association with coronary vasospasm. In some cases transient ST depressions were observed as the only ECG manifestation of ischemia. In other cases ST segment elevations were followed by ST depressions lasting from seconds to minutes. The authors postulated that the ST segment elevations were due to severe transmural ischemia whereas the ST depressions secondary to vasospasm were associated with a more diffuse regional reduction in perfusion. Support for the hypothesis that ST elevations with vasospasm reflect more severe ischemia than do ST depressions has been provided

---

*Transient ST elevations have also been described in patients with septic shock who were being treated with dopamine infusions.[72] It was suggested that this pattern, resembling the pattern of variant angina, might have resulted from drug-induced coronary vasospasm.

Yasue et al.,[79] who recorded ECGs while patients were experiencing vaso-spasm during coronary arteriography. They found that most episodes of ST eleva-tions correlated with total occlusion of a major coronary artery. By contrast, most episodes of ST depressions correlated with either subtotal spastic occlusion or diffuse narrowing of a major coronary artery. Furthermore, when ST depressions occurred with total coronary occlusion, the occlusion was in either a major coronary supplied by a collateral vessel or a small branch of the major artery.

Finally, in some cases vasospasm will be associated with transient T wave inversions,[47] with nondiagnostic ST-T changes, or rarely with an entirely nor-mal ECG.[29]

From a diagnostic viewpoint, Prinzmetal's angina may pose a number of problems. First, the ST elevations often simulate the pattern of acute infarction. Second, the condition may be overlooked or misdiagnosed because patients with vasospasm often have symptoms at rest (caused by abrupt cessation of coronary flow), in contrast to patients with typical angina, who have exertional chest dis-comfort (caused by excessive myocardial oxygen demands and fixed coronary obstructions). Third, documentation of ST changes with pain is often difficult. As shown in Fig. 8-5, ambulatory (Holter) monitoring may be useful in these patients to demonstrate intermittent ST elevations. (The uses and limitations of ambulatory ECG recording in the diagnosis of ischemic heart disease are dis-cussed further in Chapter 12.)

In susceptible individuals coronary vasospasm and associated ECG changes may be induced by a variety of factors, including drugs such as ergonovine, methacholine, or epinephrine or by hyperventilation.[79] Occasionally, although pain at rest is the classic symptom, vasospasm will be precipitated by exercise.* (See also p. 186.)

Arrhythmias and conduction disturbances may be a prominent feature in some cases, including complete heart block or ventricular tachyarrhythmias, which can result in syncope or sudden death.[61]

Ventricular wall motion abnormalities (including ventricular aneurysm). Isch-emic ST elevations are also sometimes a persistent finding after acute myocar-dial infarction[62] (Fig. 8-6).

The natural history of ST elevations following acute infarction was studied by Mills et al.[49] Of particular note was their observation that those persisting for 2 weeks did not resolve and were associated with more severe infarction. Persis-tent ST elevations were more common following anterior than inferior infarc-tion. The incidence of actual left ventricular aneurysm in this subgroup with persistent ST elevations was not studied. However, in a separate group of pa-tients with *chronic* ischemic disease documented by angiography, persistent el-

---

*References 23, 29, 39, 69, 75.

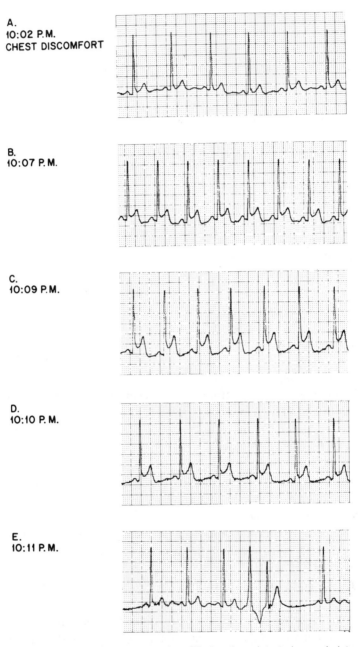

A.
10:02 P.M.
CHEST DISCOMFORT

B.
10:07 P.M.

C.
10:09 P.M.

D.
10:10 P.M.

E.
10:11 P.M.

FIG. 8-5. A modified lead II tracing shows transient ST elevations detected on ambulatory monitoring in a 68-year-old man who complained of intermittent chest discomfort primarily at rest. It was likely due to coronary vasospasm (Prinzmetal's angina), since coronary arteriography showed little more than a mild lesion in the mid–right coronary artery. With the onset of "burning chest pain," **A,** note sinus rhythm with minimal ST elevations, unchanged from baseline. This was followed by progressive ST elevations, **B** and **D,** with resolution after about 10 minutes, accompanied by ventricular ectopy, **E.**

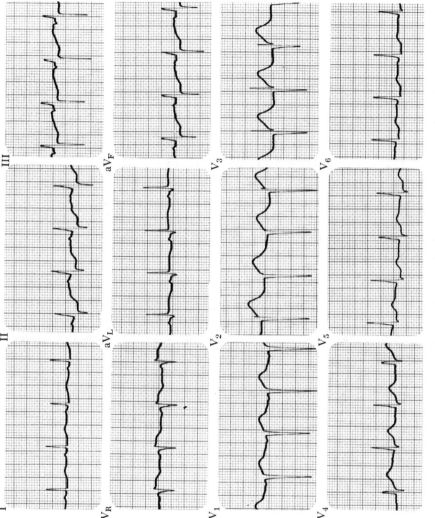

FIG. 8-6. Anterior wall aneurysm. Note the prominent Q waves in V_1 to V_3 and aV_L, with persistent ST elevations and reciprocal ST depressions in the inferior leads (II, III, and aV_F) from a patient who had sustained an infarct several months before this ECG was taken. Persistence of ST elevations more than 2 weeks after an infarction suggests the presence of ventricular wall motion abnormality and possible aneurysm.

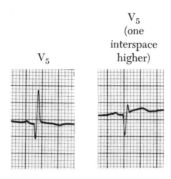

FIG. 8-7. Variable appearance of the ST segment due to slight changes in lead placement. This patient had sustained a prior anterior wall infarction and also had a probable left ventricular aneurysm. Note the marked change in ST morphology when V_5 is recorded one interspace above its usual position and also the increased depth of pathologic Q waves.

evations were noted in 40 of 65 patients (62%) with severe anterior wall asynergy. A similar incidence (64%) was reported in several other series of patients with left ventricular aneurysm. By contrast, persistent ST elevations were seen in only 1 of 30 patients (3%) with chronic coronary disease and normal left ventricular wall motion. Therefore persistent ST elevation following infarction appears to be a highly specific though relatively insensitive marker of left ventricular aneurysm.

From a clinical viewpoint the presence of persistent ST elevations following infarction may be a useful clue to an underlying ventricular wall motion disorder, for example, in patients with refractory congestive failure. However, the ECG signs do not necessarily indicate a discrete, surgically resectable, dyskinetic area.

In cases of persistent ST elevations following anterior myocardial infarction the precordial leads may show varying degrees of abnormality caused by minor changes in electrode placement. Fig. 8-7 shows an isoelectric ST segment when V_5 was recorded in the conventional position but ST elevation when it was recorded one interspace higher. Thus subtle misplacement of the chest leads can produce spurious evidence of acute or evolving ST-T changes.

Another sign of ventricular aneurysm is an rsR' or equivalent pattern in one or more of the left precordial leads.[19] The sensitivity and specificity of this pattern have not been defined. Presumably it reflects some local conduction delay in the region of the aneurysm. (The ECG in relation to ventricular aneurysm is discussed further in Chapter 21.)

ST ELEVATIONS DURING EXERCISE TESTING

The ST depression pattern (seen with coronary insufficiency or subendocardial ischemia) described in Chapter 13 is considered the classic ischemic ECG

III

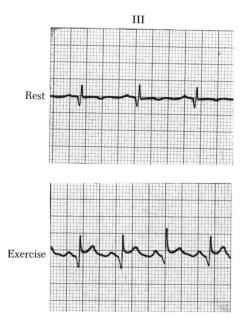

Rest

Exercise

FIG. 8-8. ST elevations during an exercise tolerance test. This patient had sustained an earlier inferior wall infarct, with complete occlusion of the circumflex and right coronary arteries, and now had residual inferior wall akinesia.

MECHANISMS OF ST ELEVATION DURING EXERCISE

Associated with chronic ventricular wall motion abnormality due to prior infarct
    Acute ischemia need not be present
    Frank aneurysm not necessarily present
Due to acute transient transmural ischemia from
    Coronary vasospasm in a normal artery or with any degree of fixed obstructive disease
    High-grade fixed coronary obstruction without vasospasm

---

response during exercise testing. Less commonly, patients with ischemic heart disease will manifest ST elevations during exercise.* *There are two major subsets of patients with exertional ST elevations: those with evidence of prior infarction (usually residual Q waves) and those without prior infarction.* The pathogenesis and clinical implications of exertional ST elevations in these subgroups are very different and are summarized in the box above.

ST elevations during exercise in patients with previous infarction are a highly specific though relatively insensitive marker of an underlying ventricular wall motion disorder[10,71] (Fig. 8-8) and sometimes a frank aneurysm.[12,26,45,70]

---

*References 2, 10, 17, 18, 39, 41, 46, 52, 69, 70, 76.

Gorlin, Klein, and Sullivan[26] initially described several patients with ventricular aneurysm who showed exercise-related ST elevations not seen on the resting ECG. Two subsequent studies[12,45] reported exertional ST elevations in 64% and 48% of patients with ventricular aneurysm.

This pattern is a variant of the well-recognized sign of persistent ST elevation after infarction on the resting ECG of patients with severe ventricular wall motion disorders (p. 181). The mechanism of exertional ST elevations with underlying wall motion disorders is uncertain but does not require active ischemia. Only a minority of patients with this pattern during exercise have concomitant angina, and thallium scintigrams may not show evidence of an acute decrease in regional perfusion.[24] Furthermore, ST elevations during exercise following Q wave infarction, though a marker of ventricular dysfunction, do not usually indicate a surgically resectable aneurysm.[46] However, the pattern is most prevalent in patients with more severe abnormalities of left ventricular function.[27]

ST elevations during exercise also occur in a small but important group of patients *without* evidence of prior infarction (Fig. 8-9). In this group they signify transient transmural ischemia that may be related to (a) coronary artery spasm in a normal vessel or one with a subcritical stenosis, (b) coronary artery spasm superimposed on a significant stenosis, or (c) high-grade stenosis without vasospasm.

Evidence for coronary artery spasm with or without significant fixed obstruction underlying coronary disease has been provided by numerous investigators.* Specchia et al.,[69] for example, studied 16 patients with exercise-induced ST elevations who did not have a history of previous infarction. All patients had coronary vasospasm induced by ergonovine. Furthermore, coronary arteriography performed at the time of the ST elevations revealed vasospasm in all patients tested: 12 of the 16 had significant (>50%) fixed luminal stenosis of one or more vessels; 1 had entirely normal-appearing arteries. The authors suggested that coronary vasoconstriction during exercise might be related to enhanced alpha-adrenergic tone. Transient ST elevations due to coronary vasospasm have also been reported during recovery from exercise,[77] probably by a similar mechanism.

Finally, exertional ST elevations due to transient transmural ischemia have been attributed to high-grade coronary blockage without actual vasospasm.[41] Strong support for this mechanism comes from dipyridamole tests performed by Picano et al.[55] in 14 patients with exercise-induced ST elevations in the absence of previous infarction. In 7 of these subjects, dipyridamole caused ST elevations in the same leads that showed such elevations on effort, along with chest pain and ventricular asynergy at echocardiographic examination. All 7 patients had nearly complete coronary stenosis. Since dipyridamole induces ischemia by causing vasodilation and a secondary coronary "steal" syndrome, coronary

---

*References 15, 23, 39, 69, 76.

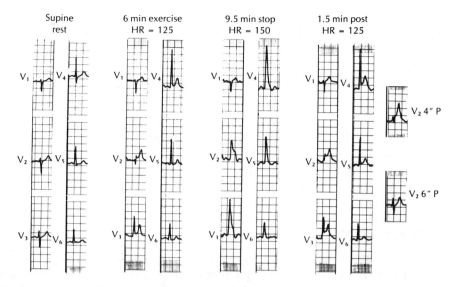

FIG. 8-9. ST elevations with exercise in a patient with a normal resting ECG and no history of infarction. Elevation of the ST segment is best seen in V_2 to V_4. Note also the increased R wave amplitude, a paradoxical sign of acute transmural ischemia (p. 31). The patient was found to have a severe subtotal obstruction of the left anterior descending coronary artery. Although vasospasm was not specifically identified in this case, it could not be positively excluded. *HR* is heart rate; *P* signifies postexercise. (From Froelicher VF: Exercise testing and training, Chicago, 1983, Year Book Medical Publishers Inc.)

spasm was highly unlikely in these patients. Of particular note, coronary arteriograms during exercise in two of the patients with ST elevations also failed to show vasospasm.

The distribution of exercise-related ST elevations may be of some value in predicting the site of coronary involvement.[41] In V_{4R}, for instance, they are specific though not particularly sensitive as a marker of right coronary artery disease.[7] In V_1 to V_3 these elevations suggest spasm of the left anterior descending coronary artery. (However, they also occur [rarely] in V_1 to V_3 with acute right ventricular ischemia.[40]) By contrast, in the inferoposterior leads they suggest right coronary or left circumflex coronary involvement. In the lateral precordial leads they do not appear to be reliable indicators of the involved coronary artery system.

Finally, it should be emphasized that when localized ST elevations occur with rest or exercise *reciprocal* ST depressions may be seen in the contralateral leads and do not necessarily imply concomitant subendocardial ischemia (Fig. 8-4).

PATHOPHYSIOLOGY OF ISCHEMIC ST ELEVATIONS

In 1909 Eppinger and Rothberger[20] observed ST segment elevations in dogs with experimental cardiac injury, and in 1920 Pardee[54] published his classic description of ST segment elevation as a clinical sign of coronary obstruction. More than 70 years have passed since these initial observations, yet the exact mechanism underlying ischemic repolarization changes is still a subject of ongoing research and debate.

Normally the ST segment is relatively isoelectric (neither positive nor negative). Myocardial cells during this early phase of repolarization (corresponding to the plateau phase of the action potential) carry the same transmembrane potential. Therefore they will not have any net current flow at the time the ST segment is inscribed. ST segment deviation from myocardial ischemia is caused by abnormal current flow (current of injury) between the boundary of normal and ischemic zones. Both *diastolic* and *systolic* injury currents have been invoked to explain ischemic ST segment elevation.

Diastolic Current of Injury Theory

Nahum, Hamilton, and Heff[50] and later Donoso, Wachtel, and Grishman[16] suggested that the ST segment elevation of infarction is caused primarily by a downward (negative) displacement of the diastolic baseline (TQ segment). This theory was based on the assumption that the ischemic myocardium loses its capacity to *repolarize* completely. During electrical diastole this ischemic muscle will remain partly or completely depolarized. Depolarized muscle carries a negative extracellular charge relative to repolarized muscle. Therefore during diastole there would be a flow of current (diastolic current of injury) between the partly or completely depolarized ischemic myocardium and the normally repolarized uninjured myocardium. The *injury current vector* (Fig. 8-10) will be directed away from the more negative ischemic zone and toward the electropositive normal myocardium.* As a result leads overlying the ischemic zone will record a negative deflection during electrical diastole, producing depression of the TQ segment (Fig. 8-10, *A*).

TQ segment depression in turn produces ST segment elevation because the ECG equipment in clinical use employs alternating current–coupled amplifiers that automatically compensate for any negative shift in the TQ segment by bringing the recording stylus back to its original baseline. As a result of this electronic compensation the ST segment will also be lifted upward. Therefore, according to the diastolic current of injury theory, ST segment elevation represents only an *apparent shift*. The true shift is the negative displacement of the TQ baseline (Fig. 8-10, *A*).

---

*There is some confusion in the ECG literature regarding the direction this injury current actually flows. In classic physical terms, current, by convention, flows from positive to negative poles. However, the standard electrocardiograph records a positive deflection when the recording electrode faces electropositive charges (positive dipole) on the outside of the myocardial cells (although current is flowing away from the positive region). Therefore it is easier to conceptualize the effect of the injury current on the surface ECG in terms of the direction of the *injury current (TQ or ST segment) vector,* which will be oriented toward electrically positive areas and away from electronegative regions.

Theoretical Basis of Ischemic ST Elevations

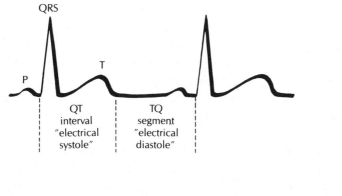

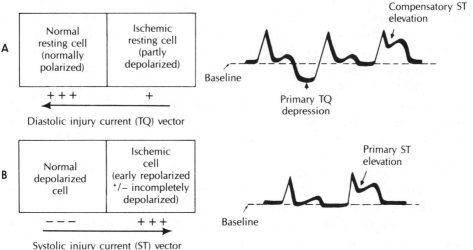

FIG. 8-10. Pathophysiology of ischemic ST elevations. Two basic mechanisms have been advanced to explain the elevations seen with acute myocardial injury. **A,** Diastolic current of injury. In this case the ST vector will be directed away from the relatively negative, partly depolarized, ischemic region during electrical diastole and the result will be primary TQ depressions. Conventional alternating current electrocardiographs compensate for the baseline shift, resulting in apparent ST elevations. **B,** Systolic current of injury. In this case the ischemic zone will be relatively positive during electrical systole because the cells are repolarized early and the amplitude and upstroke velocity of their action potentials are decreased. This vector will be oriented toward the electropositive zone, and the result will be primary ST elevations.

This theory was based on animal experiments in which direct current–coupled ECG amplifiers were used to eliminate compensatory baseline shifts. With this method the ST segment elevation recorded in acute ischemia seemed to be accounted for entirely on the basis of the TQ shifts just described.

However, other investigators[28,59] using similar experimental models have reported both a negative TQ segment shift and a primary positive ST segment elevation that has been ascribed to a systolic current of injury.

Systolic Current of Injury Theory

The original systolic current of injury theory proposed by Eyster et al.[21] was based on the assumption that ischemic myocardium is incapable of being fully depolarized during electrical systole. Such muscle would carry a positive charge on its membrane relative to normal fully depolarized muscle. This difference in potential would result in a flow of current (systolic current of injury) between uninjured muscle and the relatively more positive ischemic areas. An exploring electrode placed over the ischemic region would record this current of injury as a positive (upward) deflection at the time at which the ST segment is being inscribed.

On the basis of experimental recordings in dogs, Samson and Scher[66] proposed an alternative explanation for the systolic current of injury. By correlating intracellular electrograms with direct current–coupled ECG tracings during experimental infarction in dogs, they observed that the ST elevation was usually caused by a combination of primary negative displacement of the TQ baseline and primary positive ST displacement. However, they failed to document any evidence of incomplete depolarization of ischemic cells. Instead, by recording intracellular action potentials, they made the surprising observation that the acutely infarcted myocardium appeared to depolarize normally and actually repolarized more rapidly than the normal uninjured myocardium. The precise mechanism for this paradoxical *early repolarization* of acutely ischemic cells was not apparent.

This accelerated repolarization of acutely infarcting myocardium has been confirmed by other investigators[44,74] and appears to be a relatively transient phenomenon. With more prolonged ischemia repolarization time characteristically increases in the injured region. The longer action potential seen during the subacute or chronic phase of myocardial injury correlates with the appearance of T wave inversions and is described in Chapter 14.

The early repolarization of acutely ischemic cells will produce an electrical gradient between normal and injured cells during the latter phase of electrical systole. As a result the injury current vector will be directed toward the relatively positive, earlier repolarized, ischemic zone at the time the ST segment and T wave are inscribed (Fig. 8-10, *B*). This shift of the ST-T vector toward the ischemic zone helps explain the morphologic appearance of upsloping ST elevation and tall, positive (hyperacute) T waves during the earliest phase of infarction.

The relative contribution of diastolic and systolic injury currents to ST elevation is not certain. Samson and Scher[66] found that in most cases the primary ST segment shift caused by early repolarization occurred first and predominated over the diastolic (TQ segment) shifts that followed. By contrast, Vincent, Abildskov, and Burgess[74] subsequently reported that compensated TQ shifts were the major factor accounting for ST segment elevation in canine infarction. Kléber et al.[33] also confirmed the coexistence of primary TQ and ST segment shifts following experimental coronary artery occlusion in pigs and the role of membrane depolarization and action potential shortening in their respective genesis. However, in contrast to Samson and Scher[66] but in accord with the classic theory of Eyster et al.,[21] the data from pigs also showed evidence of decreased upstroke velocity and amplitude in the ischemic zone. Such incomplete depolarization, by rendering the infarcting cells less negative, should have contributed to the primary systolic current of injury.

In summary: The ST segment elevation that characterizes the acute phase of infarction (Fig. 8-10) appears to be the result of the combined effects of a compensated primary negative shift in the TQ segment (correlating with a primary decrease in membrane resting potential) and a primary positive displacement of the ST segment (associated with shortened action potential duration and probably decreased amplitude and upstroke velocity of the action potentials of acutely ischemic cells). Theoretically any nonischemic process that produces either membrane depolarization or accelerated repolarization could generate pseudoinfarctional ST segment elevations. Such pseudoinfarctional patterns are seen in hyperkalemic ST elevations (caused by nonischemic membrane depolarization) and in the benign early repolarization variant (possibly caused by functional accelerated repolarization). These patterns, together with the other major causes of pseudoinfarctional elevation of the ST segment, are described in detail in Chapters 9 and 10.

Ionic Basis of Diastolic and Systolic Injury Currents

Early observations by Prinzmetal et al.[57] provided important clues to understanding the electrical changes of repolarization in injured tissue in terms of the underlying ionic shifts and changes in membrane potential that occur during acute ischemia.

In their resting state myocardial cells normally have a transmembrane potential of about -90 mV; the inside of the cell is negative relative to the outside. This negative resting transmembrane potential is caused primarily by the concentration gradient of potassium (the normal intracellular to extracellular ratio is 30:1). There is also a concentration gradient for sodium (intracellular to extracellular ratio, 1:10). The transmembrane potential will be decreased (hypopolarization or depolarization) when either the extracellular concentration of potassium is increased or the intracellular concentration of sodium is increased. It has been observed experimentally that *perfusion of cardial muscle with solutions that tend to depolarize the membrane (solutions high in potassium or low in sodium) leads to ST segment elevation.* Conversely, myocardial perfusion with solutions that increase membrane resting potential (hyperpolarizing solutions) is associated with ST depression.[36]

Prinzmetal et al.[57] also observed that the ST elevation that occurs when the membrane is depolarized is caused primarily by a compensated negative displacement of the TQ segment. Samson and Scher[66] and others[34] found the same correlation between primary depression of the TQ segment and decreased membrane resting potential.

These observations suggest the following schema[57] to account in part for the ST segment elevations seen in conjunction with acute infarction:

1. Acute ischemia produces damage to myocardial cells that disrupts the normal structure and function of the cell membrane.
2. This sarcolemmal damage allows potassium to leak *out* of the cells down the potassium concentration gradient, and it allows sodium ions to flow *into* the cells down the sodium concentration gradient.
3. The consequence of these ionic shifts is a primary decrease in membrane resting potential (depolarization of the membrane).
4. This decreased membrane resting potential is associated with a primary negative shift in the TQ segment of the ECG, which will be recorded as ST segment elevation if an AC-coupled electrocardiograph is used.

The ionic basis of the accelerated repolarization and incomplete depolarization that also seem to play a role in the genesis of ischemic ST segment elevations is not known but may be, at least in part, related to local hyperkalemia (p. 133). The electrolyte and electrophysiologic perturbations accompanying acute ischemia are reviewed by Reimer and Jennings.[58]

MAGNITUDE OF ST ELEVATIONS

The magnitude (amplitude) of ischemic ST segment elevation recorded in any lead is a function of two primary variables[31]: the *spatial relation (solid angle)* between the recording electrode and the border of the ischemic zone and the *voltage gradient* between the normal and infarcting regions.

According to solid-angle theory, the geometric relation between the recording electrode and the infarcted area is a major determinant of the degree of ST elevation. The solid angle is proportional to the angle subtended by the recording electrode and the boundaries of the ischemic zone: the larger the solid angle, the greater the amplitude of ST elevation. For a precordial electrode the solid angle will be increased by enlarging the circumference of the infarct and decreased by moving the recording electrode farther from the infarct. (Paradoxically, for a direct epicardial lead the solid angle will be decreased by increasing the size of the infarct. Holland and Brooks[30] reported that the degree of ST segment elevation in direct epicardial leads placed in the center of experimental infarcts in pigs actually decreased as the infarct enlarged.)

The second major factor governing the magnitude of ST elevation is the voltage gradient between the injured and normal zones. As just described, ST segment elevation is probably the result of injury currents generated by voltage gradients between the ischemic and normal areas during both electrical diastole and electrical systole. The greater this difference of membrane potential, the greater the magnitude of ST segment elevation will be. Therefore any factors that increase the voltage gradient between normal and ischemic zones will augment the amount of ST elevation. Conversely, factors that lessen this gradient will diminish the injury current.

These considerations make it apparent that the degree of ST segment elevation recorded in any lead during acute infarction may be affected by multiple factors in addition to the degree of actual ischemia. For example, the amount of ST elevation may be influenced by drugs, conduction disturbances, electrolyte shifts, and so on, which may alter the voltage gradient between normal and injured zones independent of the degree of ischemia. Furthermore, the solid angle can also be affected by multiple factors related to infarct size and shape, wall thickness, and electrode position.[31]

Because of its complex determinants, the *absolute* magnitude of ST segment elevation cannot be used as a reliable indicator of infarct size. However, *relative* changes in ST segment amplitude recorded by multiple leads may still be useful for indirectly assessing the efficacy of interventions designed to limit acute ischemia.[2] (See also p. 175.)

From a clinical point of view it is important to recognize that ST segment elevation is a useful marker but not a direct measure of ischemic injury. In addition to the degree of ischemia, many other factors may affect the ST segment. ST segment elevation therefore is an *epiphenomenon,* a useful but indirect index of ischemic injury related to the effects of ischemia on only one aspect of myocardial function, namely, the cell membrane potential.

REFERENCES

1. Anderson JL, et al: A randomized trial of streptokinase in the treatment of acute myocardial infarction, N Engl J Med 308:1312, 1983.
2. Arora R, et al: The role of ischemia and ventricular asynergy in the genesis of exercise-induced ST elevation, Clin Cardiol 11:127, 1988.
3. Bar FW, et al: Value of admission electrocardiogram in predicting outcome of thrombolytic therapy in acute myocardial infarction. A randomized trial conducted by the Netherlands Interuniversity Cardiology Institute, Am J Cardiol 59:6, 1987.
4. Blanke H, et al: Electrocardiographic changes after streptokinase-induced recanalization in patients with acute left anterior descending artery obstruction, Circulation 68:406, 1983.
5. Boden WE, et al: Exercise-induced coronary spasm with S-T segment depression and normal coronary arteriography, Am J Cardiol 48:193, 1981.
6. Boden WE, et al: ST segment shifts are poor predictors of subsequent Q-wave evolution in acute myocardial infarction. A natural history study of early non-Q wave infarction, Circulation 79:537, 1989.
7. Braat SH, et al: Value of lead V_{4R} in exercise testing to predict proximal stenosis of the right coronary artery, J Am Coll Cardiol 5:1308, 1985.
8. Braunwald E, Maroko PR: ST-segment mapping: realistic and unrealistic expectations, Circulation 54:529, 1976.
9. Bren GB, et al: The electrocardiogram in patients undergoing thrombolysis for myocardial infarction, Circulation 76(supp II):18, 1987.
10. Bruce RA, et al: ST segment elevation with exercise: a marker for poor ventricular function and poor prognosis. Coronary Artery

Surgery Study (CASS) confirmation of Seattle Heart Watch results, Circulation 77:897, 1988.

11. Califf RM, et al: Failure of clinical measurements to predict perfusion status after intravenous thrombolysis, Ann Intern Med 108:658, 1988.

12. Chahine RA, et al: The clinical significance of exercise-induced ST-segment elevation, Circulation 54:209, 1976.

13. Chouhan L, et al: Utility of lead V_4R in exercise testing for detection of coronary artery disease, Am J Cardiol 64:988, 1989.

14. De Feyter PJ, et al: Clinical significance of exercise-induced ST elevation, Br Heart J 46:84, 1981.

15. deServi S, et al: The exercise test in variant angina: results in 114 patients, Circulation 64:684, 1981.

16. Donoso E, et al: Polarity of the S-T vector, Am J Physiol 189:219, 1957.

17. Dunn RF, et al: Exercise induced ST-segment elevation. Correlation of thallium-201 myocardial perfusion scanning and coronary arteriography, Circulation 61:989, 1980.

18. Dunn RF, et al: Exercise-induced ST-segment elevation in leads V1 or aVL: a predictor of anterior myocardial ischemia and left anterior descending coronary artery disease, Circulation 63:1357, 1986.

19. El-Sherif N: The rsR' pattern in left surface leads in ventricular aneurysm, Br Heart J 32:440, 1970.

20. Eppinger H, Rothberger CJ: Zur analyse des Electrokardiogramms, Wien Klin Wochenschr 22:1091, 1909.

21. Eyster JAE, et al: Potential changes in an injured region of cardiac muscle, Am J Physiol 124:717, 1938.

22. Fortuin NJ, Friesinger GC: Exercise-induced S-T segment elevation: clinical, electrocardiographic, and arteriographic studies in twelve patients, Am J Med 49:459, 1970.

23. Fuller CM, et al: Exercise-induced coronary arterial spasm: angiographic demonstration, documentation of ischemia by myocardial scintigraphy, and results of pharmacologic intervention, Am J Cardiol 46:500, 1980.

24. Gewirtz H, et al: Role of myocardial ischemia in the genesis of stress-induced S-T segment elevation in previous anterior myocardial infarction, Am J Cardiol 51:1289, 1983.

25. Goldberger E: Unipolar lead electrocardiography and vectorcardiography, ed 3, Philadelphia, 1953, Lea & Febiger.

26. Gorlin R, et al: Prospective correlative study of ventricular aneurysm: mechanistic concept and clinical recognition, Am J Med 42:512, 1967.

27. Haines DE, et al: Exercise-induced ST segment elevation 2 weeks after uncomplicated myocardial infarction: contributing factors and prognostic significance, J Am Coll Cardiol 9:996, 1987.

28. Hellerstein HK, Katz LN: The effects of electrical injury at various myocardial locations, Am Heart J 36:184, 1948.

29. Heupler FA: Syndrome of symptomatic coronary arterial spasm with nearly normal coronary arteriograms, Am J Cardiol 45:873, 1980.

30. Holland RP, Brooks H: Precordial and epicardial surface potentials during myocardial ischemia in the pig, Circ Res 37:471, 1975.

31. Holland RP, Brooks H: TQ-ST segment mapping: critical review and analysis of current concepts, Am J Cardiol 40:110, 1977.

32. Huey BL, et al: Acute non-Q wave myocardial infarction associated with early ST segment elevation: evidence for spontaneous coronary repolarization and implications for thrombolytic trials, J Am Coll Cardiol 9:18, 1987.

33. Kléber AG, et al: Mechanism and time course of S-T and T-Q segment changes during acute regional myocardial ischemia in the pig heart determined by extracellular and intracellular recordings, Circ Res 42:603, 1978.

34. Krucoff MW, et al: Noninvasive detection of coronary artery patency using continuous ST-segment monitoring, Am J Cardiol 57:916, 1986.

35. Krumholz HM, Goldberger AL: Reperfusion arrhythmias after thrombolysis: electrophysiology tempest or much ado about nothing? Chest [suppl]99:1355, 1991.

36. Kwoczynski JK, et al: Electrocardiographic ischemic patterns without coronary artery disease, Dis Chest 39:305, 1961.

37. Kwon K, et al: The unstable ST segment early after thrombolysis for acute infarction and its usefulness as a marker of recurrent coronary occlusion, Am J Cardiol 67:109, 1991.

38. Lange RA, et al: Cocaine-induced coronary artery vasoconstriction, N Engl J Med 321:1557, 1989.
39. Lahiri A, et al: Exercise-induced S-T segment elevation in variant angina, Am J Cardiol 45:887, 1980.
40. Lew AS, et al: Exercise-induced precordial ST segment elevation due to right ventricular ischemia, Am Heart J 111:172, 1986.
41. Longhurst JC, Kraus WL: Exercise-induced ST elevation in patients without myocardial infarction, Circulation 60:616, 1979.
42. Luchi RJ, Chahine RA: Coronary artery spasm, Ann Intern Med 91:441, 1979.
43. MacAlpin RN: Correlation of the location of coronary arterial spasm with lead distribution of ST segment elevation during variant angina, Am Heart J 99:555, 1980.
44. Mandel WJ, et al: Analysis of T-wave abnormalities associated with myocardial infarction using a theoretic model, Circulation 38:178, 1968.
45. Manvi KN, Ellestad MH: Elevated ST segments with exercise in ventricular aneurysm, J Electrocardiol 5:137, 1972.
46. Mark DB, et al: Localizing coronary artery obstruction with the exercise treadmill test, Ann Intern Med 106:53, 1987.
47. Maseri A, et al: "Variant" angina: one aspect of a continuous spectrum of vasospastic myocardial ischemia, Am J Cardiol 42:1019, 1978.
48. Meller J et al: Transient Q waves in Prinzmetal's angina, Am J Cardiol 35:691, 1975.
49. Mills RM, et al: Natural history of S-T segment elevation after acute myocardial infarction, Am J Cardiol 35:609, 1975.
50. Nahum LH, et al: The injury current in the electrocardiogram, Am J Physiol 139:202, 1943.
51. Noble RJ, et al: Normalization of abnormal T waves in ischemia, Arch Intern Med 136:391, 1976.
52. Nosratian FJ, Froelicher VF: ST elevation during exercise testing, Am J Cardiol 63:986, 1989.
53. Oliva PB, et al: Coronary arterial spasm in Prinzmetal angina: documentation by coronary arteriography, N Engl J Med 288:745, 1973.
54. Pardee HEB: An electrocardiographic sign of coronary artery obstruction, Arch Intern Med 26:244, 1920.
55. Picano E, et al: Dipyridamole-echocardiography test in patients with exercise-induced ST segment elevation, Am J Cardiol 57:765, 1986.
56. Prinzmetal M, et al: Angina pectoris. I. A variant form of angina pectoris, Am J Med 27:375, 1959.
57. Prinzmetal M, et al: Myocardial ischemia: nature of ischemic electrocardiographic patterns in the mammalian ventricles as determined by intracellular electrographic and metabolic changes, Am J Cardiol 8:493, 1961.
58. Reimer KA, Jennings RB: Myocardial ischemia, hypoxia, and infarction. In Fozzard HA, et al (editors): The heart and cardiovascular system, New York, 1986, Raven Press.
59. Reynolds EW Jr, et al: Effect of acute myocardial infarction on electrical recovery and transmural temperature gradient in left ventricular wall of dogs, Circ Res 8:730, 1960.
60. Richardson SG, et al: Relation of coronary arterial patency and left ventricular function to electrocardiographic changes after streptokinase treatment during acute myocardial infarction, Am J Cardiol 61:961, 1988.
61. Roberts WC, et al: Sudden death in Prinzmetal's angina with coronary spasm documented by angiography: analysis of three necropsy patients, Am J Cardiol 50:203, 1982.
62. Rosenberg B, Messinger WJ: The electrocardiogram in ventricular aneurysm, Am Heart J 37:267, 1949.
63. Ross AM, et al: Electrocardiographic and angiographic correlations in myocardial infarction patients treated with thrombolytic agents. A report from the NHLBI Thrombolysis in Myocardial Infarction (TIMI) trial, J Am Coll Cardiol 2:495, 1985.
64. Ross J Jr: Electrocardiographic ST-segment analysis in the characterization of myocardial ischemia and infarction, Circulation 53(suppl 1):23, 1976.
65. Rubler S, et al: Exercise testing posmyocardial infarction using right-sided chest leads (V_4R and V_6R) to detect right ventricular ischemia, Am J Noninvas Cardiol 2:355, 1988.
66. Samson WE, Scher AM: Mechanism of S-T segment alteration during acute myocardial injury, Circ Res 8:780, 1960.

67. Selzer A, et al: Clinical syndrome of variant angina with normal coronary arteriogram, N Engl J Med 295:1343, 1976.

68. Shimokawa H, et al: Variable exercise capacity in variant angina and greater exertional thallium-201 myocardial defect during vasospastic ischemic ST elevation than with ST depression, Am Heart J 103:142, 1982.

69. Specchia G, et al: Significance of exercise-induced S-T segment elevation in patients without myocardial infarction, Circulation 63:46, 1981.

70. Sriwattanakomen S, et al: S-T segment elevation during exercise: electrocardiographic and arteriographic correlation in 38 patients, Am J Cardiol 45:762, 1980.

71. Stiles GL, et al: Clinical relevance of exercise-induced S-T segment elevation, Am J Cardiol 46:931, 1980.

72. Terradellas JB, et al: Acute and transient ST segment elevation during bacterial shock in seven patients without apparent heart disease, Chest 81:444, 1982.

73. Timmis GC: Electrocardiographic effects of reperfusion, Cardiol Clin 5:427, 1987.

74. Vincent GM, et al: Mechanisms of ischemic ST-segment displacement: evaluation by direct current recordings, Circulation 56:559, 1977.

75. Waters DD, et al: Coronary artery spasm during exercise in patients with variant angina, Circulation 59:580, 1979.

76. Waters DD, et al: Clinical and angiographic correlates of exercise-induced ST-segment elevation: increased detection with multiple ECG leads, Circulation 61:286, 1980.

77. Weiner DA, et al: ST segment elevation during recovery from exercise: a new manifestation of Prinzmetal's variant angina, Chest 74:133, 1978.

78. Willich SN, et al: High-risk subsets of patients with non-Q wave myocardial infarction based on direction and severity of ST segment deviation, Am Heart J 114:1110, 1987.

79. Yasue H, et al: Comparison of coronary arteriographic findings during angina pectoris associated with S-T elevation or depression, Am J Cardiol 47:539, 1981.

ST segment elevations: normal variants

ARTIFACTUAL ST ELEVATIONS

In assessing apparently pathologic ST elevations, one must always first exclude artifactual sources of error. Several artifactual sources of ST segment elevation are commonly seen.

Probably the most frequent source is a wandering baseline, which is usually induced by either movement or poor electrode contact. Fig. 9-1 shows a typical example of ST elevation caused entirely by upward movement of the baseline.

Artifactual ST segment elevation can also be produced by an overdamped ECG stylus (Fig. 9-2). Overdamping is recognized by the slurring it produces in the standardization (calibration) pulse, which normally is "squared off" at its peak. This can cause upward slurring of the J point, simulating ST elevation.

Poor skin-to-electrode contact in the precordial leads can cause artifactual ST elevations.[22] Artifactual elevation of the ST segment may also appear in conjunction with ventricular-triggered pacemakers (Fig. 9-3) and may be induced by bedside or ambulatory cardiac monitors with an inadequate low-frequency response[2,15] (Fig. 9-4) or a nonlinear phase response (p. 248).

A pseudo–current of injury pattern with prominent localized ST elevations in the left chest leads was reported after cardiac surgery when the epicardial ventricular pacing wires came into contact with the precordial electrodes.[2a]

Finally, the wide terminal R waves of right bundle branch block can create the misleading appearance of ST elevation (Fig. 4-9, *III*).

BENIGN (FUNCTIONAL) ST ELEVATIONS: EARLY REPOLARIZATION VARIANTS

The term *early repolarization* has been applied to two distinct and apparently benign ECG variants that may simulate the ST elevations of acute infarction or pericarditis.

1. *The left precordial early repolarization variant* (Figs. 9-5 to 9-7) is characterized by ST segment elevations in the midprecordial to left precordial leads and occasionally in one or more of the extremity leads. Prominent T

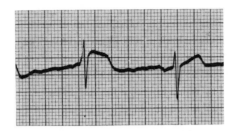

FIG. 9-1. Spurious ST elevation. In the first QRS-T complex, note that the ST is slightly elevated, suggesting acute ischemia; however, in the second QRS-T it has returned to normal. This distortion was produced by a movement artifact, which deflected the baseline upward.

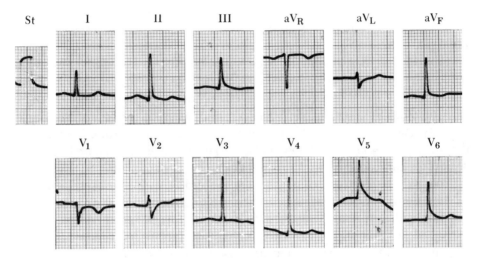

FIG. 9-2. Pseudoelevation of the ST caused by an overdamped stylus. Overdamping can be seen on the upstroke of the standardization mark *(St)*. It results in elevation and slurring of the J point (V_5 and V_6), with reciprocal J point depression in aV_L.

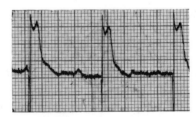

FIG. 9-3. Spurious ST elevations caused by a ventricular-triggered pacemaker. Note the similarity to a current of injury.

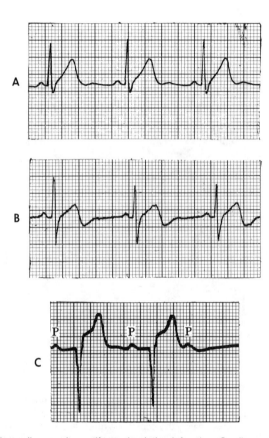

FIG. 9-4. Oscilloscopic cardiac monitor artifacts simulating infarction. Cardiac monitors used in clinical practice may produce distortions of the true ST-T morphology if their frequency response is not adequate. **A** and **B** were recorded sequentially from the same patient. The coved T wave inversions in **B** are an artifact produced by changing the balance of the electronic filters. **C** is a monitor strip showing pseudoinfarctional elevation of the ST. (The third P wave represents a blocked premature atrial depolarization.)

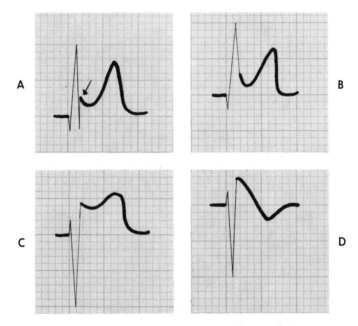

FIG. 9-5. Left and right precordial early repolarization patterns. **A** and **B,** Left precordial variants. With this benign type of early repolarization there are ST elevations in the middle to lateral precordial leads and in limb leads that have a positive QRS. The ST segment always retains its normal concave form and often is followed by a prominent T wave, simulating the hyperacute phase of infarction. The J point may be notched (*arrow* in **A**), giving the complex a qRsr′ appearance. In other cases (**B**) the ST segment may be smooth or slurred. **C** and **D,** Right precordial variants. With this pattern there are ST elevations in the right-sided chest leads. The ST may show a saddle-back or humpback morphology (**C**) or have a coved appearance with terminal T wave inversion (**D**). The QRS usually has an rSr′ configuration.

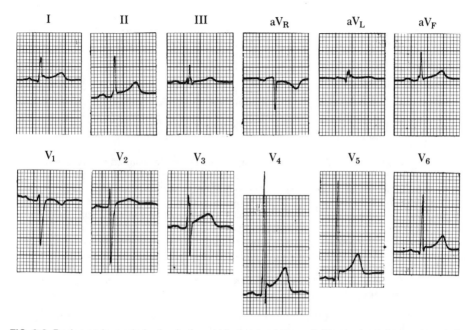

FIG. 9-6. Benign early repolarization in the middle to lateral precordial leads simulating acute anterior infarction or acute pericarditis. The patient is a healthy 20-year-old man. Note the prominent concave ST elevations in the middle to lateral leads (3 mm in V_4), with slight ST elevations in I, II, aV_L, and aV_F. Lead aV_R shows reciprocal ST depressions. Prominent QRS voltage in the precordial leads is a normal variant, particularly in young men. There is notching at the J point (seen best in V_4 and V_5), giving the QRS an Rsr' appearance. J point notching (Fig. 9-5, *A*) is characteristic of benign early repolarization, although in some cases the J point transition will have a smooth (slurred) contour (Figs. 9-5, *B,* and 9-7).

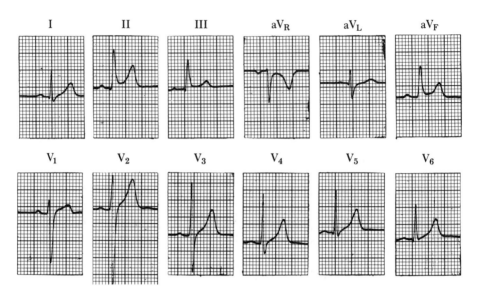

FIG. 9-7. Early repolarization ST elevations simulating acute inferior infarction in a healthy 17-year-old man. Note the smooth upwardly concave elevations in II, III, and aV$_F$, with reciprocal depressions in aV$_R$. These are a variant of the common left precordial early repolarization pattern. In most cases such elevations are best seen in the middle to lateral precordial leads. Occasionally, however, as in this case, they are most prominent in one or more limb leads where the QRS voltage is positive. ST elevations caused by benign early repolarization rarely if ever exceed 2 mm in the limb leads. (Here they are 1 mm in II.) Early repolarization ST elevations in the middle to lateral precordial leads sometimes reach about 3 mm. Benign early repolarization always produces concave elevation of the ST segment. In some cases there is characteristic notching of the QRS at the J point (Fig. 9-6); in others, such as this one, the J segment has a smooth or slurred contour. Such concave ST elevations also occur with acute infarction and acute pericarditis.

waves are also commonly associated with this pattern, simulating the hyperacute phase of infarction (see the discussion of tall positive T waves in Chapter 19).

There are also several reports of marked terminal T wave inversions associated with this pattern of early repolarization ST segment elevations (Figs. 15-2 and 15-3). This unusual pattern of benign ST elevations coupled with terminal T wave inversions is described in detail in Chapter 15.

2. *The right precordial early repolarization variant* (Figs. 9-5, 9-8, and 9-10) is characterized by ST elevations with a saddle-back (humpback) shape or ST-T complexes with a "coved" appearance in the right precordial leads.

These benign early repolarization variants are considered in detail in the following discussion.

Left Precordial Early Repolarization

Myers et al.[17] called attention to normal variant ST segment elevations (0.5 to 2 mm) in the precordial leads. Subsequently Goldman[6] reported more marked

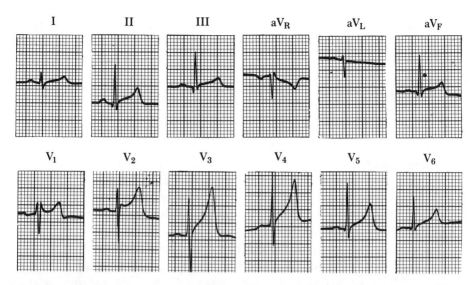

FIG. 9-8. Early repolarization ST elevations simulating acute infarction. This tracing, from a 34-year-old black man, illustrates both right and left precordial variants. V_1 and V_2 show the characteristic rSr' configuration followed by saddle-back ST elevations (Figs. 9-5, C, and 9-8). The ST segments also are elevated in the middle to lateral precordial leads and are followed by tall positive T waves simulating the hyperacute phase of infarction. Such T waves frequently occur with the left precordial early repolarization variant.

ST elevations (2 to 4 mm) in V_3 to V_6 in a group of 23 young, predominantly black, men without other clinical or laboratory evidence of cardiac disease. He suggested that these striking and apparently benign ST elevations were secondary to early repolarization. Chelton and Burchell[4] later described the same pattern in a group of predominantly white adults.

Although "early repolarization" of ventricular fibers has been cited as the basis for these normal variant ST segment elevations, their precise mechanism remains uncertain. Initially, this pattern was ascribed to early repolarization of the subepicardium.[4] Subsequent investigators[16] suggested that functional ST elevations reflected relatively earlier repolarization of the anterior wall of the ventricles compared to the posterior wall, mediated by regional differences in sympathetic tone or in sympathetic-parasympathetic balance. In dog studies[12] stimulation of the right cardiac nerve preferentially shortens refractory periods on the anterior surface of the heart and is associated with elevation of the ST segment in vector lead Y.* Further support for the theory that benign ST segment elevations reflect disparities in ventricular recovery time (probably mediated via the autonomic nervous system) is provided by the clinical observations that these

---

*The potential importance of the sympathetic nervous system in the genesis of other repolarization changes is discussed on pp. 297 to 303.

ST elevations return to isoelectric baseline during vigorous exercise or with iso-proterenol infusion but become more accentuated with propranolol administration.[16] Catecholamine stimulation, by globally shortening ventricular refractory periods, would be predicted to normalize differences in ventricular recovery time, whereas beta blockade might be expected to accentuate such regional differences. There is also a high prevalence of this pattern in subjects with intrinsic sympathetic dysfunction due to cervical spinal cord injury.[11] (See also p. 207.)

Of related interest is that ST segment elevations seen with myocardial infarction have also been ascribed to "early repolarization," based on observation of shortened action potentials in areas of acute ischemia.[24] The role, if any, of the sympathetic nervous system in the genesis of this pathologic early repolarization has not been defined (p. 190).

The concept that early repolarization is the mechanism underlying functional ST segment elevations is not without its critics. For example, Mirvis,[14] using ECG body surface mapping techniques, observed no apparent relationship between the degree of ST elevation in normal subjects and the time from the onset of ventricular recovery to the end of ventricular excitation. However, these results do not preclude regional differences in recovery time, which are related more to the termination of repolarization than to its onset.

In summary: Although functional disparities in regional ventricular repolarization appear to underlie the early repolarization variant, the exact mechanism is unresolved. The term *early repolarization pattern* should be considered synonymous with "benign" or "functional" ST segment elevations. Indeed, the two latter terms, which do not imply any mechanism, are probably preferable.

The basic characteristics of the pattern of these functional ST elevations (Figs. 9-5 to 9-7) include the following:

1. *Occurrence in the middle to left precordial leads.* ST segment elevations are typically greatest in V_3 to V_5 and may reach 3 or 4 mm. Those in V_6 tend to be less marked and rarely exceed 1 or 2 mm. More prominent ST deviations in V_6 imply acute myocardial infarction or pericarditis.[26] (See also p. 216 for a discussion of the ST segment/T wave amplitude ratio in V_6 in the differential diagnosis of early repolarization vs. pericarditis.) The limb leads may also show some degree of ST elevation. Normally this rarely if ever exceeds 2 mm; ST elevations exceeding these limits suggest either acute infarction or acute pericarditis. Occasionally the ST segment elevations are more prominent in the limb leads than in the precordial leads (Fig. 9-7). Reciprocal ST depressions in II, III, and aV_F are not a feature of benign early repolarization and suggest acute anterior infarction (Fig. 8-1). Slight reciprocal ST segment depressions, however, may be present in aV_R.

2. *Upwardly concave morphology.* The ST segments of early repolarization

appear to have been lifted evenly off the baseline, preserving the normal upward concavity of the J point,[31] as seen in Figs. 9-6 and 9-7. The ST segment elevations of both acute pericarditis and acute myocardial infarction may also retain this concave form. However, the straightened or convex ST segments (Fig. 8-2, *B* and *D*) frequently seen with acute infarction are not a feature of the benign early repolarization variant in the left precordial leads.

The J point in the early repolarization variant may show a contour that is either notched (Fig. 9-6, V_4) or smooth (Fig. 9-7).[31] The smooth J point is not distinguishable from the pattern seen with acute pericarditis or infarction. However, the notched J point is suggestive (though not diagnostic) of this pattern of benign ST elevation. Fig. 9-5 is a diagrammatic illustration of both the smooth and the notched J point variants. Note that when the notched J point is present the QRS complex has an Rsr' configuration and the ST segment has an elevated takeoff from the terminal r' wave.

3. *Prominent positive T waves.* Early repolarization ST segment elevations are frequently associated with tall vaulting T waves (Fig. 9-8), which may exceed 10 mm[30,31] and mimic the hyperacute phase of infarction (see Figs. 18-1 and 18-6).

4. *Temporal stability.* In contrast to the rapidly evolving ST-T changes of acute myocardial infarction or pericarditis, the elevated ST segments and prominent T waves seen with benign early repolarization generally remain fixed over long periods. Chelton and Burchell[4] reported one case in which they persisted for 24 years. In a longitudinal survey of subjects with the early repolarization variant,[9] 74% had some degree of ST segment elevation over many years of observation. The degree may be variable. For example, the ST segments often return to baseline transiently with exercise. Such lability caused by sympathetic tone or other factors may create the false impression of evolving ST segment changes.

5. *Response to exercise testing.* Benign early repolarization ST elevations frequently but not invariably return to the baseline transiently during treadmill testing or equivalent exercise (Fig. 9-9). This is in obvious contrast to the relatively fixed current of injury ST elevations seen with pericarditis and infarction. Goldman[6] and Chapman and Overholt[3] noted transient postexertional normalization of the ST segment in all subjects tested. Similarly, another study[17] reported "normalization" of ST elevation in 13 of 14 subjects with early repolarization pattern and normal coronary arteriograms. Fig. 9-9 illustrates the physiologic return of ST segments to baseline during exercise in a subject with the early repolarization variant. Wasserburger and Alt,[31] however, observed this effect in only about 60% of subjects.

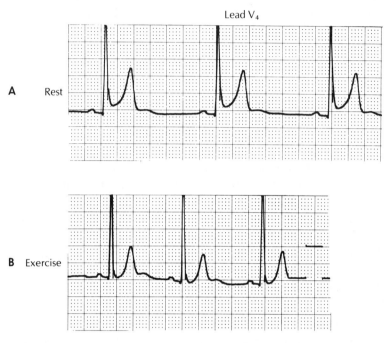

FIG. 9-9. A, Prominent normal-variant early repolarization pattern at rest. **B,** Return of the ST segments to their isoelectric baseline following exercise.

The presence of the early repolarization pattern does not preclude latent coronary artery disease. Of interest is one study[1] in which the two subjects with this pattern on their resting ECGs (which showed ≥1 mm ST depressions during exercise) were found to have significant coronary occlusions at arteriography.

6. *Response to hyperventilation.* Wasserburger and Alt[31] reported transient T wave inversions in precordial leads showing early repolarization ST elevations (Fig. 15-4). These changes were noted after brief (15-second) periods of hyperventilation in about two thirds of subjects tested. The posthyperventilatory T wave inversions had a striking coved plane appearance simulating that of ischemia, characterized by elevation of the ST segment followed by sharp, often deep, terminal inversion of the T wave. These posthyperventilatory T wave inversions in subjects with early repolarization are identical in morphology to the stable pattern of ST elevations and T wave inversions that has been reported as a normal variant (Fig. 15-2) and is described in Chapter 15. A similar pattern of deep terminal T wave inversions has been produced by applying cold packs to the chest walls of subjects with early repolarization ST elevations.[10,21]

The deep posthyperventilatory T wave inversions sometimes seen in subjects with early repolarization are much more prominent than the nonspecific ST-T changes (minimal T wave inversion or T wave flattening) most commonly observed in normal subjects after hyperventilation (Fig. 12-3). These nonspecific hyperventilatory changes are probably related to sympathetic stimulation producing an asynchronous shortening of repolarization in different areas of the myocardium (p. 246). It is not clear why such functional hyperventilatory repolarization changes should induce more marked T wave inversions in subjects with the early repolarization pattern.

7. *Effect of drugs.* Grusin[7] reported one case of transient ST "normalization" following the administration of amyl nitrite. However, Morace et al.[16] reported no change in this pattern with either amyl nitrite or atropine but noted that the ST segment became isoelectric following isoproterenol administration and more elevated with propranolol. Chelton and Burchell[4] reported no change subsequent to the administration of either atropine or methacholine (Mecholyl).

8. *Precordial QRS patterns.* The early repolarization variant is often associated with an early precordial transition zone.[31]

9. *Prevalence.* Benign ST elevations have been reported in all age groups, ranging from children[25] and adolescents[29] to adults in the seventh decade[31] or older. Seriki and Smith[25] found that the pattern is relatively rare in Nigerian children under 10 years of age and appears with increasing frequency through the second and third decades of life. The pattern is more common in males.[30]

   Benign ST elevations of varying amplitudes are a universal ECG variant and have been reported in Japanese,[18] Indians,[27] and Africans,[7,25] as well as in American blacks and whites.[30,31] The pattern appears to be most prevalent in black males for unknown reasons. For example, ST elevations of 2 mm or more were noted in 34% of young Nigerian males whose average age was 24 years[25] and in 27% of American blacks 20 to 40 years of age.[30] In contrast, a review of 50,000 ECGs from clinically normal Air Force personnel (99% white) revealed ST segment elevations in less than 3% of cases.[20]

   Benign ST elevations are a common finding in athletes.[8,12] Additional features of the athlete's ECG simulating organic heart disease are discussed on pp. 283 and 320.

   Lehmann et al.[11] reported this pattern in 13 of 20 middle-aged males with complete chronic injury to the spinal cord at the C5 to C8 level. Of note, these subjects all had total disruption of central sympathetic outflow. Decreased ST segment elevation was observed following exogenous catecholamine infusion (isoproterenol) but not with exercise (arm ergometer) in this group.

10. *Differentiation from acute pericarditis.* See pp. 211 to 216.

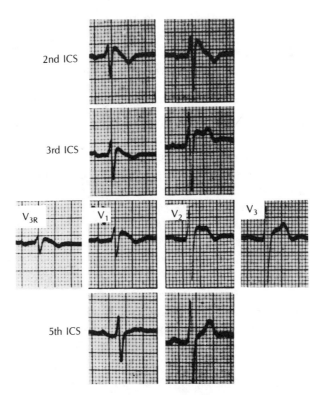

FIG. 9-10. Right precordial early repolarization variant simulating acute anteroseptal infarction. This tracing, from a healthy 32-year-old man, illustrates some morphologic variants of benign ST elevations in the right precordial leads. In some (e.g., V_1) the ST elevations have a sharp downward slope (coved appearance) with terminal inversion of the T wave. In others (V_2) there is a characteristic saddle-back or humpback shape. The QRS in some leads (e.g., V_2) has a characteristic rSr' configuration that is seen typically with this pattern. *ICS,* Intercostal space. (From Marriott HJL: Practical electrocardiography, ed 8, Baltimore, 1988, The Williams & Wilkins Co.)

Right Precordial Early Repolarization

The term *early repolarization* has also been used to describe a distinct pattern of benign ST elevations in the right precordial leads.[18,22]

The elevated ST segment in the right precordial leads may have a saddleback (humpback) appearance (Figs. 9-5, *C*, 9-8, and 9-10), or the ST-T complex may show a coved shape with terminal inversion of the T wave (Figs. 9-5, *D*, and 9-10). The coved ST-T complex is often most evident in leads taken above the normal V_1 or V_2 position, for example, the second or third interspace (Fig. 9-10). It is usually associated with an rSr′ type of complex in the right precordial leads (Figs. 9-8 and 9-10). The left precordial and limb leads show normal QRS and ST-T complexes. Occasionally both left precordial and right precordial early repolarization ST elevations are seen together (Fig. 9-8).

The pattern of benign right precordial ST elevations was first noted by Osher and Wolff[19] in three clinically normal subjects. The authors suggested that these functional ST elevations could have been produced either by early repolarization or by a right ventricular conduction defect (accounting for the rSr′ pattern). Similar examples were subsequently reported by others[5,23,28] in patients whose ages ranged from the 30s to the 80s. In one case in which an autopsy was performed,[28] the heart was entirely normal. This pattern, like that of benign left precordial ST elevations, appears to be stable over time.[5] Its prevalence has not been determined, but it appears less common than the left precordial early repolarization pattern just described.

There are no reports concerning the effect of exercise, hyperventilation, or pharmacologic agents on right precordial ST elevations, nor is there any definite substantiation for the claim that they are in fact caused by early repolarization.

Similar saddle-back ST elevations in the right precordial leads have been reported in association with poor skin-to-electrode contact,[22] improper ECG stylus damping, and hyperkalemia (Chapter 10).

REFERENCES

1. Alimurung BN, et al: The influence of early repolarization variant on the exercise electrocardiogram: a correlation with coronary arteriograms, Am Heart J 99:739, 1980.
2. Arbeit SR, et al: Dangers in interpreting the electrocardiogram from the oscilloscope monitor, JAMA 211:453, 1970.
2a. Bilazarian SD: Pseudoinfarction pattern on electrocardiogram after coronary-artery bypass, Chest 98:1271, 1990.
3. Chapman DW, Overholt E: Acute benign idiopathic pericarditis: a report of twenty cases, Arch Intern Med 99:708, 1957.
4. Chelton LG, Burchell HB: Unusual RT segment deviations in the electrocardiograms

of normal persons, Am J Med Sci 230:54, 1955.
5. Edeiken J: Elevation of the RS-T segment, apparent or real, in the right precordial leads as a probable normal variant, Am Heart J 48:331, 1954.
6. Goldman MJ: RS-T segment elevation in the mid- and left precordial leads as a normal variant, Am Heart J 46:817, 1953.
7. Grusin H: Peculiarities of the African's electrocardiogram and changes observed in serial studies, Circulation 9:860, 1954.
8. Hanne-Paparo N, et al: Common ECG changes in athletes, Cardiology 61:267, 1976.

9. Kambara H, Phillips J: Long-term evaluation of early repolarization syndrome (normal variant RS-T segment elevation), Am J Cardiol 38:157, 1976.

10. Kaminer B, Bernstein RE: Electrocardiographic and plasma potassium responses elicited on cooling the chest wall of man, Circulation 15:559, 1957.

11. Lehmann KG, et al: Altered ventricular repolarization in central sympathetic dysfunction associated with spinal cord injury, Am J Cardiol 63:1498, 1989.

12. Kralios FA, et al: Local ventricular repolarization changes due to sympathetic nerve-branch stimulation, Am J Physiol 228:1621, 1975.

13. Lichtman J, et al: Electrocardiogram of the athlete: alterations simulating those of organic heart disease, Arch Intern Med 132:763, 1973.

14. Mirvis DM: Evaluation of normal variations in S-T segment patterns by body surface isopotential mapping: S-T segment elevation in absence of heart disease, Am J Cardiol 50:122, 1982.

15. Mirvis DM, et al: Instrumentation and practice standards for electrocardiographic monitoring in special care units, Circulation 79:464, 1989.

16. Morace G, et al: Effect of isoproterenol on the "early repolarization" syndrome, Am Heart J 97:343, 1979.

17. Myers GB, et al: Normal variations in multiple precordial leads, Am Heart J 34:785, 1947.

18. Nakamoto K: The Cornell Medical Index in patients with concave RS-T elevations in the mid- and left precordial leads and new questionnaires specifically designed for actual neurosis, Jap Circ J 30:1031, 1966.

19. Osher HL, Wolff L: Electrocardiographic pattern simulating acute myocardial injury, Am J Med Sci 226:541, 1953.

20. Parisi AF, et al: The spectrum of ST segment elevation in the electrocardiograms of healthy adult men, J Electrocardiol 4:137, 1971.

21. Rahman SA, et al: Effect of cooling the anterior chest wall on the T wave of the electrocardiogram, Am Heart J 47:394, 1954.

22. Rees PH: The ST segment in the electrocardiogram of young adults, East Afr Med J 48:622, 1971.

23. Roesler H: An electrocardiographic study of high take-off of the R(R')-T segment in the right precordial leads: altered repolarization, Am J Cardiol 6:920, 1960.

24. Samson WE, Scher AM: Mechanism of S-T segment alteration during acute myocardial injury, Circ Res 8:780, 1960.

25. Seriki O, Smith AJ: The electrocardiogram in young Nigerians, Am Heart J 72:153, 1966.

26. Spodick DH: Differential characteristics of the electrocardiogram in early repolarization and acute pericarditis, N Engl J Med 295:523, 1976.

27. Srikantia SG, et al: The electrocardiogram in some Indian population groups, Circulation 29:118, 1964.

28. Stein I, Weinstein J: High RS-T take-off in patients without myocardial infarction, NY J Med 58:2213, 1958.

29. Strong WB, et al: The normal adolescent electrocardiogram, Am Heart J 83:115, 1972.

30. Thomas J, et al: Observations on the T wave and S-T segment changes in the precordial electrocardiogram of 320 young Negro adults, Am J Cardiol 5:468, 1960.

31. Wasserburger RH, Alt WJ: The normal RS-T segment elevation variant, Am J Cardiol 8:184, 1961.

ST segment elevations: abnormal noninfarctional causes

ACUTE PERICARDITIS

The classic ECG pattern of acute pericarditis consists of ST segment elevations followed during the subacute or chronic phases by T wave inversions. This sequence simulates the pattern of repolarization changes seen in conjunction with acute infarction. The ECG differential diagnosis can often be made on the basis of the following criteria:

1. *Topography (distribution) of ST-T changes* (Figs. 10-1 and 10-2).[36] The ST elevations and subsequent T wave inversions seen with pericarditis are characteristically *diffuse,* in contrast to the *localized* pattern of ST-T changes seen with acute infarction. The ST segment elevations of acute pericarditis are usually found in I, II, aV_L and aV_F, and V_2 to V_6. Reciprocal ST depression may be seen in aV_R and sometimes V_1. With acute infarction, however, the ST elevations are generally confined to either I and aV_L (anterior infarction) or II, III, and aV_F (inferior infarction), and there are often reciprocal ST depressions in the contralateral leads.

   The ST elevations of acute pericarditis, like those of acute myocardial infarction, represent a current of injury pattern. With pericarditis this pattern is caused by inflammation of the superficial epicardial layers, which usually are involved in the pericardial process. The nonlocalized distribution of ST-T changes with pericarditis reflects this diffuse epicarditis.[36] The epicardial injury current (ST segment) vector is oriented inferiorly and leftward toward the left ventricular apex, as reflected by the ST segment elevations typically seen in the lateral chest leads and in I and II as well as by the reciprocal ST depressions in aV_R.[33]

   Occasionally pericarditis will be associated with more localized ST segment elevations (Fig. 10-3) simulating the regional current of injury pattern seen with acute myocardial infarction or Prinzmetal's angina[3] (Chapter 8).

2. *Atrial injury current patterns of acute pericarditis.* Acute pericarditis not only causes inflammation of the ventricular surface, it frequently induces atrial inflammation as well. The atrial involvement, in turn, may

211

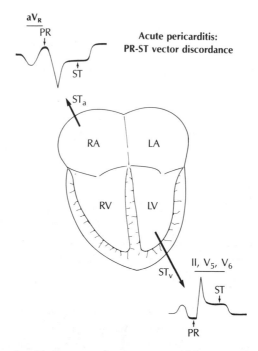

FIG. 10-1. With acute pericarditis there are often two apparent injury currents: one generated by atrial injury, the other by ventricular injury. The atrial injury current vector (ST_a) is usually directed upward and to the right, producing PR segment elevations in aV_R with reciprocal depressions in II, V_5, and V_6. The ventricular injury current (ST_v) is directed downward and to the left, causing ST elevations in II, V_5, and V_6 with reciprocal depressions in aV_R. (See Figs. 10-2 and 10-3 for examples of this characteristic PR-ST vector discordance.)

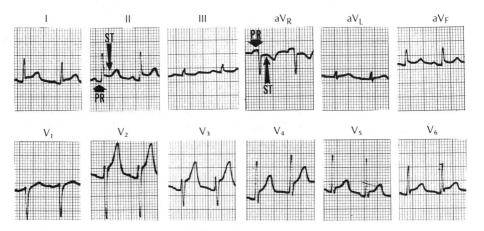

FIG. 10-2. Acute pericarditis causing diffuse ST elevations in I, II, aV_F, and V_2 to V_6, with reciprocal depressions in aV_R. The atrial current of injury, by contrast, causes PR elevations in aV_R with reciprocal depressions in the left chest leads and II.

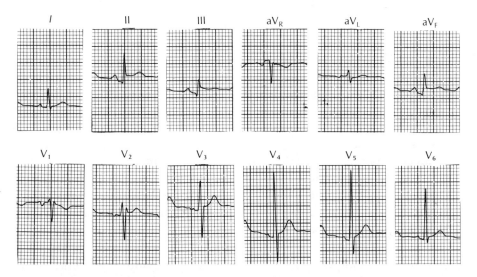

FIG. 10-3. Acute idiopathic pericarditis with more localized ST elevations in II, III, and aV$_F$ simulating an acute inferior wall infarct. Note the characteristic PR segment changes (elevation in aV$_R$, depression in the inferolateral chest leads). Compare with Fig. 10-2.

generate an atrial current of injury associated with deviation of the atrial ST segment.[3,32,33] The atrial ST segment (ST$_a$) corresponds to the PR segment (between the end of the P wave and beginning of the QRS complex). Thus the ST$_a$ deviation reflects an atrial injury current exactly analogous to the ventricular injury current responsible for ST elevation seen with pericarditis. Furthermore, acute pericarditis is associated with a characteristic *discordance* between the PR segment (up in aV$_R$, down in the left chest leads) and ST segment (down in aV$_R$, up in II and the left chest leads), as shown in Figs. 10-1 to 10-3 and 19-6.

With acute pericarditis the atrial injury current vector is oriented superiorly and to the right, accounting for the PR elevations in aV$_R$ and the reciprocal PR depressions in the inferolateral leads (e.g., II, aV$_F$, V$_5$, V$_6$). These can range from ≤0.5 to about 2 mm in the more marked examples (Fig. 10-2). In one series,[32] characteristic PR deviations were noted in 82% of cases of acute pericarditis.

Atrial repolarization changes with PR deviations are not specific for acute pericarditis, They may be seen also with atrial infarction (p. 23) or other types of atrial injury. For example, similar PR segment changes have been reported with surgical and mechanical atrial trauma[9] as well as with metastatic atrial tumor.[14,29] Slight (usually ≤1 mm or less) deviation of the PR segment may also occur in the absence of atrial disease, particularly with increased sympathetic tone and tachycardia.[37] However, the *combination* of the PR and ST segment changes described here (Figs. 10-1 to 10-3) is highly specific for acute pericarditis.

3. *Abnormal Q waves.* Acute pericarditis affects only the repolarization process. The epicardial injury that occurs does not cause enough loss of myocardial potentials to result in Q waves. The sudden appearance of Q waves with ST-T changes is usually indicative of infarction but may also occur with *acute myocarditis* (Chapter 6). Noncoronary Q waves have been described in association with chronic constrictive pericarditis[18] (Chapter 7).

4. *Amplitude of ST elevations.*[36] With pericarditis the ST elevations are usually 5 mm or less above the baseline. ST segment elevations greater than 5 mm are more common with acute infarction, reflecting the greater degree of myocardial damage. Relatively subtle ST elevations are also common with acute ischemia (Fig. 11-7). Rarely acute pericarditis will produce ST elevations with tall positive T waves simulating those of the hyperacute phase of infarction (Fig. 19-6).

5. *ST segment morphology.*[2,36,41] The ST segment with acute pericarditis is elevated at the J point and usually retains its normal concavity (Fig. 10-2). In some cases it will rise obliquely in a straight line. Similar changes may occur with acute myocardial infarction (Fig. 8-2, *A*). However, the dome-shaped (convex) ST segment of infarction (Fig. 8-2, *D*) is not characteristic of pericarditis. The basis of these morphologic differences is not known but probably relates to the greater injury current associated with infarction.

6. *T wave inversions.* The inverted T waves seen during the healing (subacute or chronic) stages of pericarditis often have a symmetric "coronary T wave" shape[22] (Fig. 10-4). This similarity probably reflects a common underlying mechanism. In both instances myocardial injury delays repolarization of the epicardium, which leads to a reversal in the normal direction of repolarization.[36] With pericarditis the inverted T waves are generally of small amplitude (less than 5 mm) (Fig. 10-4). Rarely do deeper T wave inversions occur, simulating those of infarction[41] (Fig. 10-5).

7. *Sequence of ST-T changes.* With pericarditis the evolution of repolarization abnormalities often takes place more slowly and more asynchronously than with acute infarction.[36] Leads facing an infarcted area tend to show the same stage of ST-T evolution. With pericarditis, the myocardial injury is more diffuse and different areas of myocardium reflect different stages in the pattern of repolarization abnormalities; therefore various degrees of T wave inversion or ST segment elevation can be present concurrently in different leads.

Furthermore, with pericarditis the T wave inversions generally occur after the ST segment has returned to baseline.[11] By contrast, T wave inversions with an evolving infarct frequently have an elevated ST segment, producing the characteristic deep coved plane (Fig. 14-4). However, as shown in Fig. 9-4, exceptions do occur.

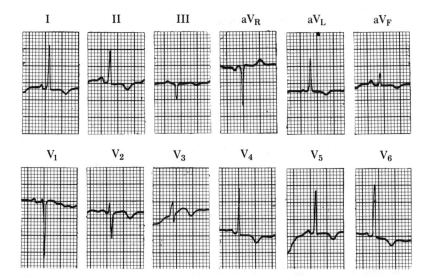

FIG. 10-4. Pericarditis simulating diffuse ischemia. This tracing from a 32-year-old woman shows symmetric T wave inversions. The patient died following acute pericardial tamponade. At autopsy a generalized pericardial and epicardial inflammation of undetermined cause was found. The coronary arteries were normal. The T wave inversions are similar in morphology to the pattern seen with subacute or chronic pericarditis (Fig. 14-4). Recall that inverted T waves with acute pericarditis are rarely deeper than 5 mm and are not associated with pathologic Q waves. (The QS in III here is a physiologic variant.)

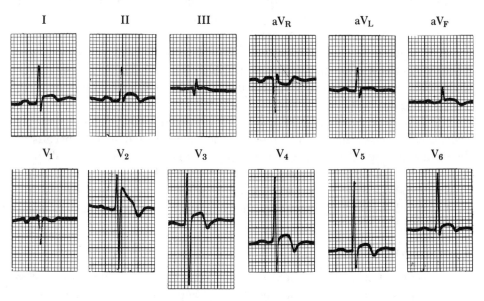

FIG. 10-5. Pericarditis simulating extensive ischemia. Note the diffuse ST elevations with reciprocal depressions in aV$_R$ and V$_1$ on this tracing from a 26-year-old black man with chest pain. Notice also the deep T wave inversions with a coved plane morphology (Fig. 14-4). The diffuse nature of these T wave inversions, plus the absence of prolonged QT intervals, makes them more typical of pericarditis than of myocardial infarction.

8. *QT interval.* Delayed repolarization caused by myocardial injury often produces deeply inverted T waves with a prolonged repolarization time (QT interval). In acute pericarditis a smaller mass of myocardium is injured, and an increased QT interval is generally not observed[11,31,36] (Fig. 10-5).

9. *Concurrent patterns.* Pericardial effusion associated with acute pericarditis may produce low voltage on the ECG or occasionally total electrical alternans. The sudden appearance of low voltage, particularly with sinus tachycardia, should always suggest possible pericardial effusion. Total electrical alternans (involving the P, QRS, and T) is diagnostic of pericardial effusion, usually with tamponade physiology.[26]

Thus pericarditis and myocardial infarction may present similar repolarization abnormalities (ST segment elevations followed by T wave inversions) caused by the direct myocardial injury occurring in both conditions. However, because a greater surface area of epicardium is involved in pericarditis, ST changes are usually more diffuse, as opposed to the localized pattern with reciprocal changes characteristic of myocardial infarction. (Occasionally pericarditis will produce localized ST elevations and deep T wave inversions indistinguishable from those that accompany infarction.) With pericarditis less of the total thickness of myocardium is injured, so the ST-T changes are of smaller amplitude and abnormal Q waves are not seen in uncomplicated cases.*

It should be noted that pericarditis may also occur as a complication of myocardial infarction. In such cases the ECG generally shows the pattern of acute infarction, including in most but not all cases new Q waves with localized ST-T changes. Sometimes (Fig. 21-2) more diffuse ST elevations reflecting a generalized pericarditis will be superimposed on the pattern of infarction. (The diagnosis of acute pericarditis complicating acute infarction is discussed in more detail in Chapter 21.)

The ECG pattern of acute pericarditis is also commonly confused with normal-variant ST elevations (early repolarization pattern, Chapter 9) because of the diffuse nature of the deflections in both settings.[34] Ginzton and Laks[13] observed that the ratio of ST segment elevation amplitude to T wave amplitude in V_6 was the single best ECG discriminator between these two patterns, with an ST/T ratio of 0.25 or greater being more suggestive of pericarditis (compare Figs. 9-6 and 10-2).

ACUTE MYOCARDITIS

As discussed on p. 127, acute myocarditis can cause ST segment elevations (and Q waves) indistinguishable from those of acute ischemia or infarction.

---

*Anterior lead Q waves with right axis deviation were reported in two patients with large posterior pericardial effusions after cardiac surgery. R wave progression normalized after pericardiocentesis.[30] It is uncertain whether this apparent pseudoinfarct pattern was caused by a positional effect or other factor. Q waves may occur with chronic constrictive pericarditis (p. 158).

HYPERKALEMIA

Severe hyperkalemia occasionally produces ST segment elevations that simulate those of acute myocardial infarction.[4,5,12,19,39] Hyperkalemia may also be associated with transient pseudoinfarctional Q waves (p. 133) and with tall positive T waves simulating the hyperacute phase of infarction (p. 334). The ST elevations with severe hyperkalemia are usually most notable in the right precordial leads and aV_R (Figs. 6-2, A, and 10-6, A); there are sometimes reciprocal ST depressions in the lateral precordial leads and, less frequently, ST segment elevations in the lateral precordial leads as well.[4]

Moderate ST depression in the left precordial leads with slight ST elevation in the right precordial leads has been described as a regular feature of the ECG in patients with moderately advanced hyperkalemia.[19,30] However, the more pronounced pseudoinfarctional changes described here are relatively rare.

The right precordial ST elevations seen with marked hyperkalemia often have a distinctive saddle-back appearance. Terminal inversion of the T wave may also be present in these leads (Fig. 10-6, A). A similar pattern of benign saddle-back ST elevations in the right precordial leads also has been described as a normal variant. (See Fig. 9-8 and the discussion of right precordial early repolarization in Chapter 9.)

Etiology. The etiology of hyperkalemic ST elevations has not been resolved. Levine et al.[19] described three cases of hyperkalemia (serum potassium levels between 7.8 and 8.6 mEq/L) with marked ST elevations in the right precordial leads and aV_R. These diminished or disappeared completely in all three cases following successful dialysis and were attributed to a transient current of injury produced by the increased extracellular potassium concentration.

Experimentally both direct local application of potassium ions to the epicardium[15] and perfusion of the coronary arteries with potassium solutions[17] have produced ST segment elevations identical to those associated with an ischemic current of injury. The noninfarctional ST elevations seen in these experimental cases have been attributed to the lowered membrane resting potential, which results from the local increase in extracellular potassium concentration. In actual infarction a similar depolarizing effect may be produced by ischemic cell membrane damage that allows a leakage of myocardial potassium ions to the extracellular fluid.[23]

However, the pattern of ST deviations most often seen with hyperkalemia (ST elevations in the right precordial leads, reciprocal depressions in the lateral leads) is not consistent with a typical current of injury pattern (diffuse ST elevations). Surawicz[35] therefore suggested that these hyperkalemic ST alterations do not represent a primary current of injury but are secondary to the intraventricular conduction disturbance usually seen with marked hyperkalemia. For example, ST segment elevations in the right precordial leads with reciprocally depressed lateral ST segments may occur with left bundle branch block, simulating the pattern of acute anteroseptal infarction (p. 103). However, the ST el-

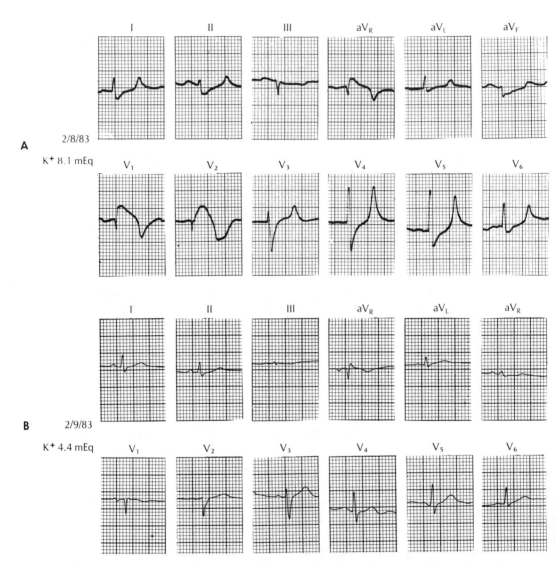

FIG. 10-6. Severe hyperkalemia associated with diabetic acidosis causing an anterior wall pseudoin-farct pattern. **A,** Note the ST elevations in V_1 and V_2 along with slightly widened QRS complexes and the peaked T waves in V_3 to V_6. **B,** Resolution of these changes the following day after correction of the serum potassium level.

evations reported with hyperkalemia are not always associated with marked widening of the QRS[19] (Fig. 10-6, A).

In some of the case reports of hyperkalemic ST elevations, other factors (hypotension, acute cor pulmonale, acute pericarditis) were also present and may have contributed to the ST alterations.[12,19]

The acidosis usually seen in patients with severe hyperkalemia probably does not contribute significantly to the current of injury pattern. In an experimental study Altschule and Sulzbach[1] observed transient ST elevations in two patients who were ventilated with 5% carbon dioxide, producing respiratory acidosis. However, subsequent observations in animals[27] and humans[25] have failed to document pseudoinfarctional ECG changes attributable to acidosis per se. Nevertheless, acidosis may act to potentiate the ECG changes of hyperkalemia since hydrogen ions are exchanged for intracellular potassium ions and this increases the extracellular concentration of potassium.

Differential diagnosis. Morphologically the ST changes seen with hyperkalemia may be indistinguishable from the pattern of true infarction. Hyperkalemia may also sometimes produce transient Q waves (Fig. 6-2) (described in Chapter 6).

Generally hyperkalemic ST elevations are most prominent in the right precordial leads. Elevations in the left precordial leads strongly suggest underlying ischemia or pericarditis. Most important, *the acute ST-T changes attributable to hyperkalemia should always resolve when serum potassium levels are restored to normal* (Fig. 10-6, B).

Although hyperkalemia may be associated with pseudoinfarctional Q waves and ST-T alterations, *hypokalemia* does not produce "transmural" infarct patterns. Occasionally the deep ST depressions associated with marked hypokalemia will mistakenly suggest subendocardial ischemia (Fig. 12-6).

HYPOTHERMIA (J WAVES)

The effect of cold on the heart has been of interest for many years. Wilson and Finch[40] described increased T wave negativity in II and III that was recorded when a patient drank 600 ml of cold water. Similarly, an increase in T wave negativity, occasionally with deep T wave inversions, has been produced in the precordial leads by applying cold packs to the chest.[16,24] These alterations are probably secondary to regional prolongation of repolarization caused by the local myocardial exposure to cold.[35]

The experimental application of cold to the heart is associated with relatively nonspecific ST-T changes. Systemic hypothermia, however, produces a distinctive ECG pattern that may be mistaken for acute myocardial ischemia (Fig. 10-7).

Extreme hypothermia (especially with body temperatures below 90° F [32°

C]) is associated with a distinctive elevation of the J segment (J wave, Osborn wave, hypothermic hump) that may simulate primary ischemic ST elevation. This J elevation is a convex waveform at the junction of the QRS deflection and ST segment (Fig. 10-7). Its amplitude is related generally to the degree of hypothermia: the wave becomes more prominent with lower internal temperatures and less prominent with rewarming. A small residual J wave may persist, however, when euthermia is restored.* Reciprocal J point depression appears in aV_R and sometimes V_1. The J wave is usually most notable in the midprecordial and lateral precordial leads, and its elevation may reach striking amplitude. For example, Emslie-Smith, Sladden, and Stirling[10] reported a J point elevation of 21 mm in V_3 in a patient whose body temperature was 88° F (31° C).

In addition to this characteristic J wave, other common ECG manifestations of profound hypothermia[7,10,38] include (1) muscle tremor artifact, (2) bradycardia, (3) prolonged PR and QT intervals, (4) T wave inversions (sometimes greater than 5 mm and usually most notable in leads with prominent J waves), and (5) serious arrhythmias including atrial fibrillation and ventricular fibrillation.

Morphologically the J wave differs from the usual current of injury pattern that causes elevation of the entire ST segment rather than just the initial J point. It has been suggested that cooling the myocardium may slow the depolarization and repolarization processes at different rates, producing a change in the balance of electrical forces when the J wave is inscribed. Such alteration in repolarization could theoretically produce J point elevation in a manner analogous to the way early repolarization is thought to produce ST segment elevation in myocardial infarction.[10]

The significance of the J wave in hypothermia is still unresolved. Debate centers on whether this waveform is part of the ST segment and reflects altered repolarization or whether it is part of the QRS complex and represents a terminal delay in depolarization. Osborn[21] suggested that J waves represent a current of injury caused by the acidosis of hypothermia. He was able to block their appearance by maintaining a normal body pH in hypothermic animals. However, J waves can appear even with a controlled pH.[10] Clements and Hurst[7] supported the view that the J wave is part of the QRS complex and represents a delay in terminal depolarization of the inferior and basal portions of the left ventricle. However, morphologically the J wave often appears to be part of the ST segment (Fig. 10-7).

Clinically the J point elevation of hypothermia must be distinguished from actual ischemic ST alterations. The Osborn wave causes elevation mainly of the initial portion of the ST segment. Infarction causes elevation of the entire ST

---

*References 7, 10, 20, 21, 35, 38.

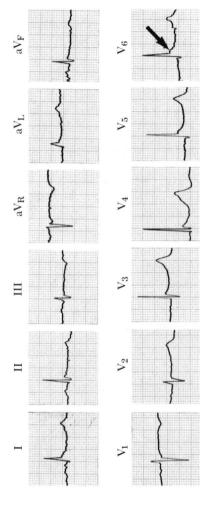

FIG. 10-7. Hypothermia simulating acute anterolateral wall infarction. This tracing is from a 52-year-old alcoholic woman who wandered away from her room on a cold night. When found, she had a rectal temperature below 92° F (33.3° C). J point elevations, best seen in the lateral precordial leads (*arrow* in V₆) are a characteristic finding (see text). Their mechanism is uncertain. However, they disappear with rewarming and must be distinguished from a true ischemic current of injury. In addition to J waves, note the sinus bradycardia (approximately 40/min), marked QT interval prolongation, and somatic tremor artifact. This combination is virtually pathognomonic of hypothermia.

segment. Furthermore, the J wave is related to internal body temperature and should always diminish in amplitude as the patient is rewarmed. The associated T wave inversions should also resolve. Finally, abnormal Q waves are *never* caused by hypothermia alone. The appearance of Q waves and ST-T changes in a hypothermic patient indicates true infarction.

By way of summary: A large J deflection is virtually pathognomonic of hypothermia. Smaller J point humps have also been reported with subarachnoid hemorrhage[8] and in normal subjects.[28] However, the combination of J waves, bradycardia, muscle tremor artifact, and QT prolongation is virtually diagnostic of systemic hypothermia (Fig. 10-7).

DC CARDIOVERSION

Transient noninfarctional ST segment elevation occurs infrequently following DC cardioversion (Fig. 10-8). Chun, Davia, and Donohue[6] reported three patients (with an age range of 22 to 68 yr) who manifested ST segment elevations following attempted cardioversion of atrial fibrillation. In all cases multiple incremental shocks were administered, with ST elevations noted after 100 to 400 joules. Myocardial infarction was excluded by negative technetium-99m-pyrophosphate scans and normal creatine kinase isoenzymes. Similarly, Zelinger, Falk, and Hood[42] reported one patient with ST segment elevation in lead II lasting only 90 seconds after multiple incremental countershocks. The ST changes were first noted after a 320-joule countershock. The mechanism of these transient repolarization changes is unknown but may be related to local depolarization of ventricular fibers leading to a current of injury.[42]

OTHER CAUSES OF ST ELEVATIONS

Other noncoronary causes of ST elevations are described elsewhere in this book—in the sections dealing with left ventricular hypertrophy (ST segment elevations in right precordial leads), acute cor pulmonale (ST elevations in inferior limb and right precordial leads), idiopathic hypertrophic subaortic stenosis (precordial ST elevations), left bundle branch block (right precordial leads), acute myocarditis, acute metabolic injury (transient ST elevations with reversible ischemia, scorpion sting toxin, etc.), cerebrovascular hemorrhage or related injury, cardiac echinococcal cyst (rarely simulates ventricular aneurysm), cardiac tumor (rarely simulates aneurysm), and cardiac sarcoidosis.

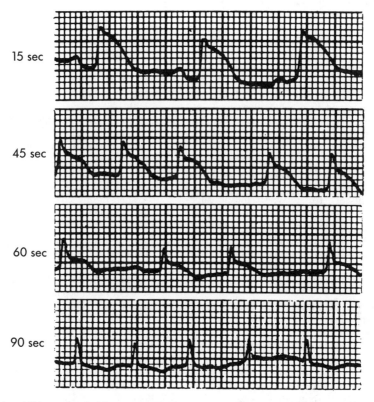

FIG. 10-8. Lead II immediately after cardioversion showing transient ST elevations and the rapid sequential return to baseline within 90 seconds. (From Zelinger AB, et al: Am Heart J 103:1073, 1982.)

REFERENCES

1. Altschule MD, Sulzbach WM: Tolerance of the human heart to acidosis: reversible changes in RS-T interval during severe acidosis caused by administration of carbon dioxide, Am Heart J 33:458, 1947.
2. Barnes AR, Burchell HB: Acute pericarditis simulating acute coronary occlusion: report of 14 cases, Am Heart J 23:247, 1942.
3. Bruce M, Spodick DH: Atypical electrocardiogram in acute pericarditis: characteristics and prevalence, J Electrocardiol 13:61, 1980.
4. Castleman L, et al: Selected electrocardiographic changes during acute renal failure and hemodialysis, Am J Cardiol 12:841, 1963.
5. Chawla KK, et al: Electrocardiographic changes simulating acute myocardial infarction caused by hyperkalemia: report of a patient with normal coronary arteriograms, Am Heart J 95:637, 1978.
6. Chun PKC, et al: ST-segment elevation with elective DC cardioversion, Circulation 63:220, 1981.
7. Clements SD, Hurst JW: Diagnostic value of electrocardiographic abnormalities observed in subjects accidentally exposed to cold, Am J Cardiol 29:729, 1972.
8. De Sweit J: Changes simulating hypothermia in the electrocardiogram in subarachnoid hemorrhage, J Electrocardiol 5:193, 1972.
9. Dicosky C, Zimmerman HA: Atrial injury, J Electrocardiol 2:51, 1969.
10. Emslie-Smith D, et al: The significance of the changes in the electrocardiogram in hypothermia, Br Heart J 21:343, 1959.
11. Friedman HH: Diagnostic electrocardiography and vectorcardiography, ed 2, New York, 1971, McGraw-Hill Book Co.
12. Gelzayd EA, Holzman D: Electrocardiographic changes of hyperkalemia simulating acute myocardial infarction: report of a case, Dis Chest 51:211, 1967.
13. Ginzton LE, Laks MM: The differential diagnosis of acute pericarditis from normal variant: new electrocardiographic criteria, Circulation 65:1004, 1982.
14. Goldberger AL, Ludwig M: Metastatic atrial tumor: case report with electrocardiographic-pathologic correlation, J Electrocardiol 11:297, 1978.
15. Hellerstein HK, Katz LN: Electrical effects of injury at various myocardial locations, Am Heart J 36:184, 1948.
16. Kaminer B, Bernstein RE: Electrocardiographic and plasma potassium responses elicited on cooling the chest wall of man, Circulation 15:559, 1957.
17. Kwoczynski JK, et al: Electrocardiographic ischemic patterns without coronary artery disease, Dis Chest 39:305, 1961.
18. Levine HD: Myocardial fibrosis in constrictive pericarditis: electrocardiographic and pathologic observations, Circulation 48:1268, 1973.
19. Levine HD, et al: Dialyzable currents of injury in potassium intoxication resembling acute myocardial infarction, Circulation 13:29, 1956.
20. Osborn JJ: Experimental hypothermia: respiratory and blood pH changes in relation to cardiac function, Am J Physiol 175:389, 1953.
21. Phillipson E, Herbert FA: Accidental exposure to freezing: clinical and laboratory observation during convalescence from near-fatal hypothermia, Can Med Assoc J 97:786, 1967.
22. Porte D, Pardee HEB: The occurrence of the coronary T wave in rheumatic pericarditis, Am Heart J 4:584, 1929.
23. Prinzmetal M, et al: Myocardial ischemia: nature of ischemic electrocardiographic patterns in the mammalian ventricles as determined by intracellular electrographic and metabolic changes, Am J Cardiol 8:493, 1961.
24. Rahman SA, et al: Effect of cooling the anterior chest wall on the T wave of the electrocardiogram, Am Heart J 47:394, 1954.
25. Reid JA, et al: The effect of variations in blood pH upon the electrocardiogram, Am Heart J 47:394, 1954.
26. Rigney DR, Goldberger AL: Non-linear mechanics of the heart's swinging during pericardial effusion, Am J Physiol 257:H1292, 1989.
27. Roberts KE, Magida MG: Electrocardiographic alterations produced by decrease in plasma pH, bicarbonate, and sodium as compared with those produced by increase in potassium, Circ Res 1:206, 1953.

28. Rothfield EL: Hypothermic hump [Letter to the editor], JAMA 213:626, 1970.

29. Rothfield EL, Zirkin RN: Unusual electrocardiographic evidence of metastatic cardiac tumor resembling atrial infarction, Am J Cardiol 10:882, 1962.

30. Salem BI, et al: Electrocardiographic pseudo-infarction pattern: appearance with a large posterior pericardial effusion after cardiac surgery, Am J Cardiol 42:681, 1978.

31. Soffer A: Electrocardiographic abnormalities in acute, convalescent, and recurrent stages of idiopathic pericarditis, Am Heart J 60:729, 1960.

32. Spodick DH: Diagnostic electrocardiographic sequences in acute pericarditis: significance of PR segment and PR vector changes, Circulation 48:575, 1973.

33. Spodick DH: Electrocardiogram in acute pericarditis: distributions of morphologic and axial changes by stages, Am J Cardiol 33:470, 1974.

34. Spodick DH: Differential characteristics of the electrocardiogram in early repolarization and acute pericarditis, N Engl J Med 295:523, 1976.

35. Surawicz B: ST-T abnormalities. In Macfarlane PW, Lawrie TDV (editors): Compre-

hensive electrocardiology. Theory and practice in health and disease, New York, 1989, Pergamon Press Inc, vol 1.

36. Surawicz B, Lasseter KC: Electrocardiogram in pericarditis, Am J Cardiol 26:471, 1970.

37. Tranchesi J, et al: Atrial repolarization: its importance in clinical electrocardiography, Circulation 22:635, 1960.

38. Trevino A, et al: The characteristic electrocardiogram of accidental hypothermia, Arch Intern Med 127:470, 1971.

39. Weintraub LR, Reynolds EW: Electrocardiographic changes simulating myocardial infarction in potassium intoxication, Univ Mich Med Bull 26:348, 1960.

40. Wilson FN, Finch R: The effect of drinking iced water upon the form of the T deflection of the electrocardiogram, Heart 10:275, 1923.

41. Wolff L: Acute pericarditis simulating myocardial infarction, N Engl J Med 230:422, 1944.

42. Zelinger AB, et al: Electrical-induced sustained myocardial depolarization as a possible cause for transient ST elevation post–DC elective cardioversion, Am Heart J 103:1073, 1982.

Review 2: Differential diagnosis of ST segment elevations (Chapters 8 through 10)

Too often ST segment elevations are assumed to be pathognomonic of acute myocardial ischemia or infarction. However, a number of other causes must be considered. The differential diagnosis of ST segment elevations is summarized as follows:

1. Artifactual or spurious (e.g., baseline movement, ventricular-triggered pacemakers)
2. Normal variants: "early repolarization" pattern
3. Myocardial ischemia or infarction
   a. Acute noninfarctional transmural ischemia (Prinzmetal's angina)
   b. Acute infarction
   c. Chronic infarction: ventricular aneurysm
4. Acute pericarditis
5. Acute myocarditis
6. Left bundle branch block or left ventricular hypertrophy (right precordial leads)
7. Miscellaneous: hyperkalemia (right precordial leads), hypothermia (J waves), acute cor pulmonale (inferior limb leads and right precordial leads), DC cardioversion, myocardial tumor, echinococcal cyst, sarcoidosis, cerebrovascular hemorrhage or related injury

There are many causes of ST elevations besides acute myocardial infarction. From a clinical viewpoint the most commonly encountered ones are normal variants ("early repolarization"), ischemic heart disease, acute pericarditis, and in the right precordial leads left bundle branch block or left ventricular hypertrophy. *Familiarity with the differential diagnosis of ST elevations is essential for all clinicians, particularly those who must decide about the indications for thrombolytic therapy.*

Even in patients with coronary artery disease, ST elevations cannot be considered diagnostic of acute infarction. Transient ST elevations may occur with coronary vasospasm (Prinzmetal's variant angina) and persistent elevations with ventricular wall motion abnormalities. ST elevations during exercise testing (stress electrocardiography) may also occur without active ischemia after a Q wave infarct or, less commonly, as a sign of acute transmural ischemia without prior infarction due to a high-grade coronary lesion or to coronary vasospasm with or without a high-grade obstructive lesion (Chapter 8).

The topography of ST elevations may be of value in their differential diagnosis. Elevations limited to the right precordial leads suggest anteroseptal ischemia or right ventricular ischemia caused by coronary artery disease or occasionally by acute cor pulmonale. Right ventricular infarction generally is accompanied by evidence of concomitant inferior or posterior ischemia (p. 358). Left bundle branch block is commonly associated with noninfarctional ST elevations in the right precordial leads, often with tall positive T waves. A similar pattern of ST segments with a high takeoff is seen with left ventricular hypertrophy. Hyperkalemia is a rarer cause of such elevations in the right precordial leads. Normal individuals commonly have benign ST elevations in the right precordium as part of the early repolarization variant.

ST elevations in the midprecordial to left precordial leads may be due to a number of factors besides anterior wall ischemia. Benign "early repolarization" is probably the most common cause of noninfarctional elevations. In contrast to acute anterior myocardial infarction, reciprocal ST depressions in II, III, and aV_F are *not* seen with benign early repolarization or acute pericarditis. Acute pericarditis typically causes diffuse ST elevations whereas systemic hypothermia may be associated with J point elevations (J waves, Osborn waves), most notable in the midprecordium to lateral precordium.

In terms of underlying electrophysiologic mechanisms, ST elevations on the surface ECG may be related to more than one factor. For example, with myocardial injury caused by infarction, pericarditis, or myocarditis, the resulting elevations have been attributed to both systolic and diastolic injury currents, reflecting early repolarization or diastolic depolarization (respectively) of ventricular fibers. Regional disparities in ventricular repolarization time may also underlie the ST elevations seen as a normal variant ("early repolarization" pattern) or accompanying hyperkalemia, left bundle branch block, and left ventricular hypertrophy.

Finally, it should be recognized that ST elevations in one or more of the inferior limb leads (II, III, aV_F) or anterior leads (I, aV_L, V_1 to V_6) *cannot* be interpreted as a reciprocal change related to the presence of ST depressions from subendocardial ischemia. The only lead that consistently shows such elevations with subendocardial ischemia is aV_R. Furthermore, as will be discussed in Chapter 11, these ST elevations are not actually reciprocal but are primary since they represent orientation of the subendocardial injury current vector superiorly and rightward (i.e., toward the positive pole of aV_R) (Fig. 11-9). Ischemic ST elevations (as opposed to depressions) should always be considered a *primary*, not a reciprocal, repolarization effect.

ST segment depressions: ischemic causes

ST segment depressions, an important sign of myocardial ischemia, appear in three major clinical settings: (1) subendocardial ischemia without infarction, (2) non–Q wave myocardial infarction (traditionally* referred to as "subendocardial" or "nontransmural" infarction), and (3) transmural ischemia or infarction associated with *primary* ST elevation and *reciprocal* ST depressions.

ST depressions are generally considered an indicator of subendocardial ischemia, in contrast to the pattern of ST elevations (with reciprocal ST depressions) that accompanies subepicardial (and transmural) ischemia. ST depressions occurring in the context of subendocardial ischemia have also been referred to as the *coronary insufficiency pattern*.[28] The pathophysiology of ischemic ST segment depressions is described in more detail later in this chapter.

SUBENDOCARDIAL ISCHEMIA WITHOUT INFARCTION

Transient ST depressions are an important sign of noninfarctional ischemia. They may occur spontaneously in typical angina pectoris attacks (Fig. 11-1) or be induced during exercise stress testing (Fig. 13-1) or other provocative interventions, such as dipyridamole- or adenosine-thallium testing. Documentation of increased ST depression during an episode of chest pain is highly suggestive of ischemic heart disease. However, not all patients with typical angina pectoris will have ST depressions during pain. Furthermore, patients may have no symptoms when their ECG shows these ischemic ST changes. The important topic of *silent ischemia* is discussed in Chapter 12. The special problems of evaluating ST segment changes in the context of exercise testing are discussed in Chapter 13. Additional problems related to the sensitivity of the ECG in detecting myocardial ischemia are discussed in Chapter 20.

As shown in Figs. 11-1 and 11-2, the ST depressions that occur with subendocardial ischemia are typically horizontal or downsloping. The ST segment and

---

*The diagnosis of subendocardial versus transmural infarction on the basis of the ECG is discussed in Chapter 2.

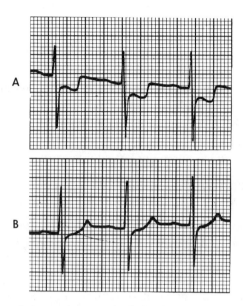

FIG. 11-1. ST depressions during angina pectoris. **A,** Lead V₄ recorded during chest pain. **B,** Five minutes later, after sublingual nitroglycerin. Note the ST normalization. (From Goldberger AL, Goldberger E: Clinical electrocardiography, ed 4, St Louis, 1990, The CV Mosby Co.)

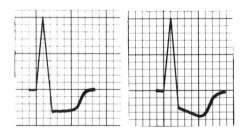

FIG. 11-2. ST depressions with subendocardial ischemia (coronary insufficiency pattern). Note that the appearance is typically squared off or downsloping. Slowly upsloping ST segments also may be seen (Chapter 13). (From Goldberger AL, Goldberger E: Clinical electrocardiography, ed 4, St Louis, 1990, The CV Mosby Co.)

T wave appear melded together, giving the ST-T complex a characteristic squared-off contour. In some cases, instead of being truly depressed the ST segment will be only subtly "straightened" during ischemic episodes (Fig. 11-3). However, transient minimal ST straightening is nonspecific and may be seen in many other settings, such as hyperventilation or digitalis effect (p. 272). In contrast to the localized pattern occurring with transmural infarction, ST depressions with subendocardial ischemia are often diffuse and present in both the anterior and the inferior leads (Fig. 11-4). ST elevations may be seen in aV_R and are traditionally considered to reflect a primary subendocardial current of injury whereas depressions in the precordial and limb leads represent reciprocal changes. ST segment depressions associated with angina pectoris are typically of short duration and resolve within 20 minutes. More prolonged ST-T changes may be seen with unstable angina or actual myocardial infarction.

NON–Q WAVE ("SUBENDOCARDIAL" OR "NONTRANSMURAL") INFARCTION

The controversial topic of electrocardiographic changes with subendocardial infarction is introduced in Chapter 2. Although pathologic Q waves may occur with nontransmural infarction, necrosis limited to the inner rind of the ventricle (roughly the inner half) often does not produce them (p. 21). However, non–Q wave infarctions may be associated with significant repolarization (ST-T) changes, including (1) ST depressions identical to the pattern just described with transient subendocardial ischemia, (2) T wave inversions with or without ST depressions, and (3) ST elevations.

The ST depressions of non–Q wave infarction[8,24,44] have the same general characteristics as those of transient ischemia (Fig. 11-5). The major difference is that with actual infarction they tend to be more persistent and may last for hours or days, in contrast to the rapid normalization seen with angina pectoris or exercise stress testing.

Another repolarization pattern that may occur with non–Q wave infarction is T wave inversions (Fig. 14-2) with or without ST depression.[8,34] (The pathogenesis of ischemic T wave inversions is described in Chapter 14.) They are thought to indicate delayed subepicardial repolarization. However, autopsy data on patients with clinical evidence of infarction and ECGs showing T wave inversions without new Q waves may reveal subendocardial infarction.[11] In such cases it seems most likely that the T wave inversions do in fact reflect subepicardial (and transmural) ischemia, but actual infarction is limited to the hemodynamically more vulnerable subendocardium[34] (p. 276). Therefore the common clinical notion that subendocardial infarction *causes* T wave inversions is not fully correct. Nevertheless, the diagnosis of infarction can be *inferred* when

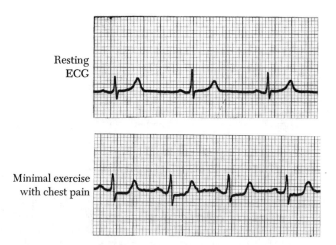

FIG. 11-3. Subtle straightening of the ST segments as a sign of ischemia. Compare the *resting* with the *exercise* ECG from this patient with coronary artery disease.

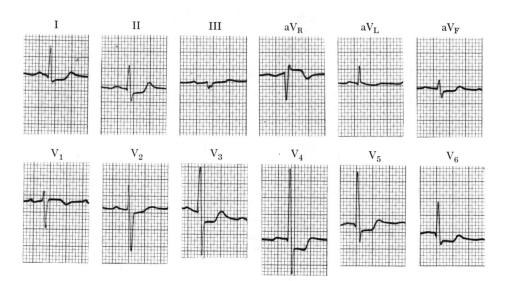

FIG. 11-4. Diffuse ST depressions during an episode of unstable angina. Note the horizontal or downsloping depressions in I, II, aV$_L$, aV$_F$, and V$_2$ to V$_6$, with ST elevations in aV$_R$.

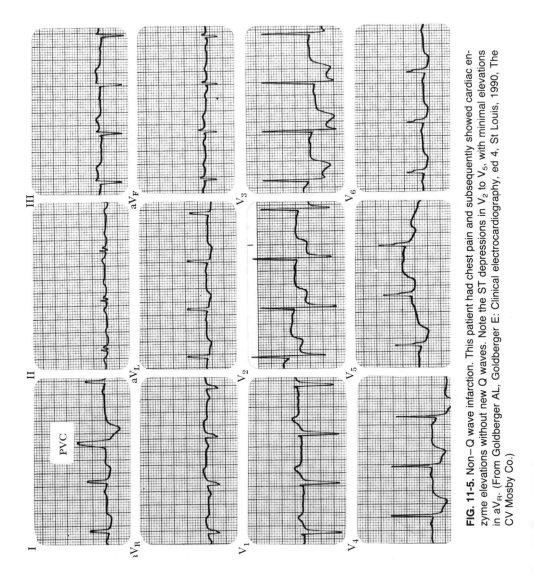

FIG. 11-5. Non–Q wave infarction. This patient had chest pain and subsequently showed cardiac enzyme elevations without new Q waves. Note the ST depressions in V_2 to V_5, with minimal elevations in aV_R. (From Goldberger AL, Goldberger E: Clinical electrocardiography, ed 4, St Louis, 1990, The CV Mosby Co.)

there is clinical evidence of myocardial necrosis (e.g., prolonged chest pain, elevated cardiac enzymes) and the ECG shows new T wave inversions without new Q waves. The T wave inversions in such cases may reflect some degree of transmural *ischemia* occurring with frank subendocardial necrosis.

Finally, the paradoxical association of ST elevations, due to transmural ischemia, with non−Q wave ("subendocardial") infarction is discussed more completely on p. 177.

TRANSMURAL INFARCTION WITH RECIPROCAL ST DEPRESSIONS

Reciprocal ST depressions are also an important feature of the ECG pattern of acute myocardial infarction[16,40] (described in Chapter 1), seen in leads facing the uninjured myocardial surface. Thus inferoposterior myocardial infarction is characterized by primary ST elevations in II, III, and aV_F and sometimes by reciprocal ST depressions in one or more of the anterior leads (I, aV_L, and V_1 to V_4) (Fig. 11-6). Conversely, acute anterior infarctions may be associated with reciprocal ST changes in II, III, and aV_F (Fig. 8-1). With a localized posterior infarct (Fig. 3-11) reciprocal ST depressions are generally recorded in the right and middle precordial leads (V_1 to V_3).

Morphologically these reciprocal ST depressions are indistinguishable from the ones seen with actual subendocardial ischemia. In both cases they have a horizontal or downsloping contour. Occasionally the reciprocal changes with acute transmural infarction will be more pronounced than the primary ST elevations (Fig. 11-7). In such cases the mistaken diagnosis of primary subendocardial ischemia can be made. Fig. 3-11, from a patient with acute posterior infarction, shows ST depressions in V_1 to V_4 that could also be misinterpreted as a sign of primary anterior subendocardial ischemia, when they are actually reciprocal to an acute posterior wall current of injury.[5]

Reciprocal ST segment depressions are *not* seen in all cases of acute infarctions.[29] The clinical and theoretical significance of repolarization changes, particularly of ST segment depression in the anterior leads with acute inferior infarction, has become the subject of intense investigation and some controversy in recent years.* The two major issues are (1) whether patients with an acute inferior wall infarction and ST depressions in the anterior leads have more extensive infarction than those without associated ST depressions and (2) whether such ST depressions are predominantly a reciprocal ("mirror image") change or indicate concomitant anterior subendocardial ischemia ("ischemia at a distance") due to multivessel disease.

---

*References 2-6, 9, 10, 12-14, 19, 20, 23, 25, 29, 30, 35-39.

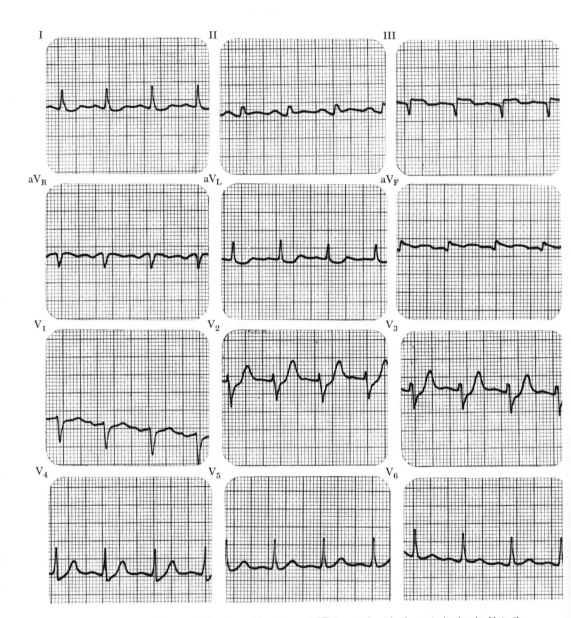

FIG. 11-6. Acute inferior wall infarction with reciprocal ST depressions in the anterior leads. Note the ST elevations and Q waves in the inferior limb leads. Reciprocal depressions occur also in I, aV_L, and V_2 to V_4. (From Goldberger AL, Goldberger E: Clinical electrocardiography, ed 4, St Louis, 1990, The CV Mosby Co.)

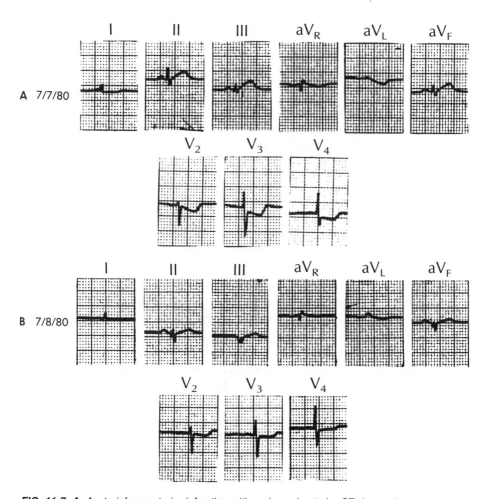

FIG. 11-7. A, Acute inferoposterior infarction with reciprocal anterior ST depressions more apparent than the subtle primary hyperacute changes evidenced by a relative increase in T wave positivity in II, III, and aV_F. The orientation of the current of injury vector in an anterior-to-posterior direction, relatively perpendicular to the frontal plane, may account for the predominance of reciprocal changes. **B,** One day later. Q waves have appeared in the inferior leads. (From Goldberger AL, Erickson R: PACE 4:709, 1981.)

Most[13,14,19,23,30] but not all[10,35] studies have suggested that acute inferior wall infarctions with prominent (e.g., >1 mm) ST depressions in the anterior leads are larger than (often with posterior and lateral involvement) and have a poorer prognosis compared to infarctions without associated ST depressions. However, differences in clinical outcome among reports are not surprising given the heterogeneity of the patient populations studied, whether the reciprocal changes were sought in more localized (e.g., V_1 to V_4) or more diffuse (V_1 to V_6, I, aV_L) lead sets, and the length of time the ST depressions persisted. For example, Lembo et al.[23] reported that ST depressions in one or more of V_1 to V_4 were only indicative of reduced left ventricular function and higher mortality if these repolarization changes persisted for 24 hours.

Clinical studies of isolated acute inferior wall infarction[10,13,14,30] as well as observations during balloon angioplasty of the right and left circumflex coronary arteries[42] have disproved the contention that anterior ST depressions imply anterior ischemia or left anterior descending coronary disease[36] (ischemia at a distance). Instead, the data are generally in accord with the classic notion that an inferoposterior-type infarct can produce purely reciprocal ST depressions in one or more anterior leads, reflecting displacement of the injury current (ST) vector away from the noninfarcted (anterior) zone. However, in the case of relatively small localized inferior wall infarcts, the ST vector will tend to be displaced relatively perpendicular to the plane of the anterior chest leads (Fig. 11-8, A), and as a result little or no reciprocal changes can be anticipated. By contrast, more extensive inferoposterior or inferolateral infarcts may displace the ST vector at greater than 90 degrees vis-à-vis the positive poles of the anterior precordial leads, resulting in more prominent reciprocal ST depressions[6,12,38,40] (Fig. 11-8, B). This theory agrees with the clinical data just cited showing that reciprocal ST depressions with inferior wall infarcts do, in fact, correlate with relatively larger infarcts that have more likelihood of lateral and posterior extension.

However, the magnitude of these reciprocal changes must always be interpreted with caution in individual patients, because numerous other factors (cardiac position, chest geometry, ventricular hypertrophy, metabolic status) can alter the orientation and magnitude of the ST vector. (See also pp. 192 and 193.) Furthermore, concomitant acute right ventricular ischemia can actually attenuate the degree of reciprocal precordial ST depressions with acute inferior infarction.[25]

Boden et al.[4] reported that precordial ST depressions during transmural inferior infarction may also be associated with a septal wall motion abnormality by radionuclide imaging. This study deliberately excluded patients with evidence of concomitant posterior or lateral involvement. The authors concluded, therefore, that selective inferior or posteroseptal ischemia or infarction in the absence of extensive posterior or lateral involvement was another explanation for the apparently "reciprocal" ST depressions observed in some of these patients.

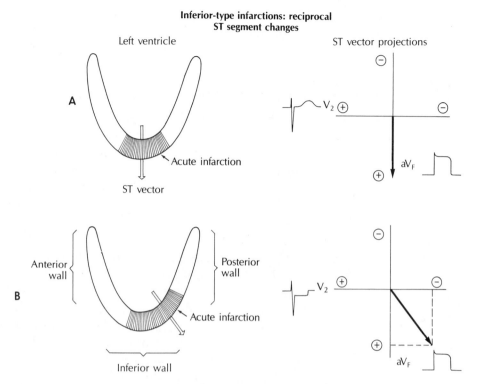

FIG. 11-8. A, With isolated inferior wall infarcts the current of injury *(ST)* vector will tend to be oriented directly toward the positive pole of aV$_F$ and at right angles to the V$_2$ axis; thus reciprocal ST depressions in that lead would not be anticipated. **B,** With more extensive inferoposterior infarcts, however, the current of injury vector will likely be displaced posteriorly so it projects onto both the negative axis of V$_2$ and the positive axis of aV$_F$; as a result, reciprocal ST depressions in V$_2$ will be recorded.

By way of review, the following points summarize the association of precordial ST segments with acute *inferior* wall infarction:

1. In most instances, ST depressions in V$_1$ to V$_3$ or V$_4$ constitute a reciprocal effect and are not the result of concomitant anterior subendocardial ischemia. (However, in *any* patient the question of whether prominent ST depressions in the anterior leads solely reflect reciprocal changes or also indicate some degree of anterior ischemia cannot usually be answered with certainty from a single ECG alone.)*

2. Reciprocal ST depressions are likely to occur with extensive inferior ischemia involving the lateral or posterior walls, but they also may occur with more limited inferior or inferoseptal infarcts.

---

*Ischemic ST depressions in V$_5$ and V$_6$ with acute inferior wall infarctions are not likely to be purely reciprocal but instead suggest concomitant lateral or apical subendocardial ischemia.

3. In some cases of acute inferoposterior or inferolateral infarcts, the reciprocal changes may be more apparent than the primary changes, leading to the mistaken diagnosis of "acute anterior subendocardial infarction."[5,38]

PATHOPHYSIOLOGY OF PRIMARY ISCHEMIC ST DEPRESSIONS

There are two conflicting theories regarding the pathogenesis of the primary ST segment depressions associated with subendocardial ischemia and non–Q wave infarction (coronary insufficiency pattern): (1) the classic theory of a subendocardial current of injury and (2) the theory advanced by Prinzmetal and his colleagues that the subendocardium is electrically silent and the ST depressions recorded by surface electrocardiography reflect relatively mild epicardial ischemia causing cellular hyperpolarization.

According to classic theory the ST depressions seen with transient or infarctional ischemia are the reciprocal of a primary subendocardial current of injury.[1,18,33,43] Recall (Chapter 8) that acute epicardial injury produces ST elevations (current of injury) in leads overlying or reflecting the injured myocardial surface. Analogously it has been suggested that primary subendocardial injury can generate a similar injury current. However, in contrast to the epicardial current of injury, the subendocardial ST vector is oriented toward the ventricular cavity and away from leads reflecting the epicardial surface (Fig. 11-9). Consequently, primary subendocardial ischemia should produce reciprocal ST depressions in the precordial leads and limb leads (except for aV_R). Actual ST elevation may be recorded in aV_R, reflecting the rightward and superior orientation of the ST vector with subendocardial injury. (Lead aV_R therefore is sometimes considered a "cavity lead," recording potentials similar to those from the atrial and ventricular cavities.)

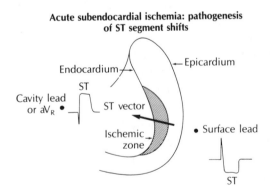

Acute subendocardial ischemia: pathogenesis of ST segment shifts

FIG. 11-9. With acute subendocardial ischemia the current of injury *(ST)* vector will be oriented away from the epicardium toward the subendocardium and ventricular cavity. As a result, cavity leads or aV_R will record ST elevations while surface leads record ST depressions. (Modified from Becker RC, Alpert JS: Am Heart J 115:862, 1988.)

This classic theory of a primary subendocardial current of injury is premised on two key assumptions: (1) that subendocardial ischemia may occur in the absence of subepicardial ischemia and (2) that the subendocardium can generate an injury current and is not electrically silent.

The subendocardium does appear to be more vulnerable to ischemia than the subepicardium. First, subendocardial vessels are "throttled" during ventricular systole by the high pressure of the subjacent cavity.[7] Therefore subendocardial perfusion is confined primarily to diastole. Second, subendocardial flow may be reduced because of limited vasodilatory reserve.[17] Normally subendocardial vessels are more dilated than those in the epicardium. With ischemia, blood may actually be shunted away from the subendocardium to the epicardium, which has greater vasodilatory capacity. Using microsphere techniques to measure coronary flow in experiments with dogs, Guyton et al.[17] found that perfusion of the subepicardial layers was maintained even when subendocardial flow was reduced to as much as 25% of its baseline level.

There are also several lines of experimental data that suggest that the ischemic subendocardium can generate a current of injury and therefore is not electrically silent. For example, an electrode pressed against the subendocardium will elicit ST elevations similar to those recorded with local epicardial injury. Early experiments by Hellerstein and Katz,[18] Pruitt, Burchell, and Essex,[33] and Wolferth et al.[43] made use of mechanical and chemical injury to the subendocardium. In these studies ST elevations were recorded by local subendocardial or cavity electrodes while reciprocal ST depressions were observed at epicardial sites. Subsequently Zakopoulos, Herrlich, and Lepeschkin[45] produced subendocardial injury with a bioptome and recorded reciprocal ST depressions at overlying precordial sites. However, in a number of these experiments the degree of reciprocal epicardial ST depressions was minimal. Furthermore, it may be misleading to extrapolate results of localized chemical or mechanical subendocardial injury in dogs to the clinical setting of ischemia.

More convincing data to support the subendocardial injury current theory were reported by Guyton et al.[17] in the experiments just mentioned. These investigators produced subendocardial ischemia with normal subepicardial flow (confirmed by microsphere measurements) by means of coronary stenosis and tachycardia in dogs. During the studies electrodes placed in the subendocardium recorded a marked current of injury whereas overlying epicardial electrodes recorded apparently reciprocal ST depressions of lesser amplitude. Similarly, MacAlpin and Cabeen[26] recorded ST elevations with intracavitary ventricular leads during atrial pacing studies in patients with ischemic heart disease. Simultaneously recorded precordial leads showed ST depressions. In some cases, however, precordial ST depressions were noted without concomitant ST elevations in the ventricular cavity.

A divergent theory of ischemic ST segment depressions was proposed by Prinzmetal et al.,[32] challenging the classic concept of a subendocardial injury current. They suggested that the subendocardium is electrically "silent" and ischemic ST depressions are caused by relatively mild epicardial injury leading to myocardial hyperpolarization. This countervailing theory was based on the following observations of experimental infarction in dogs:

1. With acute transmural infarction epicardial electrodes record ST elevations, in contrast to the relatively small injury current recorded from the "silent" subendocardial layer.[27]

2. During acute transmural infarction ST elevations were recorded by electrodes placed in the central cyanotic zone whereas ST depressions were recorded in peripheral areas of milder ischemia. With reperfusion of the central ischemic zone the ST elevations were sometimes replaced by depressions.[11]

3. During experimental hypotension "islands" of ST segment depressions were recorded by epicardial leads, whereas no injury current was recorded by simultaneous intracavitary leads.[11]

4. Increased membrane resting potential (hyperpolarization) was directly recorded by intracellular electrodes placed in areas of relatively mild ischemia associated with ST depressions on the surface ECG.[32]

5. Coronary perfusion with low concentrations of potassium chloride also produced cellular hyperpolarization and ST depressions.[11,32]

Based on these experimental findings, Toyoshima et al.[41] proposed a unified theory of ischemic ST deviations suggesting that both ST elevations and ST depressions are caused by epicardial injury currents. With severe epicardial ischemia, it was theorized that there would be potassium loss and cellular depolarization with consequent ST elevations (p. 191). By contrast, mild epicardial ischemia as a result of hypotensive episodes or coronary insufficiency or in areas peripheral to an infarct might lead to increased uptake of potassium by cells, resulting in myocardial hyperpolarization and ST depression.

This theory relating ST segment depressions to epicardial ischemia is not inconsistent with the clinical observation that ST depressions are associated with severe subendocardial ischemia or infarction. The subendocardium is more vulnerable to ischemia than the subepicardium. Therefore relatively mild epicardial ischemia sufficient to cause ST depressions will almost invariably be associated with more severe ischemia of the subendocardium and, according to Prinzmetal's theory, the surface ECG will record only indirectly evidence of subendocardial ischemia or infarction. A similar argument has been used (p. 275) to explain the apparently paradoxical correlation of T wave inversions (reflecting delayed epicardial repolarization) with the clinical finding of subendocardial ischemia.[34]

The exact cause of ischemic ST depressions remains unresolved. The classic theory that the subendocardium is *not* electrically silent and does in fact generate a current of injury with reciprocal epicardial ST depressions is most widely accepted. More recent data from simultaneous subepicardial and subendocardial recordings just described[17] are in accord with this concept. However, Kjekshus, Maroko, and Sobel[22] studied experimental infarcts in dogs and reported that ST segment depression did not correlate with decreased subendocardial blood flow as measured by microsphere techniques. Further data are therefore still needed to resolve this long-standing debate concerning the degree to which the subendocardium per se contributes to the surface ECG pattern of ischemic ST-T changes.[17,21,31]

REFERENCES

1. Bayley RH: Biophysical principles of electrocardiography, New York 1958, Paul B Hoeber Inc.
2. Becker RC, Alpert JS: Electrocardiographic ST segment depression in coronary heart disease, Am Heart J 115:862, 1988.
3. Berland J, et al: Anterior ST segment depression in inferior myocardial infarction: correlation with results of intracoronary thrombolysis, Am Heart J 111:481, 1986.
4. Boden WE, et al: Inferoseptal myocardial infarction: another cause of precordial ST segment depression in transmural inferior wall myocardial infarction? Am J Cardiol 54:1216, 1984.
5. Boden WE, et al: Electrocardiographic evolution of posterior acute myocardial infarction: importance of early precordial ST-segment depression, Am J Cardiol 59:782, 1987.
6. Boden WE, Spodick DH: Diagnostic significance of precordial ST-segment depression, Am J Cardiol 63:358, 1989.
7. Braunwald E, et al: Mechanisms of contraction in the normal and failing heart, ed 2, Boston, 1976, Little Brown & Co.
8. Cook RW, et al: Electrocardiographic changes in acute subendocardial infarction. I. Large subendocardial and large nontransmural infarcts, Circulation 18:603, 1958.
9. Crawford MH, et al: Mechanism of inferior electrocardiographic ST-segment depression during acute anterior myocardial infarction in a baboon model, Am J Cardiol 54:1114, 1984.
10. Croft CH, et al: Clinical implications of anterior S-T segment depression in patients with acute inferior myocardial infarction, Am J Cardiol 50:428, 1982.
11. Ekmekci A, et al: Angina pectoris. IV. Clinical and experimental differences between ischemia with S-T elevation and ischemia with S-T depression, Am J Cardiol 7:412, 1961.
12. Ferguson DW, et al: Angiographic evidence that reciprocal ST-segment depression during acute myocardial infarction does not indicate remote ischemia: analysis of 23 patients, Am J Cardiol 53:55, 1984.
13. Gibson RS, et al: Precordial ST-segment depression during inferior myocardial infarction: clinical scintigraphic and angiographic correlations, Circulation 66:732, 1982.
14. Goldberg HL, et al: Anterior S-T segment depression in acute inferior infarction: indicator of posterolateral infarction, Am J Cardiol 48:1009, 1981.
15. Goldberger AL, Erickson R: A subtle ECG sign of acute infarction: prominent reciprocal ST depression with minimal primary ST elevation, PACE 4:709, 1981.
16. Goldberger E: Unipolar lead electrocardiography and vectorcardiography, ed 3, Philadelphia, 1953, Lea & Febiger.
17. Guyton RA, et al: Significance of subendocardial S-T segment elevation caused by coronary stenosis in the dog, Am J Cardiol 40:373, 1977.
18. Hellerstein HK, Katz LN: Electrical effects of injury at various myocardial locations, Am Heart J 36:184, 1948.
19. Herlitz J, Hjalmarson A: Occurrence of anterior ST depression in inferior myocardial infarction and relation to clinical myocardial infarction and clinical outcome, Clin Cardiol 10:529, 1987.
20. Kilpatrick D, et al: Derived epicardial potentials differentiate ischemic ST depression from ST depression secondary to ST elevation in acute inferior myocardial infarction in humans, J Am Coll Cardiol 14:695, 1989.
21. Kisch B, et al: The predominance of surface over deep cardiac injury in producing changes in the electrocardiogram, Am Heart J 20:174, 1940.
22. Kjekshus JK, et al: Distribution of myocardial injury and its relation to epicardial ST-segment changes after coronary artery oc-

clusion in the dog, Cardiovasc Res 6:490, 1972.

23. Lembo NJ, et al: Clinical and prognostic importance of persistent precordial (V1-V4) electrocardiographic ST segment depression in patients with inferior transmural myocardial infarction, Circulation 74:56, 1986.

24. Levine HD, Ford RV: Subendocardial infarction: report of six cases and critical survey of literature, Circulation 1:246, 1950.

25. Lew AS, et al: Factors that determine the direction and magnitude of precordial ST-segment deviations during inferior wall acute myocardial infarction, Am J Cardiol 55:883, 1985.

26. MacAlpin RN, Cabeen WR: The inside-out electrocardiographic stress test: a view from the left ventricular cavity, Angiology 28: 384, 1977.

27. Massumi RA, et al: Studies on the mechanism of ventricular activity. XVI. Activation of the human ventricle, Am J Med 19:832, 1955.

28. Master AM, et al: Acute coronary insufficiency: an entity, J Mt Sinai Hosp 14:8, 1947.

29. Mukharji J, et al: Is anterior ST depression with acute transmural inferior infarction due to posterior infarction? A vectorcardiographic and scintigraphic study, J Am Coll Cardiol 4:28, 1984.

30. Ong L, et al: Precordial S-T segment depression in inferior myocardial infarction: evaluation by quantitative thallium-201 scintigraphy and technetium-99m ventriculography, Am J Cardiol 51:734, 1983.

31. Pipberger HV, Lopez EA: "Silent" subendocardial infarcts: fact or fiction? Am Heart J 100:597, 1980.

32. Prinzmetal M, et al: Myocardial ischemia: nature of ischemic electrocardiographic patterns in the mammalian ventricles as determined by extracellular electrographic and metabolic changes, Am J Cardiol 8:493, 1961.

33. Pruitt RD, et al: Deviations of the RS-T segment in acute subendocardial injuries, Circulation 4:108, 1951.

34. Pruitt RD, et al: Certain clinical states associated with deeply inverted T waves in the

precordial electrocardiogram, Circulation 11:517, 1955.

35. Rutledge JC, et al: Anterior ST-segment depression associated with acute inferior myocardial infarction: clinical, hemodynamic, and angiographic correlates, Am J Noninvas Cardiol 1:290, 1987.

36. Salcedo JR, et al: Significance of reciprocal S-T segment depression in anterior precordial leads in acute inferior myocardial infarction: concomitant left anterior descending coronary artery disease? Am J Cardiol 48:1003, 1981.

37. Sato H, et al: Right coronary artery occlusion: its role in the mechanism of precordial ST segment depression, J Am Coll Cardiol 14:297, 1989.

38. Sclarovsky S, et al: Ischemic ST segment depression in leads V2-V3 as the presenting electrocardiographic feature of posterolateral wall myocardial infarction, Am Heart J 113:1085, 1987.

39. Shah PK et al: Noninvasive identification of high risk subset of patients with acute inferior myocardial infarction, Am J Cardiol 46:915, 1980.

40. Sodi-Pallares D: New bases of electrocardiography, St Louis, 1956, The CV Mosby Co.

41. Toyoshima H, et al: Angina pectoris. VII. The nature of S-T depression in acute myocardial ischemia, Am J Cardiol 13:498, 1964.

42. Wagner NB, et al: Transient alterations of the QRS complex and ST segment during percutaneous transluminal balloon angioplasty of the right and left circumflex coronary arteries, Am J Cardiol 63:1208, 1989.

43. Wolferth CC, et al: Negative displacement of the RS-T segment in the electrocardiogram and its relationships to positive displacement: an experimental study, Am Heart J 29:220, 1945.

44. Yu PNG, Stewart JM: Subendocardial myocardial infarction with special reference to the electrocardiographic changes, Am Heart J 39:862, 1950.

45. Zakopoulos KS, et al: Effects of subendocardial injury on the electrocardiogram of intact dogs, Am J Physiol 213:143, 1967.

ST segment depressions: normal variants and nonischemic abnormal causes

A variety of nonischemic causes of ST segment depression may simulate the pattern of subendocardial ischemia (coronary insufficiency) described in Chapter 11. The differential diagnosis of ST depressions includes spurious causes, normal variants, and a number of abnormal but nonischemic patterns: left ventricular hypertrophy with strain, secondary ST-T changes caused by altered ventricular conduction, hypokalemia, and drug effects (particularly from digitalis).

SPURIOUS AND NORMAL-VARIANT ST DEPRESSIONS

ST depressions are not always a pathologic finding. In assessing them one must exclude possible artifact. A common spurious cause is downward deflection of the ECG baseline, often caused by patient movement or poor electrode contact (Fig. 12-1). As described on p. 197, cardiac monitor lead systems may be helpful in tracking ST-T changes provided lead placement is standardized and the system is adequate to record low-frequency signals without phase distortion.[23] (See also p. 248.) Finally, in some cases of right bundle branch block the deep wide terminal S wave seen in the lateral chest leads may have a squared-off appearance and be mistaken for ST depression (Fig. 12-2).

Some normal subjects will have slight (usually 1 mm or less) ST depressions as a physiologic variant (Fig. 13-3), typically most prominent at the J point (between the end of the QRS and beginning of the ST segment) and giving the ST a concave upsloping appearance. Physiologic J point depression may be related to an atrial repolarization effect. Normally, the atrial depolarization (P wave) and repolarization (T_A wave) vectors are discordant so that leads showing a positive P wave should also show a negative T_A wave. However, the atrial T wave is usually of low amplitude and obscured by the QRS complex and ST segment. On occasion the atrial T wave will be more prominent, producing slight depression of the early ST segment. Studies[25] of atrial repolarization in subjects with AV block have shown that the atrial T wave may be depressed as much as 1.2 mm in lead II at the time the ST segment is inscribed. During exercise the atrial T

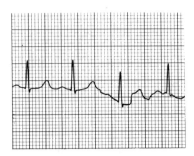

FIG. 12-1. Spurious ST depressions from downward deflection of the baseline caused by patient movement.

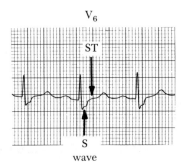

FIG. 12-2. A prominent terminal S wave in V_6 caused by right bundle branch block may be mistaken for ST segment depression.

wave negativity may cause as much as 1.9 mm of ST depression in II and account for some false-positive exercise test results (p. 256).

HYPERVENTILATION

Hyperventilation is a well-documented cause of functional ST-T changes, sometimes inducing T wave inversions (Fig. 15-4) or ST depressions (Fig. 12-3) simulating coronary disease.* As discussed on p. 206, it can cause T wave inversions in the chest and limb leads and these may be particularly notable in patients whose resting ECG shows normal variant ST elevations (early repolarization variant).[39]

Some healthy people will have horizontal ST depressions with hyperventilation[2,5,15,43] mimicking the pattern of coronary insufficiency (Fig. 12-3). In most of the reported cases these have been 2 mm or less in depth and accompanied by sinus tachycardia. The ST changes are usually transient, disappearing within seconds or minutes after the subject stops hyperventilating. Patients in whom

---

*References 2, 17, 20, 22, 40, 43.

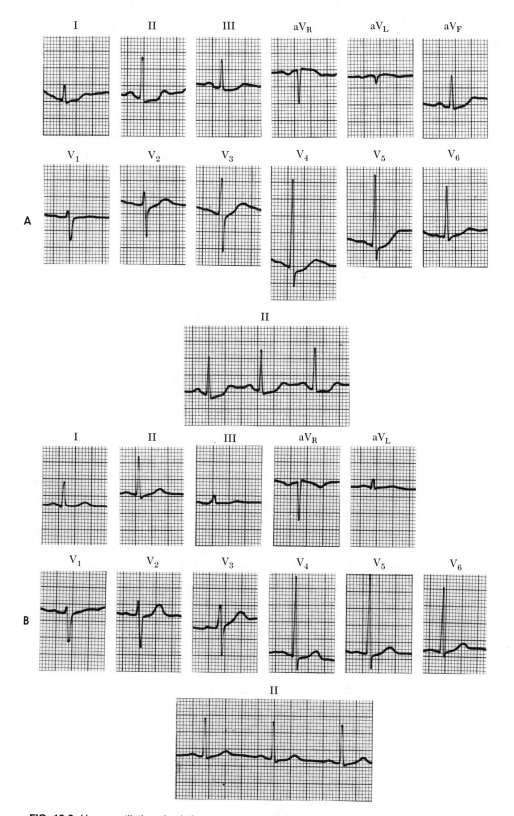

FIG. 12-3. Hyperventilation simulating coronary insufficiency. **A,** This patient had a pH of 7.6 and a P_{CO_2} of 20 mm Hg. The diffuse horizontal ST depressions suggest ischemia. **B,** One hour later, with normal respiration. The ST-T changes have resolved. Note the increased heart rate associated with hyperventilation.

ST-T changes develop with hyperventilation are particularly likely to have false-positive exercise test results.

The cause of the hyperventilatory ST depression and T wave inversions is not entirely certain but probably relates to increased sympathetic tone rather than to respiratory alkalosis or electrolyte change, as suggested by some investigators.[7,43] Biberman, Sarma, and Surawicz[3] made the following observations in a group of normal subjects during experimental hyperventilation: (1) ST-T changes occurred in 8 of 11 cases, (2) these changes were noted during rapid voluntary hyperventilation of both room air (with respiratory alkalosis) and 6% carbon dioxide (without respiratory alkalosis), (3) *slow* hyperventilation of room air sufficient to produce respiratory alkalosis but not tachycardia did not produce the changes, (4) the changes did not correlate with any change in serum electrolyte concentration, and (5) similar ST-T changes could be produced with infusion of isoproterenol.

On the basis of these findings the investigators[3] concluded that the repolarization changes associated with hyperventilation were caused by not respiratory alkalosis or electrolyte shift but probably by increased sympathetic tone induced by hyperpnea. They speculated that increased sympathetic tone in certain subjects might cause a selective shortening of the action potential of the subendocardium. The resultant shift of the ST-T vector would produce ST depressions or T wave inversions in epicardial leads. In another study[13] the ST-T changes of hyperventilation were prevented with propranolol, a sympathetic beta-blocking agent.

Other investigators[15,43] studying the basis of hyperventilatory ST-T changes have reported somewhat contradictory data. Yu, Yim, and Stanfield[43] found that the ST-T changes could be prevented by hyperventilating with carbon dioxide, implying that respiratory alkalosis does play a role in ST-T pathogenesis. Similarly, Golden, Golden, and Beerel[15] noted reversal of the ST-T changes when their subjects hyperventilated with carbon dioxide. However, in both these studies the heart rates during CO_2 breathing were lower than during room air hyperventilation. Furthermore, Yu, Yim, and Stanfield[43] recorded similar ST-T changes during intravenous infusion of epinephrine.

By way of summary: Current data suggest that the ST-T changes seen with hyperventilation are caused primarily by changes in sympathetic tone. The nonspecific repolarization changes sometimes seen with anxiety or standing (orthostatic) or after meals probably have a similar functional basis.[36]

In contrast to the purely functional ST depressions reported during hyperventilation by some normal subjects, patients with coronary vasospasm (Prinzmetal's angina) may have characteristic ischemic ST elevations after hyperventilation.[42] (See p. 181.) The exact mechanism whereby hyperventilation triggers coronary vasospasm in susceptible individuals is unknown.

ST DEPRESSIONS DURING AMBULATORY (HOLTER) MONITORING: FALSE-POSITIVES

The use of ambulatory ECG monitoring to detect "silent ischemia" has provoked intense interest as well as controversy since the initial reports by Stern and Tzivoni.[31,32] Despite the fact that subsequent reports[1,8] cast doubt on the specificity of ST depression recorded at ambulatory monitoring as an indicator of ischemia, more recent studies[9,10,33,34] have validated the utility of this finding, particularly in carefully selected patients (Fig. 12-4).

Episodes of silent ischemia have been reported in as many as half to three quarters of patients with exercise-induced ischemia.[12] Detection of silent ischemia is important because it appears to identify higher-risk subgroups of patients with stable[26] or unstable[16] angina. The clinical aspects of silent ischemia are well-reviewed elsewhere[5,6,11,27,28] and lie outside the scope of this discussion. Attention here is focused on the potential causes of false-positive ST depressions during ambulatory monitoring.

For recording and quantitating ambulatory ST changes, two channels (e.g., modified V_3 and V_5) are typically recorded with either an amplitude modulated or a frequency modulated system.[29] The usual criteria for an ischemic ECG response are generally the same as those employed for exercise testing: ≥ 1 mm of horizontal or downsloping ST depression measured 80 msec after the end of the QRS complex (p. 254) using a calibrated signal. Considerable care with skin

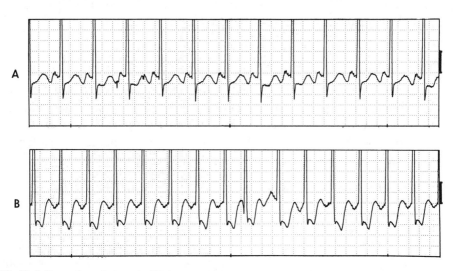

FIG. 12-4. Dynamic variations in ST depressions during ambulatory (Holter) monitoring evident on a modified lead II tracing. **A,** Sinus rhythm (97 beats/min). Note the moderate horizontal or upsloping ST depressions. **B,** Subsequently, with sinus tachycardia (118 beats/min), the depressions become more pronounced. A single premature atrial depolarization can be seen (9th beat).

preparation and lead fixation must be taken to obtain a high-quality signal free of motion artifact. Positional effects on the ECG should be assessed as well.[12]

False-positive ST deviations (e.g., depression in the absence of coronary disease) may occur for multiple reasons.[2,5,12] Electronic distortion of the ST segment may be induced by a recording system with inadequate low-frequency response[4,19] or phase distortion.[37] Spurious ST depression may occur with motion artifact. Truly ischemic ST segment shifts during ambulatory monitoring tend to increase in magnitude over several beats and then to resolve after a variable period ranging from less than a minute to over an hour. Abrupt ST shifts noted over two or three beats are usually artifactual.[12]

False-positive ST depressions during ambulatory monitoring can occur with any of the normal variants or abnormal but noncoronary conditions described elsewhere in this chapter as well as in the discussion of exercise testing in Chapter 13. For example, in certain healthy subjects they may occur with postural change or hyperventilation. Other factors include digitalis, hypokalemia, ventricular hypertrophy, and conduction disorders.

Given the multiple conditions that can alter the ST segment, ambulatory ST depressions most likely represent ischemia in a patient with either definite coronary artery disease or a high prior probability of this diagnosis. (See Bayes theorem, p. 260.) In such patients ambulatory ST recordings are likely to be of greatest value in detecting the frequency and duration of silent ischemic episodes as a guide to therapy and prognosis.

The ambulatory ECG may also be useful in detecting either symptomatic or painless episodes of ST elevation associated with coronary vasospasm[1,30] (Fig. 8-5).

LEFT AND RIGHT VENTRICULAR "STRAIN"

The "strain" pattern, consisting of T wave inversions, often with ST depressions, is described on p. 64. The cause of this pattern and its relation to actual ischemia are not resolved. In cases of more marked left (Fig. 4-1) or right (Fig. 4-4) ventricular strain, prominent ST depressions may mimic the pattern of acute subendocardial ischemia.

SECONDARY ST DEPRESSIONS

As described in Chapter 5, secondary ST-T changes are a characteristic finding in patients with altered ventricular conduction. Right bundle branch block routinely causes T wave inversions and sometimes ST depressions in the right to middle chest leads showing an rSR' morphology (Fig. 5-9). Left bundle branch block (Fig. 5-2, A) induces wide R waves generally with T wave inversions and often ST depressions. Finally, the Wolff-Parkinson-White pattern (Fig. 5-11) may produce secondary ST-T changes. These are seen with altered ventricular activation and not only may mimic ischemia but frequently also will mask true infarctional changes. Furthermore, false-positive ST depressions are sometimes recorded during stress tests in leads showing secondary ST-T changes (Chapter 13).

DIGITALIS

Numerous drugs (p. 8) can affect the ECG, usually producing relatively non-specific ST-T abnormalities. Digitalis glycosides are of particular importance because they may induce repolarization changes simulating ischemia on the resting ECG as well as false-positive ST depressions during exercise testing (p. 265). The term *digitalis effect* refers to these drug-related ST-T changes, in contrast to *digitalis toxicity,* which describes the arrhythmias and systemic side effects associated with drug excess.

Digitalis effect is characterized by slight ST depressions and T wave inversions with shortening of the QT interval. As schematized in Fig. 12-5, the ST-T complex with digitalis effect may have a distinctive "scooped" or "hammocked" shape (Fig. 12-5, *A*) or be more triangulated (Fig. 12-5, *B*). In either case the ST segment and T wave are difficult to separate. Slight downward depression of the ST segment (1 to 2 mm) may be seen.

These ST-T changes of digitalis effect are usually most prominent in leads with tall R waves (e.g., V_4 to V_6 and one or more of the limb leads depending on the electrical axis). In subjects with normal ECGs digitalis can cause reversal of T wave polarity (Fig. 12-6). In patients with baseline ST depressions or T wave inversions it may accentuate these repolarization abnormalities. The ST-T changes of digitalis effect may appear within minutes of intravenous drug administration.[21]

Electrophysiologic studies have shown that the major effect of digitalis is to shorten the duration of the ventricular action potential, reflected on the surface ECG by abbreviation of the QT interval.[36] Woodbury and Hecht[41] specifically correlated ST depressions with a shortening of the plateau phase and more negative slope of phase 3 of the action potential. The exact manner by which alteration of the duration and morphology of the action potential leads to characteristic ST-T changes is not certain. It has been suggested that digitalis may cause relatively greater shortening of subendocardial (vs. subepicardial) action poten-

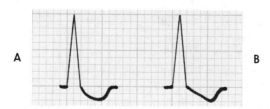

FIG. 12-5. Digitalis often produces distinctive ST-T changes: scooping of the ST-T complex, **A,** or oblique downsloping of the ST segment with T wave inversion, **B.**

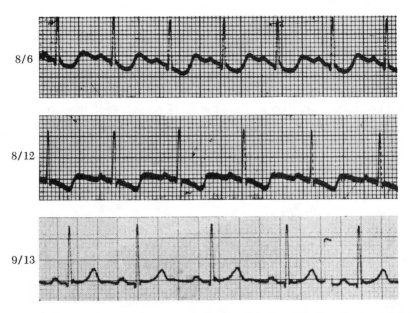

FIG. 12-6. Serial ECGs from a patient who stopped taking digitalis on 8/6. Note the pronounced ST-T changes, with downsloping ST depressions on the first two tracings and complete normalization of repolarization at follow-up (9/13). (From Surawicz B, Lasseter KC: Prog Cardiovasc Dis 13:26, 1970. Used by permission.)

tials, with consequent reversal of the normal ventricular gradient.[21]

Differentiation of digitalis effect from actual ischemic ST-T changes is often impossible. It is unusual for digitalis to produce horizontal ST depressions on the resting ECG. However, with exercise it can induce horizontal ST segment depressions simulating those of ischemia (p. 265). As a rule digitalis does not produce the coved plane or symmetric T wave inversions sometimes seen with ischemia (Fig. 14-4).

HYPOKALEMIA

Hypokalemia is an important cause of nonischemic ST segment depression. The characteristic ECG signs include ST depressions, T wave flattening or inversions, and prominent U waves.[35]

Occasionally hypokalemia produces ST segment depressions, mimicking the coronary insufficiency pattern (Fig. 12-7) usually noted with a serum potassium level of less than 3 mEq/L.[37] These depressions are generally diffuse, occurring in both the anterior and the inferior leads. Hypokalemia is also a reported cause of false-positive ST depressions during exercise tolerance tests. As described on p. 266, exercise may evoke such depressions in hypokalemic subjects with normal resting ECGs.[14]

The ST depressions with severe hypokalemia are associated with hyperpolar-

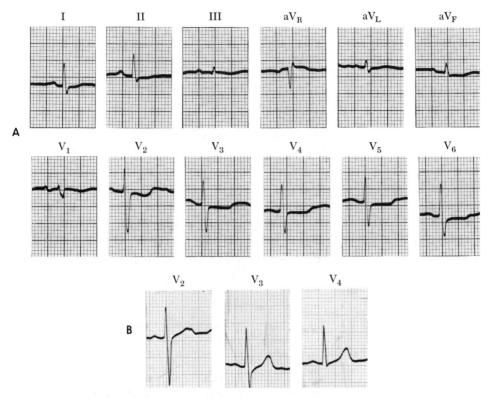

FIG. 12-7. Diffuse ST depressions simulating ischemia in a patient whose serum potassium was 2.3 mEq/L. **A,** At the time of admission. **B,** After normalization of the potassium level.

ization of the myocardial cell membranes. The electrophysiologic effects of *hypo*kalemia are opposite those of *hyper*kalemia (p. 217) (depolarization of the cell membrane leading to ST elevations). Reducing the extracellular concentration of potassium increases the resting potential of the myocardial cells. Hypokalemia also prolongs the duration of the action potential, which produces the characteristic increased repolarization time (QU prolongation) on the ECG. Experimental coronary infusion of hypokalemia solutions also leads to local ST segment depressions.[18]

Prinzmetal et al.[24] suggested that the ST depressions seen with coronary insufficiency are not reciprocal to primary subendocardial ST elevations but reflect primary epicardial ischemia. They proposed that mild degrees of ischemia could lead to increased potassium uptake by epicardial cells, with consequent membrane hyperpolarization and ST segment depression, analogous to the pattern seen with hypokalemia (p. 240).

Differentiation of hypokalemia from ischemia or other patterns causing ST depressions (digitalis effect, left ventricular strain) may be difficult. As a rule, serum potassium should be checked in any patient with unexplained nonspecific ST-T changes or ST depressions. The presence of prominent U waves is often helpful. However, quinidine, or particularly the combination of quinidine and digitalis, may produce an ECG pattern indistinguishable from that of hypokalemia, with ST depressions and U waves.[35] Hypokalemia should be corrected before the performance of an exercise tolerance test.

Besides causing ST depressions that simulate those of coronary artery disease, hypokalemia alone can produce or potentiate serious atrial and ventricular arrhythmias as well as AV conduction disturbances. Ventricular ectopy is particularly common when digitalis is given to hypokalemic patients.[35]

MISCELLANEOUS CAUSES

In addition to the patterns just mentioned, ST segment depressions occur with a variety of other noncoronary conditions, including ventricular "strain" (p. 64), mitral valve prolapse (p. 311), cardiomyopathy (Chapter 7), cerebrovascular accident (Chapter 16), and selective coronary arteriography (Chapter 17).

REFERENCES

1. Armstrong WF, et al: Prevalence and magnitude of S-T segment and T wave abnormalities in normal men during continuous ambulatory electrocardiography, Am J Cardiol 49:1638, 1982.
2. Berman DS, et al: The detection of silent ischemia: cautions and precautions, Circulation 75:101, 1987.
3. Biberman L, et al: T-wave abnormalities during hyperventilation and isoproterenol infusion, Am Heart J 81:166, 1971.
4. Bragg-Remschel DA, et al: Frequency response characteristics of ambulatory ECG monitoring systems and their implications for ST segment analysis, Am Heart J 103:20, 1982.
5. Cohn PF: Silent myocardial ischemia and infarction, New York, 1986, Marcel Dekker.
6. Cohn PF: Silent myocardial ischemia, Ann Intern Med 109:312, 1988.
7. Coy KM, et al: Silent myocardial ischemia during daily activities in asymptomatic men with positive exercise test responses, Am J Cardiol 59:45, 1987.
8. Crawford MH, et al: Limitations of continuous ambulatory electrocardiogram monitoring for detecting coronary artery disease, Ann Intern Med 89:1, 1978.
9. Deanfield JE, et al: Analysis of ST-segment changes in normal subjects: implications for ambulatory monitoring in angina pectoris, Am J Cardiol 54:1321, 1984.
10. Deanfield JE, et al: Transient ST-segment depression as a marker of myocardial ischemia during daily life, Am J Cardiol 54:1195, 1984.
11. Epstein SE, et al: Myocardial ischemia: silent or symptomatic, N Engl J Med 318:1038, 1988.
12. Feldman RL: Ambulatory monitoring: the test for ischemia in 1988? Ann Intern Med 109:608, 1988.
13. Furberg C, Tengblad C-F: Adrenergic beta-receptor blockade and the effect of hyperventilation on the electrocardiogram, Scand J Clin Lab Invest 18:467, 1966.
14. Georgopoulos AJ, et al: The effect of exercise on electrocardiograms of patients with low serum potassium, Circulation 23:567, 1961.
15. Golden GS, et al: Hyperventilation-induced T-wave changes in the limb lead electrocardiogram, Chest 67:123, 1975.
16. Gottlieb SO, et al: Silent ischemia predicts infarction and death during 2 year follow-up of unstable angina, J Am Coll Cardiol 10:756, 1987.
17. Jacobs WF, et al: False-positive ST-T-wave changes secondary to hyperventilation and exercise: a cineangiographic correlation, Ann Intern Med 81:479, 1974.
18. Kwocznyski JK, et al: Electrocardiographic ischemic patterns without coronary artery disease, Dis Chest 39:305, 1961.
19. Lambert CR, et al: Low-frequency require-

ments for recording ischemic ST-segment abnormalities in coronary artery disease, Am J Cardiol 58:225, 1986.

20. Lary D, Goldschlager N: Electrocardiographic changes during hyperventilation resembling myocardial ischemia in patients with normal coronary arteriograms, Am Heart J 87:383, 1974.

21. Lepeschkin E: Modern electrocardiography, Baltimore, 1951, The Williams & Wilkins Co, vol 1.

22. McHenry PL, et al: False positive ECG responses to exercise secondary to hyperventilation: cineangiographic correlation, Am Heart J 79:683, 1970.

23. Mirvis DM, et al: Instrumentation and practice standards for electrocardiographic monitoring in special care units: a report for health professionals by a task force of the Council on Clinical Cardiology, American Heart Association, Circulation 79:464, 1989.

24. Prinzmetal M, et al: Myocardial ischemia: nature of ischemic electrocardiographic patterns in the mammalian ventricles as determined by intracellular electrographic and metabolic changes, Am J Cardiol 8:493, 1961.

25. Riff DP, Carleton RA: Effect of exercise on the atrial recovery wave, Am Heart J 82:759, 1971.

26. Rocco MB, et al: Prognostic importance of myocardial ischemia detected by ambulatory monitoring in patients with stable coronary artery disease, Circulation 78:877, 1988.

27. Rozanski A, Berman DS: Silent myocardial ischemia. I. Pathophysiology, frequency of occurrence, and approaches toward detection, Am Heart J 114:615, 1987.

28. Rozanski A, Berman DS: Silent myocardial ischemia. II. Prognosis and implications for the assessment of patients with coronary artery disease, Am Heart J 114:627, 1987.

29. Shook TL: Comparison of amplitude-modulated (direct) and frequency-modulated ambulatory techniques for recording ischemic electrocardiographic changes, Am J Cardiol 60:895, 1987.

30. Silverman ME, Flamm MD Jr: Variant angina pectoris: anatomic findings and prognostic implications, Ann Intern Med 75:339, 1971.

31. Stern S, Tzivoni D: Dynamic changes in the ST-T segment during sleep in ischemic heart disease, Am J Cardiol 32:17, 1973.

32. Stern S, Tzivoni D: Early detection of silent ischemic heart disease by 24-hour ECG monitoring during normal daily activity, Br Heart J 36:481, 1974.

33. Stern S, et al: Diagnostic accuracy of ambulatory ECG monitoring in ischemic heart disease, Circulation 52:1045, 1975.

34. Stern S, et al: Characteristics of silent and symptomatic myocardial ischemia during daily activities, Am J Cardiol 61:1223, 1988.

35. Surawicz B: Relationship between electrogram and electrolytes, Am Heart J 73:814, 1967.

36. Surawicz B: ST-T abnormalities. In Macfarlane PW, Lawrie TDV (editors): Comprehensive electrocardiology. Theory and practice in health and disease, New York, 1989, Pergamon Press Inc, vol. 1.

37. Surawicz B, et al: Quantitative analysis of the electrocardiographic pattern of hypopotassemia, Circulation 16:750, 1957.

38. Tayler D, Vincent R: Signal distortions in the electrocardiogram due to inadequate phase response, IEEE Trans Biomed Eng 30:352, 1983.

39. Wasserburger RH, Alt WJ: The normal RS-T segment elevation variant, Am J Cardiol 8:184, 1961.

40. Wasserburger RH, et al: The effect of hyperventilation on the normal adult electrocardiogram, Circulation 13:850, 1956.

41. Woodbury LA, Hecht H: Effects of cardiac glycosides upon the electrical activity of single ventricular fibers of the frog heart and their relation to the digitalis effect of the electrocardiogram, Circulation 6:172, 1952.

42. Yasue H, et al: Coronary arterial vasospasm and Prinzmetal's variant form of angina induced by hyperventilation and Tris-buffer infusion, Circulation 58:56, 1978.

43. Yu PNG, et al: Hyperventilation syndrome, Arch Intern Med 103:902, 1959.

13

ST segment depressions: false-positive exercise tests

Exercise testing (stress electrocardiography) is routinely employed in clinical practice to help diagnose coronary artery disease. The most widely used protocols involve incremental grades of exercise on a treadmill or bicycle ergometer (multistage exercise testing).[21,28]* The increases in heart rate, myocardial contractility, and blood pressure during exercise augment cardiac oxygen requirements and may induce ischemia not present in the resting state.

Coronary perfusion can also be assessed with thallium-201 scintigraphy during exercise[47] or in association with infusion of a vasodilator (dipyridamole or adenosine).[43]

The ECG shows a number of signs of ischemia during exercise testing. The most commonly observed is depression of the ST segment. In other cases there may be ST elevation (p. 185) or U wave inversion (p. 268). (Transient Q waves during exercise testing are discussed on p. 131.)

ST segment depressions during exercise are generally thought to reflect primary subendocardial ischemia occurring in the context of increased oxygen demand and inadequate coronary flow. The subendocardium is particularly vulnerable because of its relative distance from the major coronary vessels, limited vasodilatory reserve, and proximity to the high-pressure ventricular cavity (Chapter 11).

Ischemic ST depressions during exercise testing may be accompanied by angina or be asymptomatic ("silent").[28] (See also p. 247.)

The most widely employed criterion[49] for a positive (abnormal) exercise ECG is the appearance of ≥ 1 mm (0.1 mV) horizontal (Fig. 13-1) or downsloping (Fig. 13-2) ST segment depressions occurring at least 0.08 second from the end of the QRS. These are measured with reference to the PR segment baseline. Other studies[68,78] suggest that ≥ 1 mm ST depressions, 0.08 second after the

---

*Alternatives to conventional exercise protocols or to adenosine or dipyridamole-thallium tests for evaluating coronary artery disease include atrial or external transthoracic pacing, cold pressor testing, administration of beta-adrenergic agonists, isometric exercise (handgrip), and arm ergometry.[77]

V_5

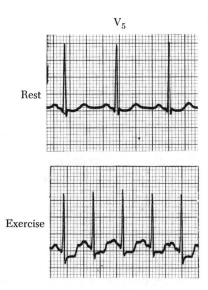

FIG. 13-1. Positive exercise tolerance test with horizontal ST segment depressions.

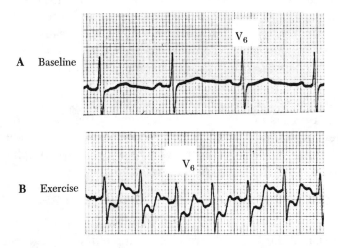

FIG. 13-2. Positive exercise tolerance test with downsloping ST segment depressions.

end of the QRS, also are a positive response even when the ST segments are *slowly* upsloping.

The significance of ST depressions during exercise in patients with an abnormal resting ECG is problematic. Generally exercise testing is of limited value in assessing the response of patients with ST depressions on their resting ECG, because the factors that cause these depressions (hyperventilation, digitalis, left ventricular hypertrophy, intraventricular conduction delays) also provoke false-positive exercise responses.[63] Stress electrocardiography may be helpful in evaluating T wave inversions with isoelectric ST segments at rest. In one study[4] 88% of patients with T wave inversions caused by ischemic heart disease had ST depressions during exercise, compared to only 4% with functional T wave inversions. Excluded from the latter group, however, were patients who had evidence of hypertrophy, digitalis use, bundle branch block, etc.*

Unfortunately, the specificity of ST depressions as an index of ischemia is limited. The specificity of a clinical test is defined as the percentage of subjects without disease who have a normal test result. Thus a test with 100% specificity will not yield any false-positive results, and the more false-positive results (e.g., ST depressions in the absence of coronary disease) the test generates the lower its specificity.

There are a number of well-documented causes of false-positive ST segment depressions during exercise electrocardiography. Familiarity with these sources of possible misinterpretation is essential for clinicians involved in the actual interpretation of exercise tests as well as in the referral of patients for such procedures.

Generally, any of the factors described in Chapter 12 (hyperventilation, digitalis, hypokalemia) that produce ST depressions on the resting ECG can result in false-positive exercise tests. It is helpful to classify the causes of false-positive exercise ECGs in four etiologic groups: (1) physiologic (functional) factors, (2) organic noncoronary heart disease, (3) altered ventricular conduction, and (4) metabolic factors.

It should also be emphasized that clinicians generally use the term *false-positive* exercise tests to refer to ST depressions in the absence of coronary artery disease, but not necessarily in the absence of myocardial ischemia. ST depressions during exercise in patients with ventricular hypertrophy and normal coronary arteries may reflect actual subendocardial ischemia.

PHYSIOLOGIC (FUNCTIONAL) FALSE-POSITIVE TEST RESULTS

During exercise normal subjects may have slight (usually less than 1 to 2 mm) depression of the J junction with upsloping of the ST segment back to the baseline (Fig. 13-3). Occasionally 2 to 3 mm of physiologic J point depression will be seen.[61] The precise cause of these is not certain but they may be related to atrial repolarization effects. As described on p. 243, the negative atrial T wave is inscribed during the early phase of ventricular repolarization. There is one report[7] of horizontal or downsloping ST depressions in 3 of 12 presumed normal patients with a short PR interval on their resting ECG. A small but clinically significant percentage of normal patients also will have horizontal or downslop-

---

*The significance of transient normalization during exercise of T waves that are inverted on the resting ECG is discussed on pp. 268 and 331.

V_5

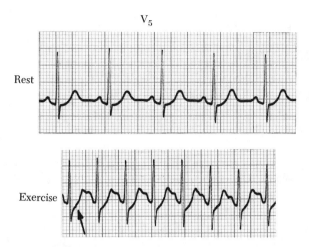

FIG. 13-3. Physiologic ST depressions with exercise. Note the J junction depression *(arrow)* with up-sloping of the ST segments.

ing ST depressions during exercise, simulating ischemia.[8,28,80] False-positive exercise test results have been reported in up to 10% of normal men.[49,75,86] The prevalence of false-positive test results in women has not been precisely defined but appears to be even higher.[28,39] Sketch et al.[70] reported positive test results in 10 of 46 women with normal coronary arteries (or less than 50% occlusion) by angiogram. In a prospective series of women 29 to 64 years old with chest pain but normal coronary arteriograms,[37] false-positive ST responses during exercise testing were noted in 34% of subjects. Weiner et al.[86] reported false-positive results in 53% of women compared to 12% of men. Cumming et al.[19] found only 10% false positive results in women under 40 years of age but 25% in women over 40 years.

There has been disagreement as to whether this decreased specificity of exercise testing merely reflects the relatively lower prevalence of coronary disease among women[86] or is an actual indication that "non-Bayesian" factors[11] (p. 260) are also contributing. The suggestion[50] that women with false-positive ST-T responses may have excessive elevations of blood pressure during exercise has not been confirmed.[11] The higher prevalence of mitral valve prolapse in women probably accounts for some false-positive results (p. 311). Thallium scintigraphy[26] (p. 266) or exercise echocardiography[69] may help in resolving their significance.

False-positive ST segment depressions have also been reported in normal subjects during sudden strenuous exertion. Barnard et al.[9] observed ischemic-appearing ST segment depression in 19 of 30 normal men (63%) following 10 to 15 seconds of treadmill exercise at 9 mph and 30% grade. These men all had normal conventional exercise test responses. The authors suggested that sudden severe exercise can cause relative subendocardial ischemia even with normal coronary arteries.[10] Comparable ST changes were not observed in a subsequent study of normal subjects during sudden strenuous exercise.[24] However, a different protocol was used.

False-positive ST depressions during exercise also may occur among normal subjects because of functional changes in autonomic tone, as in the cases of hyperventilation (p. 244), postural change,[64] and so-called "vasoregulatory lability" (discussed below).

Hyperventilation

Hyperventilation is a well-documented cause of functional ST-T abnormalities (Figs. 12-3 and 15-4). These repolarization changes are probably caused by increased sympathetic tone associated with voluntary hyperventilation and not by respiratory alkalosis or electrolyte shifts.[16]

Several studies have reported a correlation between hyperventilatory ST-T changes and false positive exercise tests. McHenry et al.[62] reported a 30-year-old patient with 1 to 2 mm of horizontal ST-T depression during hyperventilation. Similar ischemic ST changes were noted during an exercise test. A coronary angiogram was normal. Other cases have been described.[45,52] Although the authors of these studies suggested that hyperventilation during exercise directly induces the false positive ST changes, it seems more likely that the hyperventilatory and exercise-induced ST depressions in these patients were caused by a common factor: increased sympathetic tone. Hyperventilatory ST depressions in susceptible individuals can be blocked by propranolol and mimicked by isoproterenol or epinephrine infusion (p. 246). Clinically it may be helpful to hyperventilate subjects before exercise testing as well as to look for orthostatic changes or other evidence of vasoregulatory reactions that may be associated with false-positive stress tests. Of note, an association has been reported[29] between hyperventilatory ST-T changes and the presence of mitral valve prolapse (p. 311).

Vasoregulatory Lability

The term *vasoregulatory lability* has been applied to functional ST-T alterations seen in some normal individuals. Subjects with vasoregulatory lability may have nonspecific ST-T changes, with ST segment depression or slight T wave inversion, usually in the inferior limb and lateral precordial leads. These ST-T deviations occur with standing (orthostatic repolarization changes), after meals, with anxiety, or with exercise and are probably caused by functional repolarization changes associated with increased sympathetic tone (Fig. 13-4).

Friesinger et al.[27] reported false-positive exercise tolerance tests in 40 patients with vasoregulatory ECG changes. In many of these subjects prominent ST-T changes developed with standing. Propranolol blocked some of the changes. Interestingly, a few subjects with false-positive ST depressions had a

Baseline

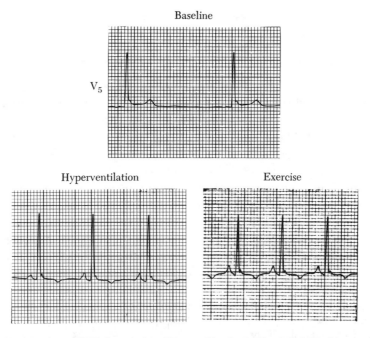

V_5

Hyperventilation   Exercise

FIG. 13-4. Vasoregulatory ST-T changes in a 25-year-old patient without clinical evidence of coronary artery disease. The resting ECG shows slight ST elevations caused by normal-variant early repolarization. With both hyperventilation and exercise there is an increase in the heart rate. The ST segments return to baseline, with inversion of the T waves. Such ST-T lability is probably due to increased sympathetic tone, which causes functional repolarization changes.

normal ECG with further increases in heart rate. A similar ST "walk-through" phenomenon has been described in patients who have false-positive ST depressions caused by digitalis.[3]

Vasoregulatory ST-T changes are most likely due to increased sympathetic tone, which in the setting of exercise, postural changes, anxiety, etc. may produce asynchronous repolarization changes in selected individuals. The same mechanism also may underlie the labile ST-T changes seen with hyperventilation and possibly after meals in certain healthy persons.

Clinically the recognition of functional repolarization variants is important. Patients should be screened for vasoregulatory lability before exercise testing by checking for orthostatic ST-T changes and, where appropriate, for hyperventilatory effects. However, it also needs to be remembered that patients with coronary disease can have similar changes on their ECG.

In summary: Physiologic and functional factors are important causes of false-positive ST depression during exercise. Morphologically such patterns may be indistinguishable from the horizontal or downsloping ST depressions seen with actual ischemia. Generally, however, normal subjects will rarely have more marked ST depressions (e.g., 3 to 4 mm). The presence of typical anginal pain or a drop in systolic blood pressure during exercise can also be used to identify true ischemic responses.[66a,66b] (See p. 268).

Implications of Physiologic False-positive Tests: Bayes Theorem

The clinical usefulness of any test depends not only on its diagnostic accuracy (sensitivity and specificity) but also on the prevalence of the disease being investigated. According to statistical principles (Bayes theorem of conditional probability) the likelihood that a patient has a particular disease *after* a test is the product of the probability that the disease was present *before* the test (prior probability) and the diagnostic accuracy of the test.[23,49,73,74]

The importance of these statistical considerations can be illustrated in the following examples. Assume that the overall specificity of exercise testing is about 90% in men, with a sensitivity of about 70%. Now compare the results of testing a group of young adults with a predicted prevalence of coronary artery disease of only 5% to the results of testing a group of middle-aged men with atypical chest pain and a predicted prevalence of coronary artery disease of 50%.

Group 1: *1000 young adults with 5% prevalence of coronary artery disease (CAD)*
Results of exercise testing, if one assumes 90% specificity (10% false-positives) and 70% sensitivity (30% false-negatives):
50/1000 with CAD
35/1000 with true-positive test
950/1000 with normal coronary arteries
95/1000 with false-positive result
   Therefore the predictive value of an abnormal (positive) test in this group equals

$$\frac{\text{True-positive results}}{\text{Total true- and false-positive results}} \times 100$$

$$= \frac{35}{35 + 95} \times 100 \ (\text{or } 27\%)$$

Group 2: *1000 middle-aged men with atypical chest pain with 50% predicted prevalence of CAD*
Results of exercise testing, if one assumes 90% specificity (10% false-positives) and 70% sensitivity (30% false-negatives):
500/1000 with CAD
350/1000 with true-positive test
500/1000 with normal coronary arteries
50/1000 with false-positive result
Therefore the predictive value of an abnormal (positive) test in this group equals

$$\frac{350}{350 + 50} \times 100 \ (\text{or } 87.5\%)$$

These examples illustrate important limitations inherent in exercise testing. In populations with a low percentage of coronary artery disease, screening with treadmill or similar exercise tests will result in an unacceptably high percentage of false positive results. In groups with a relatively high prevalence of coronary

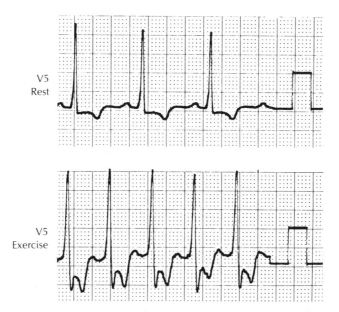

FIG. 13-5. Positive ST segment response in a 65-year-old man with hypertrophic cardiomyopathy and normal coronary arteries. The resting ECG shows ST-T changes consistent with left ventricular strain or ischemia. During exercise, very marked ST depressions are noted. The patient had complained of exertional dyspnea and chest pain. (Courtesy Dr. Howard Dittrich.)

artery disease, the predictive value of exercise testing is higher. However, even in such settings, not all patients at risk will be identified and a clinically significant number of false-positive tests will still be generated.

ORGANIC NONCORONARY HEART DISEASE

Exercise-related ST depressions have been reported in a variety of noncoronary types of organic heart disease. Harris et al.[38] studied a group of patients with normal coronary angiograms and ECG signs of left ventricular hypertrophy caused by a number of different conditions, including hypertension, valvular disease, and cardiomyopathy. False-positive ST responses were observed in 6 of 16 patients (38%). In another study[6] positive exercise test results were reported in 7 of 19 patients (37%) with aortic stenosis and no ECG evidence of left ventricular hypertrophy. The same study also noted false-positive results in 3 of 15 patients (20%) with mitral stenosis. A subsequent investigation[89] confirmed the importance of false-positive results in patients with left ventricular hypertrophy not apparent on ECG but detectable on echocardiogram. Positive exercise test results in patients with left ventricular hypertrophy or valvular disease and normal coronary arteries probably reflect relative myocardial ischemia with increased oxygen requirements (caused by exercise and cardiomegaly) or inadequate cardiac output (caused by aortic or mitral stenosis).

Fig. 13-5 shows pronounced ST depressions during exercise in a patient with hypertrophic cardiomyopathy and normal coronary arteries.

PRE-EXERCISE   POST-EXERCISE

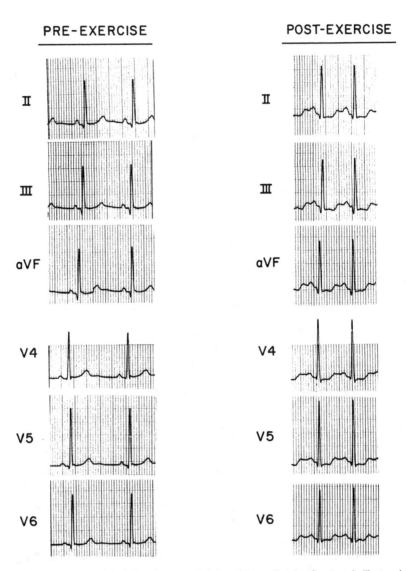

FIG. 13-6. ST depressions (1 mm deep) that developed immediately after treadmill exercise in an 18-year-old woman with mitral valve prolapse and no evidence of coronary artery disease. The pre- and postexercise recordings shown here were obtained with the patient standing. (The test was performed to rule out exertional arrhythmias.)

Patients with mitral valve prolapse commonly have abnormal ST-T changes on their resting ECG, simulating the findings with ischemia (p. 311). False-positive exercise test responses have also been reported in a variable percentage of patients with this syndrome, ranging from 28% to 53%,[3,22,31,60,71] including some individuals with a normal resting ECG (Fig. 13-6). Increased ventricular ectopy, sometimes with ventricular tachycardia, may also occur during exercise in subjects with mitral prolapse, in the absence of coronary heart disease.[71]

The cause of false-positive exercise test results with mitral valve prolapse is uncertain. There is no firm evidence of actual ischemia. Massie et al.[60] reported normal radionuclide perfusion studies (primarily with thallium-201) during exercise in a group of patients with mitral valve prolapse, chest pain, and normal coronary arteriograms. Perfusion scintigraphy during exercise stress therefore may be of help in differentiating false-positive ST-T changes associated with mitral valve prolapse from actual coronary disease. The association between mitral valve prolapse and functional repolarization changes caused by hyperventilation[29] or orthostatic change suggests a possible mediating role for the autonomic nervous system.[22] Finally, some patients with mitral valve prolapse and significant mitral regurgitation will have false-positive stress test results caused by left ventricular hypertrophy.

ALTERED VENTRICULAR ACTIVATION

Major alterations in ventricular activation, as with left and right bundle branch blocks (LBBB, RBBB) and Wolff-Parkinson-White preexcitation (WPW) typically produce secondary ST-T abnormalities on the resting ECG (Chapter 4). During exercise, subjects with these patterns may also have prominent ST segment depressions in the absence of coronary disease.* Whinnery et al.[87] observed up to 10 mm (1 mV) of ST segment depression in a lateral chest lead during exercise testing of subjects with LBBB and normal coronary arteries (Fig. 13-7). Similarly, patients with RBBB may have false-positive ST depressions in the right precordial leads with rsR′ morphology during stress testing. However, ST depressions in the left chest leads with RBBB are suggestive of ischemia.[81] Finally, false-positive ST-T changes are routinely observed in patients with a WPW type of preexcitation pattern.[30,76]

METABOLIC FACTORS

False-positive exercise test results may be caused by several metabolic factors, particularly drug effect (digitalis) and electrolyte imbalance (hypokalemia). In addition, they have been ascribed to anemia and hypoxemia. However, the effect of low hematocrit on the exercise ECG of otherwise normal individuals has not been systematically evaluated. Furthermore, hypoxemia by itself is

---

*References 30, 67, 76, 81, 87, 88.

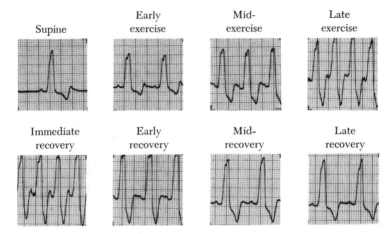

FIG. 13-7. False-positive ST depressions caused by left bundle branch block in a patient with normal coronary arteries. During exercise, note the pronounced downward deflection of the ST segments as recorded with a bipolar chest lead. Similar false-positive responses (from secondary repolarization changes) occur with right bundle branch block (right precordial leads) and Wolff-Parkinson-White pre-excitation. (Courtesy Dr. Victor Froelicher Jr.)

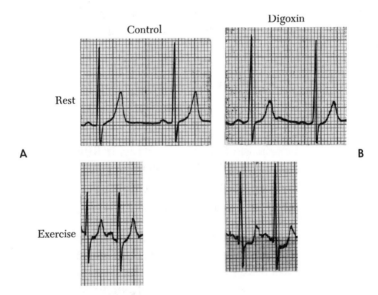

FIG. 13-8. False-positive ST depressions caused by digitalis in a normal individual before and during an exercise stress test. **A,** Before digoxin (control state). **B,** After digoxin. Note the spurious downward deflections of the ST segments when the patient repeated the test. (Courtesy Dr. Martin LeWinter.)

probably not a significant cause of false-positive exercise test results. In one study[36] only a single person (of 16) breathing 10% oxygen with a mean P_{O_2} of 31 mm Hg manifested ischemic ST-T changes during maximal exercise. Similarly, no ST depressions were reported in young male subjects exercising in a hypobaric chamber at several simulated altitudes up to the equivalent of Mt. Everest (8848 m).[57]

Digitalis

Digitalis often produces diffuse ST-T changes on the resting ECG (slight ST depressions, T wave inversions) (Figs. 12-5 and 12-6). These are referred to as *digitalis effect*. Digitalis is also an important cause of false-positive exercise results[46,48,53] (Fig. 13-8). For example, Kawai and Hultgren[48] observed ischemic ST depressions during a Master double two-step test in 8 of 16 normal subjects given digitalis. In two subsequent treadmill studies, false-positive results caused by digitalis were noted in 4 of 8[54] and 4 of 15[65] subjects. Other studies [3,40,66,82] have confirmed a variable but important incidence of false-positive exercise results induced by digitalis. Besides causing false-positive ST responses during exercise, digitalis may increase the degree of ST depression in patients with coronary disease.[48,54]

Morphologically the ST segment changes sometimes observed during exercise in normal digitalized subjects are indistinguishable from true ischemic changes. Horizontal or downsloping ST depressions lasting 0.08 second or more occur in both cases. In most instances the false-positive depressions induced by digitalis are less than 2.5 mm below the resting ST baseline.[48,65,79] However, some normal individual will have 3 to 4 mm of ST depression during exercise caused by digitalis alone.[40,66] Furthermore, the resting ECG may not show evidence of digitalis effect in persons who subsequently manifest these false-positive exercise responses.

The ST-T changes associated with digitalis effect on the resting ECG relate to shortening of the action potential. Presumably this is more pronounced in subendocardial than in epicardial regions, reversing the normal repolarization gradient and ST-T polarity (p. 249). Tachycardia also shortens the action potential. Thus the synergistic effect of digitalis and exercise-related tachycardia may explain the prominent false-positive ST depressions recorded in some cases.[40] Administration of potassium salts has prevented the false positive response to digitalis in some patients[48] but not others.[40] Hirsch noted that digitalis-induced ST segment depressions in two subjects could be blocked by giving potassium and insulin prior to exercise, possibly reversing the extracellular potassium flux caused by digitalis.[40]

From a clinical viewpoint, awareness of false-positive exercise test results caused by digitalis is essential. Ideally the drug should be withheld before exercise testing to allow sufficient time for full excretion. If the patient must be exercised while taking digitalis, ST depressions cannot be reliably interpreted. However, negative (normal) test results or the appearance of typical anginal chest pain or exertional hypotension would still be clinically significant. Thallium scintigraphy can be performed to increase the specificity.

Hypokalemia

Hypokalemia is an important cause of ST depression on the resting ECG, simulating the pattern of coronary insufficiency (Chapter 13). Hypokalemic patients may also have false-positive ST depressions during exercise testing. Soloff and Fewell,[72] using double Master tests, studied nine patients with serum potassium concentrations between 3.3 and 3.9 mEq/L and noted only nonspecific ST-T changes with no pseudoischemic responses. However, Georgopoulos, Proudfit, and Page[32] reported 0.5 to 2 mm ST depressions in another group of hypokalemic patients with normalized exercise tests following potassium repletion. False-positive depressions were recorded even when the resting ECG showed no evidence of hypokalemia. The mechanism whereby exercise unmasks or exaggerates the repolarization changes of hypokalemia is uncertain.

EXERCISE THALLIUM SCINTIGRAPHY: FALSE-POSITIVES

Cardiac imaging with the radionuclide thallium-201 during exercise is commonly performed in an attempt to enhance the sensitivity (Chapter 21) or specificity of the conventional stress ECG in detecting coronary artery disease and to localize zones of ischemia.[35,47] Thallium is distributed to the myocardial cells in linear proportion to the blood flow. A reduction in thallium uptake therefore may reflect either myocardial necrosis or decreased perfusion of still viable cells. These two possibilities can often be distinguished by injecting thallium at peak exercise. The heart is imaged about 5 minutes thereafter and then again after 2 to 4 hours. A *persistent* defect, one present on both early and delayed images, is seen with myocardial infarcts or other causes of irreversible cell damage or replacement. By contrast, a region of viable myocardium that has received less thallium initially because of diminished coronary perfusion will continue to take up thallium over time, while normally perfused regions will show a progressive loss of thallium. As a result of this "redistribution," the initial disparity in radionuclide counts between normal and transiently ischemic zones will partially or completely resolve on the delayed images.[47]

Although thallium scintigraphy can augment the diagnostic accuracy of the stress ECG, important limitations must be kept in mind. Pooled data from multiple studies analyzed by Detrano et al.[20] indicate that both the overall sensitivity and the specificity of exercise thallium tests are about 85%. False-positive results (apparent redistribution in the absence of coronary disease) may occur from a variety of technical, physiologic, and pathologic causes.[14,15,47] For example, regional attenuation of counts simulating ischemia may be due to overlying left breast or adipose tissue or to physiologic thinning of the apex or upper septum. Counts from the inferior wall may be attenuated by the diaphragm or an enlarged right ventricle. In addition, false-positive test results have been reported with certain cardiac conduction abnormalities (including WPW preexcitation[5] and left bundle branch block[41]) associated with altered ventricular activation. With left bundle branch block the false-positive region of hypoperfusion is typically in the ventricular septum. Redistribution of thallium with exercise testing has also been reported in patients with noncoronary heart disease, including hypertrophic cardiomyopathy[84] and sarcoidosis.[56]

FALSE-POSITIVE AND FALSE-NEGATIVE EXERCISE TESTS: SUMMARY

The box below presents a summary of the numerous factors that have been documented as definite (or probable) causes of false-positive (ST segment depression) exercise test results. Not listed are a number of other factors mentioned in the literature, including pericarditis, pectus excavatum, and barbiturate use, which are unproved or anecdotal causes of false-positive responses. Furthermore, although many normal subjects may exhibit nonspecific postprandial ST-T changes, there are no firm data to support the claim that a recent meal can cause a false-positive ischemic pattern during exercise. However, in patients with coronary artery disease, a recent meal may decrease exercise tolerance and increase the degree of actual ischemia. For this reason and because of the enhanced risk in resuscitating a patient who has recently eaten, exercise testing is usually performed in the postabsorptive state.

The new appearance or increased frequency of ventricular premature beats during exercise is also not necessarily an indicator of coronary disease.[34] Ventricular ectopy, including nonsustained ventricular tachycardia, may occur in normal subjects and is sometimes observed with organic noncoronary heart dis-

---

DOCUMENTED CAUSES OF FALSE-POSITIVE EXERCISE TEST RESULTS*

Physiologic (functional) factors†
Atrial repolarization
Hyperventilation
Vasoregulatory lability

Organic noncoronary heart disease
Aortic stenosis
Cardiomyopathy
Left ventricular hypertrophy (e.g., caused
  by valvular disease, hypertension)
Mitral stenosis
Mitral valve prolapse

Altered ventricular activation
LBBB (left precordial leads)
RBBB (right precordial leads)
WPW syndrome

Metabolic factors
Drug effect (digitalis)
Electrolyte imbalance (hypokalemia)

*Defined as ST depressions in the absence of coronary artery disease.
†False-positive responses are more common in women than in men.

ease (e.g., cardiomyopathy or mitral valve prolapse). Rate-related (tachycardia-dependent) left bundle branch block is also *not* a specific indicator of underlying coronary artery disease.[83]

To be complete, it is important to note several factors that can mask true ischemic ST-T changes and produce false-negative results. Not all patients with coronary artery disease will have ST depressions during exercise testing. The sensitivity (p. 350) of such testing is related primarily to the extent of the disease. Data pooled from several studies of exercise testing[49] have shown that with single-vessel disease the sensitivity is only 43%, with two-vessel disease 67%, and with three-vessel disease up to 86%.* In addition, normal exercise tests may be seen in patients with prior myocardial infarction. The use of antianginal drugs can also delay or prevent the appearance of exercise-induced ischemia in patients with coronary disease.[34] Sometimes, ischemic ST depression will occur only in the immediate postexercise period ("recovery only" ST depression).[51]

In addition to ST depressions, the ECG during exercise may show other signs of ischemia. ST segment elevations induced by exercise are discussed in Chapter 8. Inversion of U waves during exercise has also been reported.[33,59] As described on p. 331, normalization of baseline T wave inversions during exercise may sometimes reflect acute ischemia.[58] However, functional T wave inversions also frequently normalize during exercise; so this finding is not of diagnostic value.[4] Similarly, it was initially reported[12,17,18] that an increase in R wave amplitude during exercise might be a useful sign of abnormal left ventricular function and possible ischemia. However, subsequent studies[13,25,42,85] have demonstrated that R wave amplitude changes during exercise lack sensitivity and specificity in the diagnosis of coronary artery disease and also do not correlate with exercise-induced changes in left ventricular function or volume. Finally, recent studies indicate that heart rate adjustment of ST depression during exercise can reduce the number of false-positive test responses in men who have no symptoms while preserving test sensitivity[66a] and can improve coronary heart disease risk stratification in both men and women.[66b]

---

*Left main coronary disease is discussed briefly in Chapter 21.[53]

REFERENCES

1. Abboud S, et al: High frequency electrocardiography of three orthogonal leads in dogs during a coronary artery occlusion, PACE 12:547, 1989.
2. Abinader EG, Shahar J: Exercise testing in mitral valve prolapse before and after beta-blockade, Br Heart J 48:130, 1982.
3. Adair RF, et al: Digoxin induced exercise ECG changes in young men: ST-T walk through phenomenon above 80% maximal heart rate, Circulation 46(suppl 2):11, 1972.
4. Aravindakshan V, et al: Electrocardiographic exercise test in patients with abnormal T waves at rest, Am Heart J 93:706, 1977.
5. Archer S, et al: Exercise thallium testing in ventricular preexcitation, Am J Cardiol 59:1103, 1987.
6. Aronow WS, Harris CN: Treadmill exercise test in aortic stenosis and mitral stenosis, Chest 68:507, 1975.
7. Astrand I, et al: ST changes at exercise in patients with short P-R interval, Acta Med Scand 185:205, 1969.
8. Barlow JB: The "false positive" exercise electrocardiogram: value of time course patterns in assessment of depressed ST-seg-

ments and inverted T waves, Am Heart J 110:1328, 1985.

9. Barnard RJ, et al: Cardiovascular responses to sudden strenuous exercise: heart rate, blood pressure, and ECG, J Appl Physiol 34:833, 1973.

10. Barnard RJ, et al: Ischemic response to sudden strenuous exercise in healthy men, Circulation 48:936, 1973.

11. Barolsky SM, et al: Differences in electrocardiographic response to exercise of women and men: a non-Bayesian factor, Circulation 60:1021, 1979.

12. Baron DW, et al: R wave amplitude during exercise: relation to left ventricular function and volumes and the diagnosis of coronary artery disease, Br Heart J 44:512, 1980.

13. Battler A, et al: Relationship of QRS amplitude changes during exercise to left ventricular function and volumes and the diagnosis of coronary artery disease, Circulation 60:1004, 1979.

14. Beller GA, Bibson RS: Sensitivity, specificity, and prognostic significance of non-invasive testing for occult or known coronary disease, Prog Cardiovasc Dis 29:241, 1987.

15. Berger BC, et al: Abnormal thallium-201 scans in patients with chest pain and angiographically normal coronary arteries, Am J Cardiol 52:365, 1982.

16. Biberman I, et al: T-wave abnormalities during hyperventilation and isoproterenol infusion, Am Heart J 81:166, 1971.

17. Bonoris PE, et al: Evaluation of R wave amplitude changes versus ST-segment depression in stress testing, Circulation 57:904, 1978.

18. Bonoris PE, et al: Significance of changes in R wave amplitude during stress testing: angiographic correlation, Am J Cardiol 41:846, 1978.

19. Cumming GR, et al: Exercise electrocardiogram patterns in normal women, Br Heart J 35:1055, 1973.

20. Detrano R, et al: Factors affecting sensitivity and specificity of a diagnostic test: the exercise thallium scintigram, Am J Med 84:699, 1988.

21. Ellestad MH: Stress testing: principles and practice, ed 3, Philadelphia, 1986, FA Davis Co.

22. Engel PJ, et al: The nature and prevalence of the abnormal exercise electrocardiogram in mitral valve prolapse, Am Heart J 98:716, 1979.

23. Epstein SE: Limitations of electrocardiographic exercise testing, N Engl J Med 301:264, 1979.

24. Foster C, et al: Left ventricular function during sudden strenuous exercise, Circulation 63:592, 1981.

25. Fox K, et al: Inability of exercise-induced R wave changes to predict coronary artery disease, Am J Cardiol 49:674, 1982.

26. Friedman TD: Exercise thallium-201 myocardial scintigraphy in women: correlation with coronary arteriography, Am J Cardiol 49:1632, 1982.

27. Friesinger GC, et al: Exercise electrocardiography and vasoregulatory abnormalities, Am J Cardiol 30:733, 1972.

28. Froelicher VF: Exercise and the heart: clinical concepts, ed 2, Chicago, 1987, Year Book Medical Publishers Inc.

29. Gardin JM, et al: Pseudoischemic "false positive" S-T segment changes induced by hyperventilation in patients with mitral valve prolapse, Am J Cardiol 45:952, 1980.

30. Gazes PC: False positive exercise test in the presence of the Wolff-Parkinson-White syndrome, Am Heart J 78:13, 1969.

31. Gentzler RD, et al: Congenital absence of the left circumflex coronary artery in the systolic click syndrome, Circulation 52:490, 1975.

32. Georgopoulos AJ, et al: The effect of exercise on electrocardiograms of patients with low serum potassium, Circulation 23:567, 1961.

33. Gerson MC, et al: Exercise-induced U wave inversion as a marker of stenosis of the left anterior descending coronary artery, Circulation 60:1014, 1979.

34. Gianelly RE, et al: The effect of propranolol on exercise-induced ischemic S-T segment depression, Am J Cardiol 24:161, 1969.

35. Goldman L, Lee TH: Non-invasive tests for diagnosing the presence and extent of coronary disease: exercise electrocardiography, thallium scintigraphy, and radionuclide ventriculography, J Gen Intern Med 1:258, 1986.

36. Guenter CA: The effects of acute severe arterial hypoxemia on the electrocardiogram during exercise, Chest 68:149, 1975.

37. Guiteras P, et al: Diagnostic accuracy of exercise lead systems in clinical subsets of women, Circulation 65:1465, 1982.

38. Harris CN, et al: Treadmill stress test in left ventricular hypertrophy, Chest 63:353, 1973.

39. Heinsimer JA, DeWitt CM: Exercise testing in women, J Am Coll Cardiol 14:1448, 1989.

40. Hirsch EZ: The effects of digoxin on the electrocardiogram after strenuous exercise in normal men, Am Heart J 70:196, 1965.

41. Hirzel HO, et al: Thallium-201 scintigraphy in complete left bundle branch block, Am J Cardiol 53:764, 1984.

42. Iskandrian AS, et al: Changes of R wave amplitude during exercise: correlation with left ventricular function and volumes, Cardiovasc Rev Rep 3:245, 1982.

43. Iskandrian AS, et al: Dipyridamole cardiac imaging, Am Heart J 115:432, 1988.

44. Iskandrian AS, et al: Role of exercise thallium-201 imaging in decision making, Arch Intern Med 146:1098, 1986.

45. Jacobs WF, et al: False-positive ST-T wave changes secondary to hyperventilation and exercise: a cineangiographic correlation, Ann Intern Med 81:479, 1974.

46. Kattus AA: Exercise electrocardiography: recognition of the ischemic response, false positive and negative patterns, Am J Cardiol 33:721, 1974.

47. Kaul S: A look at 15 years of planar thallium-201 imaging, Am Heart J 118:581, 1989.

48. Kawai C, Hultgren HN: The effect of digitalis upon the exercise electrocardiogram, Am Heart J 68:409, 1964.

49. Koppes G, et al: Treadmill exercise testing. I-II, Curr Probl Cardiol, Nov-Dec, 1977.

50. Kusumi F, et al: Elevated arterial pressure and post-exertional ST-segment depression in middle-aged women, Am Heart J 92:576, 1976.

51. Lachterman B, et al: "Recovery only" ST-segment depression and the predictive accuracy of the exercise test, Ann Intern Med 112:11, 1990.

52. Lary D, Goldschlager N: Electrocardiographic changes during hyperventilation resembling myocardial ischemia in patients with normal coronary arteriograms, Am Heart J 87:383, 1974.

53. Lee TH, et al: Prospective evaluation: a clinical and exercise test model for the prediction of left main coronary artery disease, Med Decis Making 6:136, 1986.

54. LeWinter MM, et al: The effects of oral propranolol, digoxin, and combination therapy on the resting and exercise electrocardiogram, Am Heart J 93:202, 1977.

55. Liebow IM, Feil H: Digitalis and the normal work electrocardiogram, Am Heart J 22:683, 1941.

56. Makler PT, et al: Redistribution on the thallium scan in myocardial sarcoidosis: concise communication, J Nucl Med 22:428, 1981.

57. Malconian M, et al: The electrocardiogram at rest and exercise during a simulated ascent of Mt. Everest (Operation Everest II), Am J Cardiol 65:1475, 1990.

58. Marin JJ, et al: Significance of T wave normalization in the electrocardiogram during exercise stress tests, Am Heart J 114:1342, 1987.

59. Mark DB: Painless exercise ST deviation on the treadmill: long-term prognosis, J Am Coll Cardiol 14:885, 1989.

60. Massie B, et al: Myocardial perfusion scintigraphy in patients with mitral valve prolapse, Circulation 57:19, 1978.

61. McHenry PL, Morris SN: Exercise electrocardiography—current state of the art. In Schlant R, Hurst JW (editors): Advances in electrocardiography, New York, 1976, Grune & Stratton Inc, vol 2.

62. McHenry PL, et al: False positive ECG responses to exercise secondary to hyperventilation: a cineangiographic correlation, Am Heart J 79:683, 1970.

63. Meyers DG, et al: The effect of baseline electrocardiographic abnormalities on the diagnostic accuracy of exercise-induced ST segment changes, Am Heart J 119:272, 1990.

64. Murayama M, et al: Different recovery process of ST depression on postexercise electrocardiograms in women in standing and supine positions, Am J Cardiol 55:1474, 1985.

65. Nasrallah A, et al: Treadmill exercise testing in the presence of nonspecific ST-T changes or digitalis effect: correlation with coronary angiography [Abstract], Am J Cardiol 35:160, 1975.

66. Nördstrom-Öhrberg G: Effects of digitalis glycosides on the electrocardiogram and exercise test in healthy subjects, Acta Med Scand 176(suppl 42):1, 1964.

66a. Okin PM, et al: Heart rate adjustment of ST segment depression for reduction of false positive electrocardiographic responses to exercise in asymptomatic men screened for coronary artery disease, Am J Cardiol 62:1043, 1988.

66b. Okin PM, et al: Heart rate adjustment of exercise-induced ST segment depression. Improved risk stratification in the Framingham Offspring Study, Circulation 83:866, 1991.

67. Orzan F, et al: Is the treadmill exercise useful for evaluating coronary artery disease in patients with complete left bundle branch block? Am J Cardiol 42:36, 1978.

68. Rijneke RD, et al: Clinical significance of upsloping ST segments in exercise electrocardiography, Circulation 61:671, 1980.

69. Sawada SG, et al: Exercise echocardiographic detection of coronary artery disease in women, J Am Coll Cardiol 14:1440, 1989.

70. Sketch MH, et al: Significant sex differences in the correlation of electrocardiographic exercise testing and coronary angiograms, Am J Cardiol 36:169, 1975.

71. Sloman G, et al: Arrhythmias on exercise in patients with abnormalities of the posterior leaflet of the mitral valve, Am Heart J 83:312, 1972.

72. Soloff LA, Fewell JW: Abnormal electrocardiographic responses to exercise in subjects with hypokalemia, Am J Med Sci 252:724, 1961.

73. Sox HC Jr: Probability theory and the interpretation of diagnostic tests. In Sox HC Jr (editor): Common diagnostic tests: uses and interpretation, ed 2, Philadelphia, 1990, American College of Physicians.

74. Sox HC Jr, et al: The role of exercise testing in screening for coronary artery disease, Ann Intern Med 110:456, 1989.

75. Spirito P, et al: Prevalence and significance of an abnormal S-T segment response to exercise in a young athletic population, Am J Cardiol 51:1663, 1983.

76. Strasberg B, et al: Treadmill exercise testing in the Wolff-Parkinson-White syndrome, Am J Cardiol 45:742, 1980.

77. Stratmann HG, Kennedy HL: Evaluation of coronary artery disease in the patient unable to exercise: alternatives to exercise stress testing, Am Heart J 117:1344, 1989.

78. Stuart RJ, Ellestad MH: Upsloping S-T segments in exercise stress testing, Am J Cardiol 37:19, 1976.

79. Sundqvist K, et al: Effect of digoxin on the electrocardiogram at rest and during exercise in healthy subjects, Am J Cardiol 57:661, 1986.

80. Taggart P, et al: Electrocardiographic changes resembling myocardial ischemia in asymptomatic men with normal arteriograms, Br Heart J 41:214, 1979.

81. Tanaka T, et al: Diagnostic value of exercise-induced S-T segment depression in patients with right bundle branch block, Am J Cardiol 41:670, 1978.

82. Tonkon MJ, et al: Influence of digitalis on the exercise stress electrocardiogram in patients with angiographically normal coronary arteries, Clin Res 23:85A, 1975.

83. Vasey C, et al: Exercise-induced left bundle branch block and its relation to coronary artery disease, Am J Cardiol 56:892, 1985.

84. Von Dohlen TW, et al: Significance of positive or negative thallium-201 scintigraphy in hypertrophic cardiomyopathy, Am J Cardiol 64:498, 1989.

85. Wagner S, et al: Unreliability of exercise-induced R wave changes as indexes of coronary artery disease, Am J Cardiol 44:1241, 1979.

86. Weiner D, et al: Exercise stress testing: correlations among history of angina, ST-segment response, and prevalence of coronary-artery disease in the coronary-artery surgery study (CASS), N Engl J Med 301:230, 1979.

87. Whinnery JE, et al: The electrocardiographic response to maximal treadmill exercise of asymptomatic men with left bundle branch block, Am Heart J 94:316, 1977.

88. Whinnery JE, et al: The electrocardiographic response to maximal treadmill exercise of asymptomatic men with right bundle branch block, Chest 71:335, 1977.

89. Wroblewski EM, et al: False positive stress tests due to undetected left ventricular hypertrophy, Am J Epidemiol 115:412, 1982.

Review 3: Differential diagnosis of ST segment depressions (Chapters 11 through 13)

The differential diagnosis of ST depressions includes the following major categories:

1. Spurious and artifactual causes
   a. ECG baseline movement
   b. Inadequate frequency or phase response
   c. S wave in the right bundle branch block pattern
2. Normal-variant patterns
   a. Physiologic ST depressions (e.g., caused by atrial repolarization effect)
   b. Functional ST depressions (associated with autonomic effects [e.g., hyperventilation, exercise, orthostatic change])
3. Ischemic patterns
   a. Acute subendocardial ischemia or infarction (coronary insufficiency)
   b. Reciprocal changes with acute transmural ischemia or infarction
4. Abnormal noncoronary patterns
   a. Left or right ventricular hypertrophy ("strain" pattern)
   b. Secondary ST-T changes (with left bundle branch block, right bundle branch block, and Wolff-Parkinson-White)
   c. Digitalis effect (or combination of digitalis and quinidine)
   d. Hypokalemia
   e. Miscellaneous (e.g., mitral valve prolapse, cerebrovascular hemorrhage, cardiomyopathy, selective coronary arteriography)

In some cases differentiating among these causes will be difficult or impossible. For example, it is not uncommon for ST depressions to reflect a combination of left ventricular hypertrophy, subendocardial ischemia, and digitalis effect. In apparently normal subjects with transient unexplained ST depressions, attempts can be made to reproduce these abnormalities with hyperventilation and orthostatic change. Slight ST depressions, sometimes with associated T wave inversions, in the inferolateral leads are not uncommon with mitral valve prolapse and usually can be confirmed by careful auscultation and echocardiography (p. 311). Exercise testing of patients with ST depressions on their resting ECG is of limited value because virtually all the factors responsible for the resting ST changes can also cause false-positive exercise responses. Thallium scanning may increase the specificity of the exercise test in these circumstances (p. 266).

14

Deep T wave inversions: ischemic causes

Deep T wave inversions may be seen in three major ischemic settings:

1. *Evolving (subacute, chronic) stage of Q wave infarction* (Fig. 14-1). The prominent T waves and ST segment elevations seen during the hyperacute-acute stage of infarction are followed after a variable time (usually hours to days) by deep ischemic T wave inversions. Tall reciprocally positive T waves may be seen in leads facing uninjured areas (Chapters 2 and 18). The T wave inversions begin to resolve after days, weeks, or months, or in some cases they persist indefinitely.[15]

2. *Non–Q wave infarction.* In the past this was often inappropriately equated with "subendocardial" or "nontransmural" infarction (see Chapters 2 and 11). It may be associated with a variety of ST-T patterns. Sometimes (Fig. 14-2) myocardial infarction will produce T wave inversions in the absence of Q waves.[19]* Other times, as described in Chapter 11, ST segment depressions will be seen. In still other cases both ST segment depressions and T wave inversions will occur.

3. *Noninfarctional ischemia.* Deep T wave inversions may be a transient finding in episodes of ischemia without acute infarction. The significance of T wave inversions in the setting of unstable angina pectoris is discussed later.

PATHOPHYSIOLOGY

The deep T wave inversions seen during the chronic or subacute phase of infarction are caused by delayed repolarization in the ischemic area.[16,22] As described in Chapter 8, the hyperacute-acute phase of infarction, marked by tall positive T waves and ST elevations, correlates with a paradoxical shortening of repolarization in the acutely ischemic myocardium. However, during the chronic stage of infarction, repolarization time becomes prolonged in the isch-

---

*As noted on p. 177, contrary to classical teaching, ST elevations, indicative of transient transmural ischemia, may also occur at the onset of non–Q wave infection and be followed by deep T wave inversions in these leads (Figs. 2-1 and 8-3).

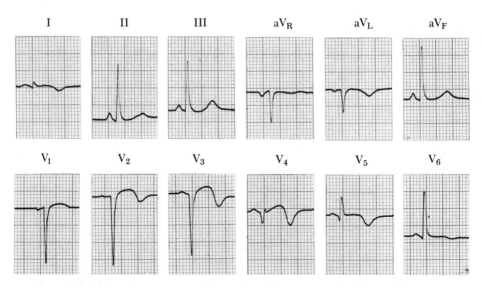

FIG. 14-1. Coved plane T wave inversions with an evolving anterior wall infarct. These are most notable in the anterior precordial leads (especially V_3 and V_4). Note also the pathologic Q waves in V_1 to V_4. The characteristic coved plane morphology is illustrated diagrammatically in Fig. 14-4, *A*.

emic area. Mandel et al.[16] observed that this delay in repolarization (measured by an increase in functional recovery periods) usually occurred within hours to days following acute coronary ligation in dogs. Clinically, relative shortening of the QT interval has been noted in association with ST segment elevations after acute infarction, followed by QT prolongation when T wave inversions appear.[2]

Depolarized muscle is electrically negative relative to repolarized muscle, and as a general rule the repolarization (ST-T) vector will be oriented from areas of extracellular negativity toward areas of positivity. Therefore the T wave vector will point away (negative T wave) from a region of chronic ischemia in which repolarization is prolonged. This delayed repolarization also accounts for the increase in the QT interval seen during the stage of T wave inversions.

The exact ionic changes underlying such prolongation of repolarization during the chronic phase of infarction are unclear. However, *deep T wave inversions and myocardial ischemia are not synonymous.* T wave inversions can theoretically come from any process (functional or organic, temporary or irreversible) that results in a relative delay in regional ventricular repolarization.[16] Normal variant patterns and abnormal but noninfarctional conditions that may be associated with deep T wave inversions are discussed later.

As mentioned earlier, subendocardial (nontransmural) infarction is sometimes associated with deep T wave inversions in the absence of pathologic Q waves. However, according to the model of T wave inversions presented here, ischemic damage located exclusively in the subendocardium should not be ex-

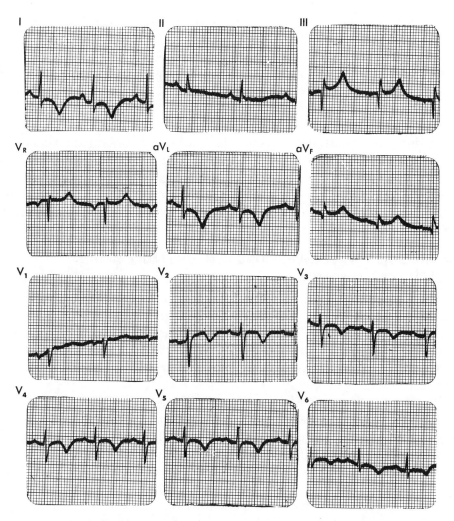

FIG. 14-2. Deep T wave inversions with myocardial infarction. This strip from a patient who complained of chest pain and had elevated cardiac enzymes shows T wave inversions with no Q waves in the anterior leads (V_2 to V_6, I, and aV_L). The reciprocally positive T waves in II, III, and aV_F with Q waves reflect a prior inferior wall infarction.

pected to cause T wave inversions in leads overlying the epicardium. Instead, subendocardial infarction should theoretically produce delayed repolarization in the inner layers of the myocardium, resulting in orientation of the T wave vector toward the epicardium (positive epicardial T waves). In 1955 Pruitt, Klakeg, and Chapin[19] suggested a reasonable explanation for the apparently paradoxical appearance of deep T wave inversions in some cases of nontransmural infarction. They proposed that these T wave inversions actually reflect transmural ischemia involving both the subepicardium and the subendocardium; however, in such cases only the hemodynamically more vulnerable subendocardium becomes necrotic (p. 239). This postulate is supported by the important observation that T wave inversions with non–Q wave infarction are sometimes preceded by transient ST elevations, indicative of transmural ischemia[12] (Figs. 2-1 and 8-3). This ECG sequence may be a marker of spontaneous thrombolysis, aborting the evolution of a frank Q wave infarct (p. 177).

It should be reemphasized, however, that T wave inversions without Q waves do not necessarily indicate subendocardial or nontransmural infarction. Q waves may, in fact, appear with nontransmural infarcts. On the other hand, not all transmural infarcts are associated with pathologic Q waves.

Deep T wave inversions also occur with ischemia (transient or persistent) without infarction. In such cases they probably reflect a degree of transmural ischemia without actual infarction.

PRECORDIAL T WAVE INVERSIONS WITH UNSTABLE ANGINA
(the LAD–T wave syndrome)

The term *unstable angina pectoris* has been used to describe a variety of clinical subsets of patients—including some with angina of increasing frequency or severity, some with angina of recent onset or occurring only at rest, and some with angina associated with profoundly ischemic ST-T changes. Older terms used in this context are *crescendo angina* and *preinfarction angina*.

An important group (14% in one series of patients with unstable angina[5]) will present with deep T wave inversions in the precordial leads (V_1 or V_2 to V_4) without enzymatic evidence of acute infarction* (Fig. 14-3). The T wave inversions may extend as far left as V_6 and may also be present in I and aV_L. Sometimes they persist for days or even weeks. Subsequent episodes of ischemia may be associated with ST elevations or paradoxical T wave normalization (p. 238).

The ECG-clinical syndrome is important for two reasons:
1. First, it is highly specific for stenosis of the left anterior descending (LAD) coronary artery. Figueras et al.[6] reported that 14 of 16 patients had 90% or more stenosis of the proximal LAD. Of the remaining two patients, one had a 60% and the other less than a 50% stenosis. Haines et al.[11] reported that 25 of 29 patients with the pattern had a 70% or greater LAD stenosis. In a large prospective study of 180 patients with unstable angina and precordial T wave inversions, de Zwaan et al.[5] noted complete LAD occlusion in 33 patients and 50% to 90% (mean 85%) stenoses in the remaining 147.

   Similarly, in an early series of 18 retrospectively identified patients with precordial T wave inversions and unstable angina, all of whom had

---

*References 3-6, 8, 10, 11, 19, 20.

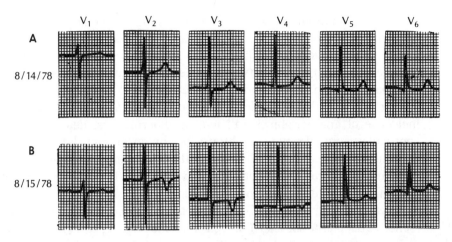

FIG. 14-3. Deep anterior T wave inversions with unstable angina. **A,** This ECG from a patient with prolonged episodes of chest pain is nondiagnostic. **B,** Note the T wave inversions recorded on the following day. Although cardiac enzymes were negative, cardiac catheterization revealed high-grade stenosis of the left anterior descending coronary artery along with anterior wall asynergy.

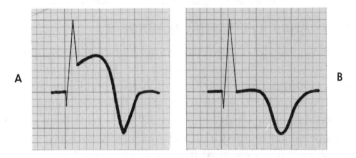

FIG. 14-4. Major morphologic variants of deep T wave inversions. **A,** The coved plane variant is characteristic but not pathognomonic of an evolving infarction. Note the ischemic ST segment (elevated) followed by the convex (coved) descending limb of the T wave, which reaches a sharply inscribed nadir and rises obliquely (in a plane) to the baseline. **B,** Coronary (Pardee) T waves are also characteristic, though not pathognomonic, of an evolving infarct. The ST segment is isoelectric but bowed slightly upward, and the T wave is relatively narrow with sharply inscribed and symmetric limbs.

undergone cardiac catheterization,[9] significant narrowing ($\geq 50\%$) of the LAD was noted in every individual and all but one had a critical lesion in this vessel (i.e., $\geq 90\%$).

The T waves with this syndrome are typically symmetric, with an isoelectric or slightly elevated ST segment (Figs. 14-3 and 14-4). Indeed, they are identical to the T waves seen during the evolving phase of an acute transmural infarct. It is not known how often such T wave inversions actually are preceded by ST elevations due to transient transmural ischemia (Fig. 8-3; see also Fig. 2-1).

2. Second, the syndrome identifies a high-risk subgroup of patients with angina who often have a poor prognosis when treated solely by medical therapy.[4,5] Patients with precordial T wave inversions and unstable angina who do not undergo coronary revascularization have a worse prognosis than patients with angina and no ECG changes.[10,11]

Furthermore, this unstable anginal syndrome is associated with a high incidence of anterior-apical wall motion abnormalities, detected by left ventriculography, despite the absence of any enzyme evidence of acute infarction.[5,6] Successful reperfusion of the left anterior descending coronary (e.g., by coronary angioplasty) may result in T wave normalization and improved anterior anterior wall motion.[20]

Thus, even without precordial Q waves or acute cardiac enzyme elevations, the presence of deep anterior lead T wave inversions (e.g., V_1 to V_4) with unstable angina is a specific predictor of severe stenosis of the left anterior descending coronary artery, often with anterior wall asynergy. The association of T wave inversions with ST elevations in the same leads and segmental ventricular wall motion abnormalities supports the theory[19] that such repolarization changes reflect some degree of transmural, and not just subendocardial, ischemia.*

MORPHOLOGY AND DIFFERENTIAL DIAGNOSIS

The morphology of the T wave inversions produced by ischemia is of some importance in differential diagnosis. Usually the T wave inversions seen in the three ischemic settings mentioned on p. 273 are notable for their relative narrowness† and symmetry. These features are shown diagrammatically in Fig. 14-4. The terms *coronary T wave* and *coved T wave* have been used to describe the classic T inversions seen with an evolving myocardial infarction.

In 1925 Pardee[18] first described the classic coronary T wave (Figs. 14-2 and 14-4, *B*), which consists of an isoelectric ST segment that is usually bowed upward and is followed by a sharp symmetric downstroke. In some cases the ST segment will be perfectly flat rather than bowed upward, and occasionally it will be slightly depressed.

The coved plane T wave described by Rothschild, Mann, and Oppenheimer[21] consists of an elevated ST segment followed by a terminal inversion (Figs. 14-1 and 14-4, *A*). The descending limb has a slight curve (coving); it then forms a sharp nadir and rises back to the baseline with a straight (planed) ascending limb.

The coved T wave and coronary T wave are morphologic variants of the

---

*The presence of inferior lead T wave inversions with unstable angina suggests right coronary or left circumflex coronary artery obstruction.[11]

†Inverted T waves can be considered relatively narrow if their descending and ascending limbs subtend less than half the Q-T interval.

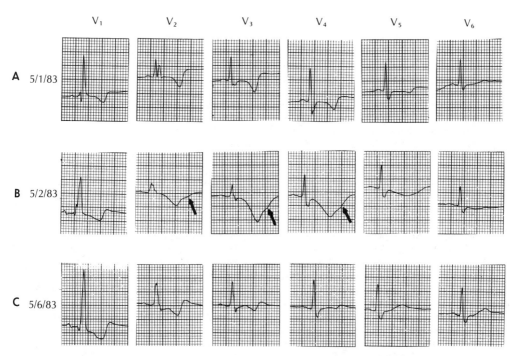

FIG. 14-5. Very deep T wave inversions associated with myocardial infarction and quinidine therapy. **A,** A right bundle branch block pattern with primary T wave inversions (V_3 to V_5) consistent with evolving anterior wall infarction in a patient with prolonged chest pain and elevated cardiac enzymes. **B,** After quinidine administration, note that the T waves are more prominently inverted with marked prolongation of repolarization. There are also two other characteristic features: widening of the QT interval and a large negative U wave (*arrows* in V_2 to V_4). **C,** Following the withdrawal of quinidine, the QT narrows and the negative U wave disappears; however, the ischemic T wave inversions remain.

same basic theme, and they have the same pathologic significance. Indeed, both can be seen in different leads on the same tracing. In concert with these T wave inversions the QT interval is usually prolonged.[16,22]

The relative narrowness and symmetry of ischemic T wave inversions have been emphasized. Less commonly myocardial ischemia produces massive, inverted, *wide* T waves.[7,8] Wide inverted T waves have the same clinical significance as the coronary and coved T waves just described. They may occur in patients with prominent ischemic T wave inversions who subsequently are treated with quinidine or related drugs[17] (Fig. 14-5). However, very deeply inverted and widely splayed T waves are more characteristic of some of the conditions discussed later, particularly cerebrovascular accident, posttachycardia pattern, postpacemaker pattern, and Stokes-Adams syndrome (Chapter 16).

The differential diagnosis of prominent T wave inversions is described in the next three chapters and summarized on pp. 319 to 320.

REFERENCES

1. Boden WE, et al: ST segment shifts are poor predictors of subsequent Q wave evolution in acute myocardial infarction. A natural history study of early non–Q wave infarction, Circulation 79:537, 1989.
2. Cinca J, et al: Time course and rate dependence of Q-T interval changes during noncomplicated acute transmural myocardial infarction in human beings, Am J Cardiol 48:1023, 1981.
3. Cutts FB, et al: Chest pain with inverted T waves, predominantly in the precordial leads, as the only electrocardiographic abnormality, Circulation 16:599, 1957.
4. de Zwaan C, et al: Characteristic electrocardiographic pattern indicating a critical stenosis high in left anterior descending coronary artery in patients admitted because of impending myocardial infarction, Am Heart J 103:730, 1982.
5. de Zwaan C, et al: Angiographic and clinical characteristics of patients with unstable angina showing an ECG pattern indicating critical narrowing of the proximal LAD coronary artery, Am Heart J 117:657, 1989.
6. Figueras J, et al: Prolonged angina pectoris and persistent negative T waves in the precordial leads: response to atrial pacing and to methoxamine-induced hypertension, Am J Cardiol 51:1599, 1983.
7. Fisch C: Giant negative T wave, J Indiana State Med Assoc 54:1664, 1961.
8. Garcia-Palmieri MR, et al: The significance of giant negative T waves in coronary artery disease, Am Heart J 52:521, 1956.
9. Goldberger AL, et al: Unpublished data, 1981.
10. Granborg J, et al: Diagnostic and prognostic implications of transient isolated negative T waves in suspected acute myocardial infarction, Am J Cardiol 57:203, 1986.
11. Haines DE, et al: Anatomic and prognostic significance of new T-wave inversions in unstable angina, Am J Cardiol 52:14, 1983.
12. Huey BL, et al: Acute non–Q wave myocardial infarction associated with early ST segment elevation: evidence for spontaneous coronary reperfusion and implications for thrombolytic trials, J Am Coll Cardiol 9:18, 1987.
13. Kloner RA: Inverted T waves. An electrocardiographic marker of stunned or hibernating myocardium in man? Circulation 82:1060, 1990.
14. Leclercq JF, et al: Correlation between angiographic and ECG signs location in unstable angina, Eur J Cardiol 9:181, 1979.
15. Lepeschkin E: Modern electrocardiography, Baltimore, 1951, The Williams & Wilkins Co, vol 1.
16. Mandel WJ, et al: Analysis of T-wave abnormalities associated with myocardial infarction using a theoretic model, Circulation 38:178, 1968.
17. Marriott HJL: Practical electrocardiography, ed 7, Baltimore, 1983, The Williams & Wilkins Co.
18. Pardee HEB: Heart disease and abnormal electrocardiograms, with special reference to coronary T wave, Am J Med Sci 169:270, 1925.
19. Pruitt RD, et al: Certain clinical states and pathologic changes associated with deeply inverted T waves in the precordial electrocardiogram, Circulation 11:517, 1955.
20. Renkin J, et al: Reversal of segmental hypokinesis by coronary angioplasty in patients with unstable angina, persistent T wave inversion, and left anterior descending coronary stenosis. Additional evidence for myocardial stunning in humans, Circulation 82:913, 1990.
21. Rothschild MA, et al: Successive changes in the electrocardiogram following acute coronary artery occlusion, Proc Soc Exp Biol Med 23:253, 1926.
22. Surawicz B: The pathogenesis and clinical significance of primary T-wave abnormalities. In Schlant RD, Hurst JW (editors): Advances in electrocardiography, New York, 1972, Grune & Stratton Inc.

 **Deep T wave inversions: normal variants**

ARTIFACTUAL AND SPURIOUS T WAVE INVERSIONS

Occasionally inversion of the T wave will be due to artifactual or spurious causes. For example, Fig. 9-4, *B,* shows the distortion of the ST-T complex with coved inversion of the T wave produced by the filter in a cardiac monitor. As emphasized earlier (p. 197), the frequency and phase responses of cardiac monitors must be adequate to ensure accurate representation of the repolarization waveform.

Littmann[17] has described artifactual T wave inversions in patients with left rib resections. Precordial leads placed over the chest wall defect in such cases may show huge inverted T waves and prominent U waves that are reminiscent of the pattern seen with cerebrovascular injury (p. 291).

Spurious T wave inversions (with poor R wave progression) have also been noted when electrode paste is applied in a confluent band across the precordium. In such cases right precordial potentials may be transmitted across the precordium, occasionally producing T wave inversions in the middle to left chest leads.[10]

Finally, T wave lability with slight inversions has been noted during ambulatory ECG recordings in healthy subjects. (See also p. 247).

JUVENILE T WAVE PATTERN

Inverted T waves in the right to middle precordial leads are a normal finding in children. On the ECGs of older adolescents and adults, T wave inversions in the precordial leads (if present) do not usually extend beyond V_2. However, in some instances the juvenile T wave pattern will persist as a normal variant.* The term *juvenile T wave pattern* should be used specifically to describe normal-variant inverted T waves in the right precordial to midprecordial leads with an rS or RS type of complex.[6] Some authors have inappropriately broadened the use of the term to include T wave inversions in the left precordial leads

---

*References 8, 16, 25, 27.

as well. However, in normal children T waves in the left precordial leads become upright during the first hours after birth.

The depth of juvenile inverted T waves is generally less than 5 mm (Fig. 15-1). They are included in this discussion because they are sometimes misinterpreted as a sign of anteroseptal ischemia or right ventricular strain. Abnormal T wave inversions in the limb leads, however, are not a feature of the juvenile T wave variant.

The pattern appears to be most common in young black adults, especially black women. Thomas, Harris, and Lassiter,[25] for example, studied 320 healthy black students between the ages of 20 and 40 years and found the juvenile T wave pattern in 4.6% of the women but only 0.3% of the men. It is apparently less common in whites. Most subjects are in their second or third decade. Upper age limits for this variant have not been clearly established.*

The juvenile T wave pattern should be distinguished from the early repolarization pattern, another normal variant sometimes associated with benign T wave inversions (Chapter 9).

Etiology. Although the persistent juvenile T wave pattern is accepted as a normal variant, its cause is not known. Goldberger[6] demonstrated the transient

---

*The failure of two studies[7,11] to document the occurrence of persistent juvenile T waves probably reflects the relative rarity of this pattern.

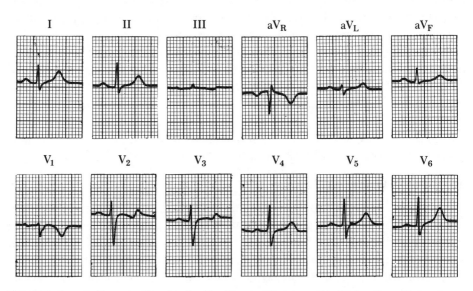

FIG. 15-1. Juvenile T wave pattern in a healthy 19-year-old woman. This tracing shows T wave inversions in V_1 and biphasic T waves in V_2 and V_3. Persistence of the juvenile pattern of T wave inversions in the right precordial to midprecordial leads is a normal variant. It must be distinguished from the pattern characteristic of anteroseptal ischemia or right ventricular strain. With the juvenile variant there should be normal R wave progression in the precordial leads and the T waves in the left precordial and extremity leads should show normal polarity.

reversibility of precordial T wave inversions in children and adults with the juvenile pattern following the oral administration of potassium. Wasserburger[27] confirmed the temporary normalizing effect of potassium and described the same type of response following the intravenous administration of propantheline (Pro-Banthine). Hyperventilation caused an increase in T wave negativity.

Presumably the juvenile T wave inversions reflect a functional delay in regional repolarization. Moderate increases of extracellular potassium levels tend to shorten repolarization and therefore might be expected to normalize these inversions. Through its effect on sympathetic tone, hyperventilation may also accentuate this relative delay in repolarization (p. 206).

BENIGN T WAVE INVERSIONS ASSOCIATED WITH THE EARLY REPOLARIZATION VARIANT

The left precordial "early repolarization" pattern described previously is marked by functional ST elevations that are usually most prominent in the middle to left chest leads (Chapter 9). A variant of this pattern has also been reported, characterized by apparently benign T wave inversions associated with precordial ST elevations (Figs. 15-2 and 15-3). The inverted T waves, which may exceed 5 mm in depth, often have a striking coved appearance that simulates the pattern seen with an evolving infarct. They are usually most notable in the midprecordial leads (V_3 and V_4). In the limb leads they may be normal or slightly inverted. The pattern usually is stable over time or may be associated with T wave lability (Fig. 15-3). Rarely it will be present in the right chest leads (Fig. 15-3).

In one reported case[18] the T waves transiently normalized following potassium infusion, after the administration of amyl nitrite, with exercise, and during a Valsalva maneuver. Following termination of the Valsalva, they became even more inverted (Fig. 15-3).

The pattern of ST elevations with benign T wave inversions is relatively uncommon and has been noted primarily in young black men.[3,7] The same racial prevalence has also been observed with the more common benign ST elevations without T wave inversions described earlier. ST elevations and T wave inversions are sometimes seen in trained athletes.[12,15]

The cause of this unusual normal variant is not known. Grant[9] described a comparable syndrome of isolated T wave negativity in young adult men that consisted of T wave inversions localized in V_3 and V_4. He attributed these to negative repolarization forces of small magnitude that were recorded only by leads directly overlying the cardiac apex.

Goldman[7] first called specific attention to the association of ST elevations and terminal T wave inversions as an apparently benign normal variant. A number of these patients were initially diagnosed incorrectly as having coronary artery disease because of this pattern. His original description was confirmed by

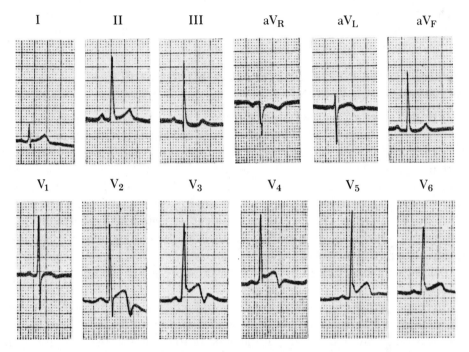

FIG. 15-2. Benign T wave inversions associated with early repolarization ST elevations simulating an anterior wall infarction. This patient, a 16-year-old athletic black youth with no history of cardiac disease, was studied because of a systolic murmur and apparently abnormal ECG. The precordial leads show ST elevations with sharp terminal T wave inversions in V_2 to V_4. The inverted T waves transiently normalized following the ingestion of potassium and after exercise. Results of cardiac catheterization and coronary arteriography were entirely normal. This tracing also shows an R/S ratio greater than 1 in V_1 and tall R waves in the middle to lateral precordial leads compatible with biventricular hypertrophy. A similar pattern simulating that of left and right ventricular hypertrophy has been reported in athletes with no organic heart disease and may reflect "physiologic" hypertrophy. (From Rafailzadeh M, et al: Dis Chest 52:101, 1967.)

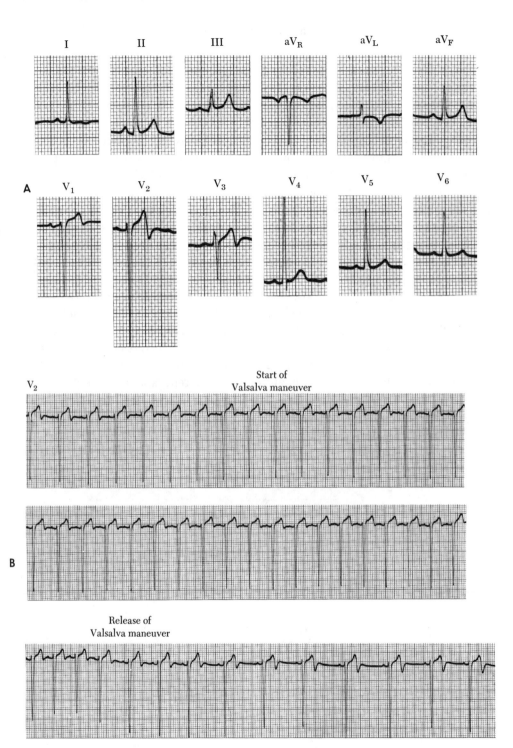

FIG. 15-3. Early repolarization variant with deep T wave inversions in a 32-year-old black man with atypical chest pain and a normal coronary arteriogram. **A,** On the resting ECG, note the ST elevations and deep terminal T wave inversions in the right precordial leads as well as the T wave inversions in I and aV$_L$. **B,** During the tachycardic phase of a Valsalva maneuver there is normalization of T wave inversions in V$_2$; after the Valsalva, with slowing of the heart rate, the T wave inversions become more pronounced. Notice the ST-T lability, which is probably related to changes in autonomic tone.

other reports[3,18,31] that also emphasized the apparent benignity of these T wave inversions. Precordial systolic murmurs[3,18,31] have been noted in a number of subjects with this pattern in whom there was no other evidence of cardiac pathology. A coronary arteriogram in one case[18] was entirely normal.

Individuals with early repolarization ST elevations in the midprecordial to lateral precordial leads often show marked terminal T wave inversions identical to the pattern just described during brief hyperventilation[28] (Fig. 15-4). Similar ST elevations with deep terminal T wave negativity have also been noted following the application of a cold pack to the chest wall of subjects with the early repolarization pattern.[13,19] These observations strongly suggest that T wave inversions associated with ST elevations represent an early repolarization variant.

Such T wave inversions would presumably reflect a slight delay in regional repolarization. The paradoxical combination of T wave inversions (associated with delayed repolarization) and ST segment elevations (associated with early repolarization) might occur if repolarization began earlier on the anterior surface of the ventricles (causing ST elevations in the overlying leads) but terminated earlier on the posterior surface (producing T wave inversions in the anterior leads). Experimental data[14,32] suggest that such functional alterations in repolarization may be mediated through regional differences in sympathetic tone (see also pp. 206 and 207). However, the exact mechanism remains unknown.

Echocardiography may be useful in the differential diagnosis of prominent unexplained T wave inversions in the midprecordial leads of young adults as a

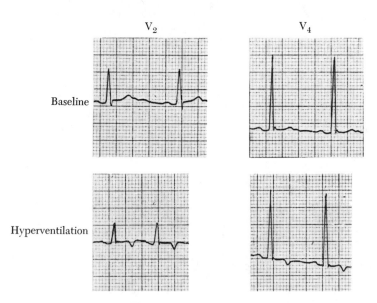

FIG. 15-4. T wave inversions induced by hyperventilation in a 20-year-old man with slight ST elevations in V_2 as part of an early repolarization variant. With hyperventilation there is a notable inversion of the T waves, simulating that seen with ischemia. Note the increase in heart rate.

means of excluding other causes (e.g., apical hypertrophic cardiomyopathy, p. 84), right or left ventricular enlargement, or regional wall motion disorders that could be due to occult myocarditis or coronary disease.

USE OF POTASSIUM SALTS AND PHARMACOLOGIC AGENTS TO DIFFERENTIATE FUNCTIONAL AND ORGANIC T WAVE INVERSIONS

For many years there has been interest in developing clinical tests that would help distinguish between functional and organic repolarization changes. The use of potassium salts will be described in more detail, together with a brief review of pharmacologic agents that have also been used for diagnostic purposes. These tests are primarily of historical and physiologic interest. They have not been adopted clinically because of limitations (discussed below).

Potassium Salts

As a general rule potassium salts normalize functional T wave inversions but not organic repolarization abnormalities. For example, Wasserburger and Corliss[29] found that T wave inversions attributable to functional disturbances (e.g., hyperventilation and anxiety) reverted transiently to normal in all cases following an oral test load of 10 g of potassium salts (5 g of potassium acetate and 5 g of potassium bicarbonate = 96 mEq of K^+). T wave inversions caused by myocardial ischemia either were unaffected or became more pronounced. Similarly, ST-T abnormalities associated with left bundle branch block, digitalis, and subacute pericarditis remained unchanged. Schneider and Lyon[22] reported comparable differentiation of functional and organic T wave abnormalities following an oral test load of 10 g of potassium chloride.

These results contrast with the findings of earlier investigators who observed T wave normalization in some patients with organic heart disease following the oral administration of potassium.[21,23] However, Schneider and Lyon[22] have criticized those and similar early studies, suggesting that the false-positive results may have been attributable to excessive doses of potassium in some experiments and to the lack of rigid criteria for T wave normalization.

The mechanism whereby potassium transiently normalizes functional T wave inversions is not known with certainty. Surawicz[24] speculated that the effect might be caused by a shortening of repolarization that occurs with slight increases in extracellular potassium concentration.

The clinical utility of the potassium-loading test in patients with ST-T alterations is limited. The use of potassium for diagnostic purposes is obviously contraindicated in patients with renal failure and may be dangerous when underlying heart disease is present. Asystole, ventricular tachycardia, and other arrhythmias have been reported[22] following the administration of a standard oral potassium test dose. Wendkos[30] specifically advised against using this test in patients over 60 years of age. Thomsen, Corliss, and Wasserburger[26] were unenthusiastic about the use of potassium loading as a routine clinical test because of its potential toxicity and the possibility of false-positive results. For these reasons potassium loading cannot be recommended in the routine differential diagnosis of functional versus organic T wave inversions.

Ergotamine Tartrate

Wendkos[30] reported temporary abolition of functional but not organic ST-T abnormalities 10 to 15 minutes after a 0.5 mg intravenous dose of ergotamine tartrate. However, in an earlier study Scherf and Schlachman[20] unexpectedly observed a reversion of

T wave abnormalities caused by myocardial infarction and hypertension after the administration of ergotamine. The coronary vasoconstricting action of ergot alkaloids contraindicates their use in patients with underlying ischemic heart disease; therefore, ergotamine should not be used as a diagnostic test for T waves.

Propranolol

Nonspecific ST-T changes sometimes reflect functional alterations in autonomic tone. Such repolarization changes might be normalized by the use of a beta-adrenergic blocking agent. Preliminary studies[2,5] have suggested that propranolol (Inderal) may be useful in differentiating ischemic from nonischemic ST-T changes; however, the sensitivity and specificity of propranolol remain to be determined. Furthermore, beta-blocking agents, by decreasing myocardial oxygen demands, are often associated with normalization of ST depressions due to acute ischemia. This test therefore is unlikely to be of definitive value in separating functional from organic repolarization patterns.

Isoproterenol

Surawicz and colleagues[4,24] have studied the effects of intravenously administered isoproterenol on both normal and abnormal T waves. Their data suggest a possible clinical use for this isoproterenol test in helping to distinguish among different types of T wave abnormalities.

In subjects with *normal* T waves, isoproterenol infusion has a biphasic temporal effect.[24] When isoproterenol is infused at a rate of 3 to 6 μg/min for 4 to 6 minutes, within the first minute the normally upright T waves become diffusely depressed and inverted in some leads, then after approximately 2 minutes they become upright again.

In a second study[4] isoproterenol was infused at 1 to 9 μg/min for 90 seconds in subjects with T wave inversions from a variety of causes. It did not reverse the primary T wave inversions associated with myocardial infarction or pericarditis or the secondary T wave changes associated with QRS prolongation of 0.1 second or more. However, it did induce a reversal of the primary T wave inversions caused by a number of other factors, in patients both with and without underlying heart disease. Specifically it reversed the T wave inversions in 50 of 52 patients with ST-T changes due to left ventricular hypertrophy, diabetes mellitus, cerebrovascular accident, cryohypophysectomy, radical neck dissection, and juvenile T wave and posttachycardia T wave patterns.

The effects of isoproterenol on T wave polarity were not rate related; similar rate increases due to atropine did not cause T wave reversion in most cases.

The normalizing effect of isoproterenol on certain primary T wave inversions may be caused by an asynchronous shortening of repolarization. Isoproterenol, a beta-adrenergic agonist, shortens the action potential of cardiac muscle fibers by accelerating repolarization time. This effect is usually reflected on the ECG as a shortening of the QT_c (rate-corrected QT) interval.[4]

In summary: The effects of isoproterenol on T wave polarity can be divided into three categories:
1. *Normal T waves.* These become initially flattened or negative, followed by a return to normal positivity.
2. *Abnormal T wave inversions with QRS prolongation, myocardial infarction, and pericarditis.* There is no change in polarity.
3. *Primary T wave inversions with other types of organic heart disease and functional T wave inversions.* A transient reversal of T wave polarity is obtained.

Based on these findings, Daoud et al.[4] suggested that isoproterenol infusion might prove clinically useful in separating patients in the second and third categories. However, this test may be dangerous with underlying heart disease or arrhythmias.

REFERENCES

1. Armstrong WF, et al: Prevalence and magnitude of S-T segment and T wave abnormalities in normal men during continuous ambulatory electrocardiography, Am J Cardiol 49:1638, 1982.
2. Behar S, Kariv I: Effect of propranolol on "nonspecific" S-T segment and T wave changes: differentiation of coronary from non-coronary ECG changes, Chest 63:376, 1973.
3. Blackman N, Kuskin L: Inverted T waves in the precordial electrocardiogram of normal adolescents, Am Heart J 67:304, 1964.
4. Daoud FS, et al: Effect of isoproterenol on the abnormal T wave, Am J Cardiol 30:810, 1972.
5. Furberg C: Effects of repeated work tests and adrenergic beta-blockade on electrocardiographic ST and T changes, Acta Med Scand 183:153, 1968.
6. Goldberger E: Significance of downward T waves in precordial leads of normal children, Am J Dis Child 71:618, 1946.
7. Goldman MJ: Normal variants in the electrocardiogram leading to cardiac invalidism, Am Heart J 59:71, 1960.
8. Gottschalk CW, Craige E: A comparison of the precordial ST and T waves in the electrocardiograms of 600 healthy young Negro and White adults, South J Med 49:453, 1956.
9. Grant RP: Clinical electrocardiography, New York, 1957, McGraw-Hill Book Co.
10. Grayboys TB, Majzoub JA: "Smudge" ECG. [Letter to the editor], N Engl J Med 292:49, 1975.
11. Greene CR, Kelly JJ Jr: Electrocardiogram of the healthy adult Negro, Circulation 20:906, 1959.
12. Henne-Paparo N, et al: T wave abnormalities in the electrocardiograms of top-ranking athletes without demonstrable organic heart disease, Am Heart J 81:743, 1971.
13. Kaminer B, Bernstein RE: Electrocardiographic and plasma potassium responses elicited on cooling the chest wall of man, Circulation 15:599, 1957.
14. Kralios FA, et al: Local ventricular repolarization changes due to sympathetic nerve–branch stimulation, Am J Physiol 228:1621, 1975.
15. Lichtman J, et al: Electrocardiogram of the athlete: alterations simulating those of organic heart disease, Arch Intern Med 132:763, 1973.
16. Littmann D: Persistence of the juvenile pattern in the precordial leads of healthy adult Negroes with report of electrocardiographic survey of three hundred Negro and two hundred White subjects, Am Heart J 32:370, 1946.
17. Littmann D: Textbook of electrocardiography, New York, 1972, Harper & Row Publishers.
18. Rafailzadeh M, et al: Physiologic studies in a healthy adolescent with inverted precordial T waves, Dis Chest 52:101, 1967.
19. Rahman SA, et al: Effects of cooling the anterior chest wall on the T wave of the electrocardiogram, Am Heart J 47:394, 1954.
20. Scherf D, Schlachman M: Electrocardiographic studies on the action of ergotamine tartrate and dihydroergotamine 45, Am J Med Sci 216:673, 1948.
21. Schlachman M, Rosenberg B: The effect of potassium on inverted T waves in organic heart disease, Am Heart J 40:81, 1950.
22. Schneider RG, Lyon AF: Use of oral potassium salts in the assessment of T-wave abnormalities in the electrocardiogram: a clinical test, Am Heart J 77:721, 1969.
23. Sharpey-Schafer EP: Potassium effect on T wave inversion in myocardial infarction and preponderance of a ventricle, Br Heart J 5:80, 1943.
24. Surawicz B: The pathogenesis and clinical significance of primary T-wave abnormalities. In Schlant RD, Hurst JW (editors): Advances in electrocardiography, New York, 1972, Grune & Stratton Inc.
25. Thomas J, et al: Observations on the T wave and S-T segment changes in the precordial electrocardiograms of 320 young Negro adults, Am J Cardiol 5:468, 1960.
26. Thomsen JH, et al: Potassium-loading test in the differentiation of T wave abnormalities, Am J Cardiol 30:298, 1972.
27. Wasserburger RH: Observations of the "juvenile pattern" of adult Negro males, Am J Med 18:428, 1955.
28. Wasserburger RH, Alt WJ: The normal RS-T segment elevation variant, Am J Cardiol 8:184, 1961.
29. Wasserburger RH, Corliss RJ: Value of oral potassium salts in differentiation of functional and organic T wave changes, Am J Cardiol 9:673, 1962.
30. Wendkos MH: The use of pharmacological agents to differentiate between organic and functional changes in the T-wave electrocardiogram, Triangle 7:177, 1966.

31. Wiener L, et al: T-wave inversion with elevated RS-T segment simulating myocardial injury, Am Heart J 67:684, 1964.
32. Yanowitz F, et al: Functional distribution of right and left stellate innervation to the ventricles: production of neurogenic electrocardiographic changes by unilateral alteration of sympathetic tone, Circ Res 18:416, 1966.

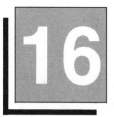

Deep T wave inversions: noninfarctional causes associated with cerebrovascular accident and related patterns

In Chapters 16 and 17 the major abnormal but noninfarctional causes of deep T wave inversions are discussed.

Chapter 16 deals primarily with the deep T wave inversions that may occur in association with cerebrovascular accidents and several related conditions, including truncal vagotomy, radical neck dissection, bilateral carotid endarterectomy, and the Stokes-Adams syndrome. These causes are grouped together because their patterns probably reflect common pathogenetic interactions between the heart and the nervous system.

CEREBROVASCULAR ACCIDENT

In some cases cerebrovascular accident produces tall positive T waves (Chapter 19), mimicking the hyperacute phase of infarction. Paradoxically in other cases it can produce some of the deepest T wave inversions encountered in clinical electrocardiography.

The classic ECG pattern of cerebrovascular accident is the triad of deep T wave inversions, prominent U waves, and marked QT(QU) prolongation.[3,12,20,71] Called the "CVA T wave pattern," it has the following characteristics:

1. *Morphology*. T wave inversions are often striking. Typically they have widely splayed arms and are blunted at the nadir (Figs. 16-1 to 16-4). Occasionally they will be so wide that their arms subtend almost the entire ST interval (Fig. 16-1, *B*). The ascending limb may display a distinctive outward "bulge" (Fig. 16-3), giving the T wave a bizarre asymmetric appearance. This convexity probably represents a large inverted U wave fused with the terminal limb of the T wave.[74]

    Widely splayed, blunted, sometimes irregular T waves contrast with the narrower, sharply inscribed, and relatively symmetric T wave inversions characteristic of infarction. However, these differences are not absolute. Widely splayed T wave inversions at times occur in conjunction with ischemia (Chapter 14). Conversely, cerebrovascular accident may be associated with narrow T wave inversions exactly mimicking those observed

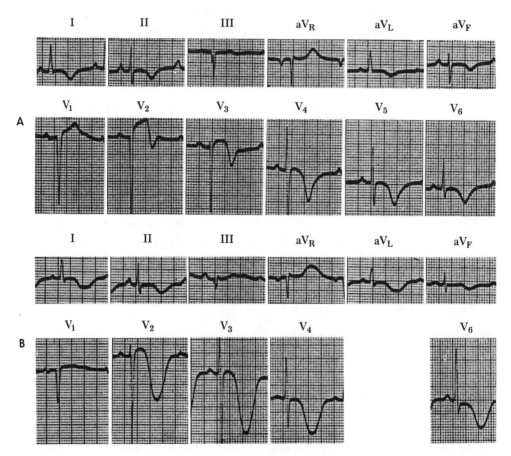

FIG. 16-1. Intracranial hemorrhage simulating myocardial infarction in a 63-year-old black woman with a history of hypertension. **A,** On the first day after admission, note the diffuse T wave inversions. The coved plane ST-T complexes in V_2 and V_3 are indistinguishable from those occurring with an evolving infarct (Fig. 14-1). There is poor R wave progression in V_1 to V_3. Voltage criteria for left ventricular hypertrophy are present in the precordial leads. **B,** Two days after admission, note that the ST-T complexes have changed: the T waves are more deeply inverted, especially in the precordial leads; reciprocal T wave positivity is present in aV_R; the widely splayed T waves have blunt nadirs. Notice the U wave in III. The QT (or QU) interval is prolonged. There is also improved R wave progression in the right precordial leads, probably due to differences in lead placement. The patient died a short time after this tracing was obtained, and at autopsy there was mild left ventricular hypertrophy with dilation, which could have accounted for the prominent precordial voltage and poor R wave progression on the initial ECG. Although several microscopic foci of necrosis were found, there was no evidence of actual infarction. The brain was not examined. Deep, widely splayed, and blunted T waves like these are unusual with myocardial infarction. (From Chou TC, Susilavorn B: J Electrocardiol 2:193, 1969.)

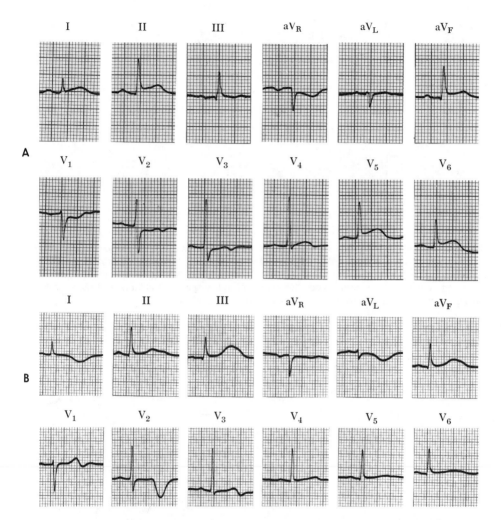

FIG. 16-2. Subarachnoid hemorrhage simulating acute myocardial infarction. **A,** The initial ECG from a comatose patient shows ST elevations in I, II, aV_F, V_5, and V_6 with slight T wave inversions in V_2 and V_3. **B,** One day later, notice the classic cerebrovascular accident pattern, with massive T wave inversions and markedly prolonged QT intervals. There is a prominent U wave in II, making the downslope of the T wave slightly irregular.

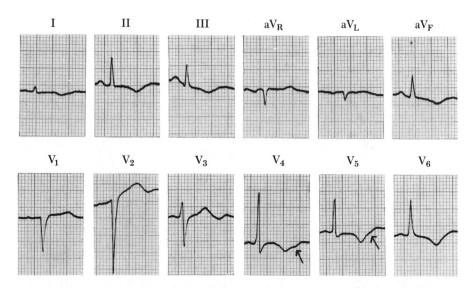

FIG. 16-3. Diffuse T wave inversions with subarachnoid hemorrhage in a 63-year-old woman. Note the prominent positive U wave in V_3. Negative U waves *(arrows)* in V_4 and V_5 are fused with the preceding T wave, giving the entire ST-T complex a characteristically irregular morphology. Although underlying ischemia cannot be ruled out, this pattern of widely splayed and irregular T waves is particularly characteristic of cerebrovascular hemorrhage.

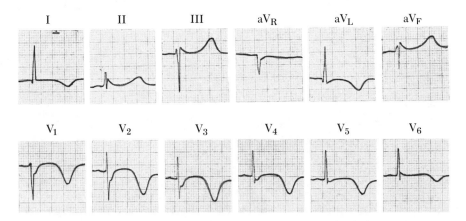

FIG. 16-4. Acute subarachnoid hemorrhage simulating extensive ischemia. This patient, a 69-year-old woman, died 3 days after this tracing was obtained. No autopsy was performed. The ECG shows massive diffuse T wave inversions with distinct prolongation of the QT interval and sinus bradycardia (40 beats/min).

with infarction (Fig. 16-1, *A*). In some cases an initial tracing taken immediately after a cerebrovascular accident will show ischemic-appearing coved T wave inversions that subsequently evolve into the widely splayed T wave pattern[17] (Fig. 16-1). The ST segment may be elevated (suggesting acute ischemia), isoelectric, or slightly depressed. Fig. 16-2 is from a patient with subarachnoid hemorrhage whose initial tracing showed diffuse ST elevations followed by broad T wave inversions with prominent U waves. In one report of two patients with subarachnoid hemorrhage and a "current of injury" pattern with prominent ST elevations,[58] actual infarction or coronary vasospasm could not be excluded.

2. *Distribution of T wave inversions.* Usually deeply and diffusely inverted in the midprecordial to lateral precordial leads and in the limb leads. This gives the appearance of massive anterior wall ischemia with inferior wall extension (Figs. 16-1 and 16-2). The T waves generally are deepest in the middle to lateral precordial leads, at times exceeding 15 mm. Reciprocally positive T waves are seen in aV_R, V_1, and III. The pattern of localized T wave inversions characteristic of infarction is less common with cerebrovascular accident.

3. *Duration of T wave inversions.* Appearing within hours after the initial cerebral injury and becoming progressively deeper over the next few hours to days. Usually they then begin to regress, and there is a gradual return to baseline over the next several weeks,[74] although residual nonspecific ST-T and QT abnormalities may persist.[66]

4. *QT prolongation and U waves.* Marked prolongation,[34] often with prominent U waves. The U waves may be either positive or negative and will at times be buried in the T wave, giving the T wave its characteristic irregular appearance. The QT(U) interval may be prolonged to over 60% of its normal value.[12] QT prolongation is also frequently seen with the deep T wave inversions of infarction but rarely if ever reaches the degree seen with cerebrovascular accident.

5. *Arrhythmias.*[20,23] Sinus bradycardia is common with the classic cerebrovascular accident pattern. Other arrhythmias (atrial and ventricular extrasystoles, wandering pacemaker, AV junctional rhythm, even complete AV block[20,33]) also have been reported. Torsade de pointes, an important variant of ventricular tachycardia, may occur in the setting of QT(U) prolongation.[15,23]

6. *Q waves.* As a general rule, only repolarization abnormalities (ST-T changes) occur. Q waves are not a typical feature of this pattern. However, there are several reports alleging new Q waves in patients with cerebrovascular accident and no autopsy evidence of infarction. Pfister and de Pando[59] reported an unusual case of extensive Q waves with ST elevations in a 53-year-old woman who died of subarachnoid hemorrhage. The

heart was entirely normal at autopsy. Abnormal Q waves without patho-logic evidence of infarction have been reported in other cases of intracra-nial hemorrhage* and in one patient with basilar artery thrombosis.[61]

The significance of Q waves with cerebrovascular accident is not cer-tain. In two cases[38,59] the patients were moderately hypotensive and the Q waves could have resulted from transient ischemia without infarction. In one experimental preparation[35] midbrain stimulation in the cat caused Q waves and histologic examination revealed localized noninfarctional myocardial degeneration.

It is of interest that the deep T wave inversions classically associated with cerebrovascular injury were not present in any of the case reports of Q waves. Conversely, none of the other cases of deep cerebrovascular T wave inversions have been associated with the appearance of new Q waves. Therefore, Q waves should not be considered a typical finding in patients with cerebrovascular accident and those that appear acutely with deep T wave inversions should be interpreted as a sign of actual infarc-tion.

7. *Incidence.* Most frequent with subarachnoid hemorrhage† though also re-ported with cerebral artery occlusion,[26] intracerebral hemorrhage,[12] and suspected cerebral embolism with infarction.[43] Deep but narrower T wave inversions occurred with probable cerebral venous occlusion in a 17-year-old woman.[39] T wave inversions have also been observed follow-ing surgery for left frontotemporal lobe tumor, meningioma of the orbital surface, and falx meningioma.[40] Massive T wave inversions indistin-guishable from the classic CVA pattern have been reported following rad-ical neck dissection,[44] bilateral carotid endarterectomy,[8] extensive cervi-cal laminectomy,[7] truncal vagotomy,[29] and Stokes-Adams attacks.[50] These are described separately later in the chapter.

Other types of central nervous system injuries may produce related ECG abnormalities. Finkelstein and Nigaglioni[28] described prominent U waves and increased QT intervals (without specific mention of deep T wave inversions) during neurosurgical procedures. Similarly, QT prolon-gation and nonspecific ST-T changes have been noted following head in-juries[41] and in association with space-occupying lesions.[42] Nonspecific ECG abnormalities were reported following cerebral angiography, pneu-moencephalography, and ventriculography.[54]

The exact incidence of deep pseudoinfarctional T wave inversions in patients with cerebrovascular accident has not been clearly determined. Kreus, Kemila, and Takala[54] found a variety of ECG abnormalities in 25 of 35 patients with subarachnoid hemorrhage. T wave inversions were noted in six (17%). However, the authors did not specifically report the

---

*References 11, 24, 31, 38, 76.
†References 4, 5, 9, 12, 20, 26, 32, 53, 55, 56, 66, 69, 73, 75.

incidence of massive T wave inversions. In a prospective study of 20 patients with subarachnoid hemorrhage and no history of underlying cardiac disease, Hunt, McRae, and Zapf[47] observed only one patient with massive diffuse T wave inversions. In a subsequent prospective study[30] ECG abnormalities were found in 62% of patients with subarachnoid hemorrhage and in 68% with intracranial space-occupying lesions. However, once again, the specific incidence of pseudoinfarct patterns was not mentioned. Yamour et al.[76] reported QT prolongation and presumed neurogenic T wave changes in three of six patients with frontal lobe hemorrhage.

Etiology. The significance of the giant T wave inversions seen with cerebrovascular injury is a subject of current investigation and debate. There is general agreement that they are the result of cerebrocardiac neural stimuli. Debate has centered on (1) whether these stimuli are primarily *vagal* or *sympathetic* and (2) whether the T wave inversions always represent *structural* cardiac injury or may be due to only *functional* repolarization disturbances.

Most of the autopsies initially reported on patients with this neurogenic T wave pattern were remarkable for the apparent absence of gross and histologic evidence of myocardial injury. Koskelo, Punsar, and Sipilä[53] observed small left ventricular subendocardial hemorrhages in three patients with intracranial bleeding and ECG alterations. Similar hemorrhages have been reported by others,[52,67] but they appeared to be a sporadic finding that would not account for the ECG changes commonly seen in their absence.

More significant, however, are reports of microscopic myocardial lesions in the absence of gross cardiac damage. Connor[18] found random areas of *myocytolysis* in patients with intracranial lesions (chiefly intracranial hemorrhage). Myocytolysis was defined as a distinct type of histologic injury marked by cell death with *contraction bands*. This type of lesion has been termed myofibrillar degeneration or contraction band necrosis.[63] Connor[19] also noted a milder form of myocardial damage, termed *fuchsinophilic* degeneration. In no case did intracranial hemorrhage produce the typical coagulative necrosis of myocardial infarction. Hammermeister and Reichenbach[38] reported focal myocytolysis-type lesions in patients dying of subarachnoid hemorrhage. The significance of all these subtle histologic changes is not known, nor has there been any definite relationship established between them and the ECG alterations seen in certain patients.

Experimental evidence suggests that both vagal and sympathetic hyperstimulation can lead to ECG abnormalities and sometimes myocardial damage. Manning, Sall, and Banting[57] produced focal myocardial degeneration and T wave alterations in dogs by continual vagal stimulation. These pathologic changes were blocked by atropine and potentiated by eserine. Cropp and Manning[20] speculated that the unusual ECG pattern observed with intracranial hemorrhage might result from similar vagocardiac reflexes caused by stimulation of vagal centers in the cortex. The ECGs of some patients with the cerebrovascular T wave pattern have reportedly shown a certain degree of normalization after the administration of atropine.[66]

Intracranial ischemia or injury may also be associated with sympathetic activation,[21,71] which in turn may cause functional and possibly organic myocardial alterations. Porter, Kamikawa, and Greenhoot[63] produced variable repolarization changes and arrhythmias by stereotactically stimulating temporal lobe foci in cats. The changes disappeared following midcervical spine transection, a finding that suggests a sympathetic reflex. Autopsy examination of the hearts of these cats revealed neither gross nor histologic abnormalities.

Yanowitz, Preston, and Abildskov[77] were able to produce marked and predictable repolarization changes in dogs by altering stellate ganglion tone; right stellate ganglionectomy or left stellate stimulation led to prolongation of the QT interval and an increase in T wave amplitude. Right stellate stimulation or left ganglionectomy produced QT prolongation with increased T wave negativity. The authors noted that right stellate ganglionectomy specifically delayed repolarization on the anterior surface of the heart whereas left ganglionectomy produced a delay in posterior repolarization. These findings suggested that the anterior and posterior aspects of the canine heart receive a differential sympathetic input and that unilateral increases or decreases in sympathetic tone can alter the repolarization vector.

On the basis of these animal studies, Abildskov[2] suggested that the T wave changes seen clinically in cerebrovascular accident might be produced entirely by functional, centrally mediated changes in sympathetic tone in the absence of any myocardial damage. Hammer, Luessenhop, and Weintraub[37] demonstrated transient normalization of deep T wave inversions in a patient with subarachnoid hemorrhage during intraoperative manipulation of the circle of Willis. They suggested that the primary repolarization changes and alterations during the surgical procedure also reflected functional changes in autonomic tone.

Other data, however, suggest that neurogenic ECG changes may, at least in some conditions, be associated with myocardial lesions attributable to increased sympathetic stimulation.

Of note, Klouda and Brynjolfsson[52] demonstrated subendocardial hemorrhages and focal myocardial necrosis with marked ECG changes following prolonged left stellate ganglion stimulation in dogs. Other data also suggest the possibility of autonomically mediated myocardial damage in central nervous system injury. Histologic evidence of myocardial degeneration, most pronounced around adrenergic terminals, has been observed in mice with intracranial hemorrhage[13,14] and in cats following midbrain stimulation.[38] Hunt and Gore[46] noted focal myocardial lesions in rats following intracranial hemorrhage. Pretreatment of these animals with a beta-blocking agent, propranolol, decreased the incidence of these lesions. Shanlin et al.[65] increased intracranial pressure in rats by inflating a subdural balloon and noted a significant rise in serum catecholamines, with undefined ECG changes and widespread patches of myocardial contraction band necrosis.

Burch et al.[13] and subsequently others[63] have attributed these neurogenic myocardial lesions and concomitant ECG changes to a "sympathetic storm" initiated by central stimulation of autonomic centers and mediated by the local release of norepinephrine at cardiac adrenergic terminals. The deep T wave inversions seen clinically with cerebrovascular accident may reflect similar organic myocardial damage induced by sympathetic hyperstimulation. The toxic myocardial effects of excessive sympathetic stimulation are well known. In one early experimental study[6] coronary artery perfusion of canine hearts with epinephrine produced peaking of the T waves followed by deep T wave inversions, without myocardial lesions at autopsy. However, both epinephrine[60] and isoproterenol[27] may cause myocardial damage. On the basis of this kind of evidence, Connor[18] and others have suggested that some patients with intracranial bleeding might benefit from treatment with adrenergic blocking agents or atropine to help shield the heart from possible autonomic hyperactivity. The observation of deep T wave inversions after truncal vagotomy,[29] bilateral carotid endarterectomy,[8] radical neck dissection,[44] and pheochromocytoma[16] also supports the claim that repolarization alterations may be associated with changes in autonomic tone. A detailed argument for sympathetic hyperactivity as the *primary* cause of the ECG changes, arrhythmias and myocardial lesions (contraction band necrosis) observed with intracranial hemorrhage and other neurologic castastrophes has been compellingly advanced by Samuels.[64] Reports of an elevated CK-MB fraction[47,51] and left ventricular wall motion abnormalities detected by two-dimensional echocardiography[62] in patients with subarachnoid hemorrhage also support the hypothesis of neurogenically induced myocardial injury.[64]

By way of summary: Current data on the genesis of ST-T changes in patients with cerebrovascular injury are still inconclusive. There is no evidence suggesting actual myocardial ischemia and infarction. However, whether the T wave inversions may, at least in certain cases, reflect purely functional repolarization changes or whether they invariably indicate actual organic cardiac damage induced by autonomic overactivity remains to be established.

The following schema summarizes proposed mechanisms underlying the ECG changes seen with cerebral injury:

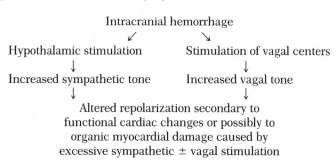

Differential diagnosis. The differential diagnosis of ischemic T wave inversions versus the T wave pattern of CVA is made primarily on the basis of differences in T wave morphology, absence of Q waves, and the clinical setting. However, in some cases the ST-T pattern seen with cerebrovascular injury will be nonspecifically abnormal or indistinguishable from that seen with infarction. In such cases serial tracings may be helpful (Fig. 16-1). On the other hand, broad deep T wave inversions are occasionally seen with acute myocardial infarction (Fig. 14-5).

It must be emphasized that deeply inverted neurogenic T waves are seen for the most part in the setting of intracranial hemorrhage. Therefore clinicians should not, in general, ascribe profound ST-T changes solely to an embolic or thrombotic type of cerebrovascular accident.

The differential diagnosis of subarachnoid hemorrhage (the most common cause of neurogenic T wave inversions) and infarction is further complicated by the fact that subarachnoid hemorrhage may produce elevations in the CK-MB fraction as noted above.[47,51]

Massively inverted wide T waves have also been noted in some patients following open heart surgery with cardiopulmonary bypass.[45] They may reflect underlying myocardial ischemia or injury. However, the possibility that they also may be related to cerebrocardiac reflexes initiated by cerebral hypoxia has been raised.[45]

TRUNCAL VAGOTOMY

Gallivan, Levine, and Canzonetti[29] noted deep widely splayed T wave inversions with QT prolongation following truncal vagotomy. This pattern was observed in 9% of patients studied. The repolarization abnormalities were noted on the first postoperative day, persisted for as long as several weeks, and were not associated with serum enzyme elevations or other clinical evidence of ischemia or infarction.

Morphologically these widely splayed postvagotomy T wave inversions bore a striking resemblance to the CVA pattern just described, a finding that suggests a common underlying mechanism. Gallivan, Levine, and Canzonetti[29] speculated that surgical manipulation of the vagal fibers might have induced retrograde vagal conduction, which in turn might have activated sympathetic centers.

RADICAL NECK DISSECTION, BILATERAL CAROTID ENDARTERECTOMY, AND CERVICAL LAMINECTOMY

Hugenholtz[44] reported an interesting case of a 56-year-old woman who underwent right radical neck dissection for metastatic carcinoma of the tongue. An ECG taken postoperatively showed massive diffuse T wave inversions identical to those associated with cerebrovascular accident. He attributed this to sympathetic nervous system perturbations secondary to operative manipulations in the neck. As noted earlier, Yanowitz, Preston, and Abildskov[77] observed pronounced repolarization changes following stellate ganglion stimulation and stellate ganglionectomy in dogs. These observations support the theory that the deep T wave inversions associated with cerebral injury are caused at least in part by alterations in sympathetic tone.

Similarly deep T wave inversions have been described in a group of patients following bilateral carotid endarterectomy.[8] The ECG changes consisted of deep diffusely inverted T waves in the precordial leads and in one or more of the limb leads, appearing on about the second postoperative day. They resolved within 3 months and were not associated with abnormal Q waves or clinical evidence of myocardial ischemia. The similarity of these T wave changes to those seen with the classic cerebrovascular injury pattern is notable; the authors suggested that altered sympathetic tone might also be responsible for the ECG abnormalities following bilateral carotid endarterectomy.

The appearance of deep T wave inversions in one patient following extensive cervical laminectomy was attributed to similar neurogenic reflexes.[7]

STOKES-ADAMS SYNDROME

Ippolito, Blier, and Fox[48] were the first to call attention to the massive T wave inversions that appear in some cases of complete heart block following Stokes-Adams attacks (Fig. 16-5). Subsequently, similar inversions have been reported in association with complete heart block and Stokes-Adams episodes[10,49,68]

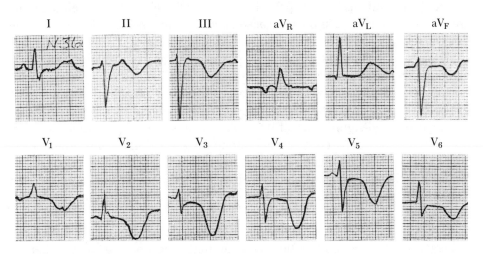

FIG. 16-5. T wave inversions possibly associated with the Stokes-Adams syndrome in an 85-year-old man with a 3-day history of dizziness secondary to pacemaker failure. Complete heart block was present, with an idioventricular rate of 35 beats/min. Although there was no definite history of actual syncope, deeply inverted and blunted T waves are typical of the pattern that follows Stokes-Adams. Almost identical massive inverted T waves occur with cerebrovascular hemorrhage (Figs. 16-1, 16-3, and 16-4). Compare these with the narrower, more sharply inscribed, inversions characteristic of actual ischemia (Figs. 14-1 and 14-2). Prominent T wave inversions may also occur after electronic ventricular pacing (postpacemaker T wave pattern, Chapter 17).

and also in one case of partial heart block with syncope.[72] Aber and Wyn Jones[1] found prominent T wave inversions in three patients with complete heart block and one with partial heart block during treatment with steroids. Van Bruggen, Sebus, and van Heys[73] reported an unusual case of similarly massive T wave inversions following syncopal episodes in an 8-year-old girl with the Jervell Lange-Nielsen syndrome (QT prolongation, syncope, and deafness; discussed in more detail on p. 310). The T wave inversions in this case (although not specifically explained by the authors) may be related to the phenomenon described with heart block and syncope.

The T wave inversions in all of these cases are identical morphologically to those occurring with cerebrovascular accident. In some cases the Stokes-Adams T waves, like the cerebrovascular accident T waves, are asymmetric because of an inverted U wave that produces a characteristic outward bulge on the ascending limb of the repolarization wave.

The T wave inversions following Stokes-Adams syncope may disappear after a few days[49] or persist for a few months.[48] They usually are most prominent in the midprecordial to lateral precordial leads. Deep T wave inversions may be present in other leads, simulating the pattern of diffuse ischemia (Fig. 6-5). Their broad, widely splayed, and sometimes irregular appearance contrasts with the narrower and more sharply inscribed T wave inversions usually encountered in ischemia and infarction (Figs. 14-2 and 14-3). Furthermore, abnormal Q waves or ST elevations never appear acutely with the Stokes-Adams syndrome.

The Stokes-Adams T wave pattern appears to be relatively rare, although its precise incidence is not known. Jacobson and Schrire[50] noted only one example in a survey of ECGs from 140 patients with heart block. Careful prospective study of patients immediately following Stokes-Adams episodes may reveal a higher incidence of T wave changes. Aber and Wyn Jones[1] noted T wave inversions in 4 of 30 patients with heart block during treatment with steroids. The inversions disappeared following discontinuance of steroid therapy.

The cause and significance of the Stokes-Adams T wave pattern are still unresolved, but they apparently are not due to myocardial infarction. Autopsy examination of one patient with syphilis and complete heart block revealed cardiac gummas without significant coronary disease.[68] In none of the other reported cases have there been clinical signs or enzyme changes consistent with infarction.

However, it is still possible that these T wave inversions reflect myocardial ischemia without actual infarction. Ippolito, Blier, and Fox[48] attributed them to bradycardia with underlying ischemia. Bradycardia prolongs diastole and therefore might further delay repolarization in ischemic areas. Szilagyi and Solomon[72] reported a patient with partial heart block whose T wave inversions varied directly with the length of the preceding diastole. However, these repolarization alterations appear to reflect more than simple rate-dependent changes. Their obvious similarity to the T wave inversions of cerebrovascular accident suggests a possible common mechanism. Jacobson and Schrire[49] proposed that cerebral hypoxia due to Stokes-Adams syncope might trigger cerebrocardiac reflexes resulting in the same type of repolarization changes seen with subarachnoid hemorrhage and other types of cerebral injury.

REFERENCES

1. Aber CP, Wyn Jones E: Steroid-induced T wave changes in heart block, Br Heart J 27:56, 1965.
2. Abildskov JA: Central nervous system influence upon electrocardiographic waveforms. In Schlant RC, Hurst JW (editors): Advances in electrocardiography, New York, 1972, Grune & Stratton Inc.
3. Abildskov JA, et al: The electrocardiogram and the central nervous system, Prog Cardiovasc Dis 13:210, 1970.
4. Ananthachari MD, Anto CD: A study of ECG changes in 20 cases of subarachnoid hemorrhage, Indian Heart J 19:105, 1967.
5. Ashby DW, Chadha JS: Electrocardiographic abnormalities simulating myocardial infarction in intracerebral haemorrhage and cerebral thrombosis, Br Heart J 30:732, 1968.
6. Barger AC, et al: Chronic catheterization of the coronary artery: infusion of autonomic drugs in the unanesthetized dog, Fed Proc 20:101, 1961.
7. Baur HR, et al: Electrocardiographic changes after cervical laminectomy, Int J Cardiol 1:37, 1981.
8. Baur HR, Pierach CA: Electrocardiographic changes after bilateral carotid endarterectomy, N Engl J Med 291:1121, 1974.
9. Beard EF, et al: Spontaneous subarachnoid hemorrhage simulating acute myocardial infarction, Am Heart J 58:755, 1959.
10. Birke G, Ström G: Attacks of ventricular fibrillation with subsequent massive T wave inversion in a case of complete A-V block, Acta Med Scand 152:479, 1955.
11. Brunninkhuis LG: Electrocardiographic abnormalities suggesting myocardial infarction in a patient with severe cranial trauma, PACE 6:1336, 1983.
12. Burch GE, et al: A new electrocardiographic pattern observed in cerebrovascular accidents, Circulation 9:719, 1954.
13. Burch GE, et al: Acute myocardial lesions following experimentally induced intracranial hemorrhage in mice: a histological and

histochemical study, Arch Pathol 84:517, 1967.
14. Burch GE, et al: Effects of experimental intracranial hemorrhage on the ultrastructure of the myocardium of mice, Am Heart J 77:427, 1969.
15. Carruth JE, Silverman ME: Torsade de pointe atypical ventricular tachycardia complicating subarachnoid hemorrhage, Chest 78:886, 1980.
16. Cheng TO, Bashour TT: Striking electrocardiographic changes associated with pheochromocytoma masquerading as ischemic heart disease, Chest 70:397, 1976.
17. Chou TC, Susilavorn B: Electrocardiographic changes in intracranial hemorrhage, J Electrocardiol 2:193, 1969.
18. Connor RCR: Heart damage associated with intracranial lesions, Br Med J 3:29, 1968.
19. Connor RCR: Fuchsinophilic degeneration of myocardium in patients with intracranial lesions, Br Heart J 32:81, 1970.
20. Cropp GJ, Manning GW: Electrocardiographic changes simulating myocardial ischemia and infarction associated with spontaneous intracranial hemorrhage, Circulation 22:25, 1960.
21. Cruickshank JM, et al: Possible role of catecholamines, corticosteroids, and potassium in production of electrocardiographic abnormalities associated with subarachnoid haemorrhage, Br Heart J 36:697, 1974.
22. Dimant J, Grob D: Electrocardiographic changes and myocardial damage in patients with acute cerebrovascular accidents, Stroke 8:448, 1977.
23. Di Pasquale G, et al: Holter detection of cardiac arrhythmias in intracranial hemorrhage, Am J Cardiol 59:596, 1987.
24. Düren DR, Becker AE: Focal myocytolysis mimicking the electrocardiographic pattern of transmural anteroseptal myocardial infarction, Chest 69:506, 1976.
25. Fabinyi G, et al: Myocardial creatine kinase isoenzyme in serum after subarachnoid

hemorrhage, J Neurol Neurosurg Psychiatry 40:818, 1977.

26. Fentz V, Gormsen J: Electrocardiographic patterns in patients with cerebrovascular accidents, Circulation 25:22, 1962.
27. Ferrans VJ, et al: Isoproterenol-induced myocardial necrosis: a histochemical and electron microscopic study, Am Heart J 68:71, 1964.
28. Finkelstein D, Nigaglioni A: Electrocardiographic alterations after neurosurgical procedures, Am Heart J 62:772, 1961.
29. Gallivan GJ, et al: Ischemic electrocardiographic changes after truncal vagotomy, JAMA 211:798, 1970.
30. Galloon S, et al: Prospective study of electrocardiographic changes associated with subarachnoid hemorrhage, Br J Anaesthesiol 44:511, 1972.
31. Gascon P, et al: Spontaneous subarachnoid hemorrhage simulating acute transmural myocardial infarction, Am Heart J 105:511, 1983.
32. Goldfinger P: Recurrent electrocardiogram changes in subarachnoid hemorrhage, NY J Med 72:2771, 1972.
33. Goldman MR, et al: Subarachnoid hemorrhage: association with unusual electrocardiographic changes, JAMA 234:957, 1975.
34. Goldstein DS: The electrocardiogram in stroke: relationship to pathophysiological type and comparison with prior tracings, Stroke 10:253, 1979.
35. Greenhoot JH, Reichenbach DD: Cardiac injury and subarachnoid hemorrhage: a clinical, pathological, and physiological correlation, J Neurosurg 30:521, 1969.
36. Hackenberry LE, et al: Biochemical evidence of myocardial injury after severe head trauma, Crit Care Med 10:641, 1982.
37. Hammer WJ, et al: Observations on the electrocardiographic changes associated with subarachnoid hemorrhage with special reference to their genesis, Am J Med 59:427, 1975.
38. Hammermeister KE, Reichenbach DD: QRS changes, pulmonary edema, and myocardial necrosis associated with subarachnoid hemorrhage, Am Heart J 78:94, 1969.
39. Harrison MT, Gibb BH: Electrocardiographic changes associated with a cerebrovascular accident Lancet 2:429, 1964.
40. Hayashi S, et al: Studies of electrocardiographic patterns in cases with neurosurgical lesions, Jap Heart J 2:92, 1961.

41. Hersch C: Electrocardiographic changes in head injuries, Circulation 23:853, 1961.
42. Hersch C: Electrocardiographic changes in subarachnoid hemorrhage, meningitis, and intracranial space-occupying lesions, Br Heart J 26:785, 1964.
43. Hugenholtz PG: Electrocardiographic abnormalities in cerebral disorders: report of six cases and review of the literature, Am Heart J 63:451, 1962.
44. Hugenholtz PG: Electrocardiographic changes typical for central nervous system disease after right radical neck dissection, Am Heart J 74:438, 1967.
45. Hultgren HN, et al: Ischemic myocardial injury during cardiopulmonary surgery, Am Heart J 85:167, 1973.
46. Hunt D, Gore I: Myocardial lesions following experimental intracranial hemorrhage: prevention with propranolol, Am Heart J 83:232, 1972.
47. Hunt D, et al: Electrocardiographic and serum enzyme changes in subarachnoid hemorrhage, Am Heart J 77:479, 1969.
48. Ippolito TL, et al: Massive T-wave inversion, Am Heart J 48:88, 1954.
49. Jacobson D, Schrire V: Giant T wave inversion, Br Heart J 28:768, 1966.
50. Jacobson D, Schrire V: Giant T wave inversion associated with Stokes-Adams syndrome, S Afr Med J 40:641, 1966.
51. Kaste M, et al: Heart type creatine kinase isoenzyme (CK MB) in acute cerebral disorders, Br Heart J 40:802, 1978.
52. Klouda MA, Brynjolfsson G: Cardiotoxic effects of electrical stimulation of stellate ganglia, Ann NY Acad Sci 156:271, 1969.
53. Koskelo P, et al: Subendocardial hemorrhage and ECG changes in intracranial bleeding, Br Med J 1:1479, 1964.
54. Kreus KE, et al: Electrocardiographic changes in cerebrovascular accidents, Acta Med Scand 185:327, 1969.
55. Levine HD: Non-specificity of the electrocardiogram associated with coronary artery disease, Am J Med 15:344, 1953.
56. Levine HJ, White NW: Unusual ECG patterns in rupture of vertebral artery aneurysm, Arch Intern Med 110:523, 1962.
57. Manning GW, et al: Vagus stimulation and the production of myocardial damage, Can Med Assoc J 37:314, 1937.
58. Nakamura Y, et al: Transient ST-segment elevation in subarachnoid hemorrhage, J Electrocardiol 22:133, 1989.

59. Pfister CW, de Pando B: Cerebral hemorrhage simulating acute myocardial infarction, Dis Chest 42:206, 1962.

60. Piscatelli RL, Fox LM: Myocardial injury from epinephrine overdosage, Am J Cardiol 21:735, 1968.

61. Poliakoff H: Basilar artery thrombosis: electrocardiogram simulating acute infarction, NY J Med 72:2891, 1972.

62. Pollick C, et al: Left ventricular wall motion abnormalities in subarachnoid hemorrhage: an echocardiographic study, J Am Coll Cardiol 12:600, 1988.

63. Porter RW, et al: Persistent electrocardiographic abnormalities experimentally induced by stimulation of the brain, Am Heart J 64:815, 1962.

64. Samuels MA: Neurogenic heart disease: a unifying hypothesis, Am J Cardiol 60:15J, 1987.

65. Shanlin RJ, et al: Increased intracranial pressure elicits hypertension, increased sympathetic activity, electrocardiographic abnormalities in rats, J Am Coll Cardiol 12:727, 1988.

66. Shuster S: The electrocardiogram in subarachnoid hemorrhage, Br Heart J 22:316, 1960.

67. Smith RP, Tomlinson BE: Subendocardial haemorrhages associated with intracranial lesions, J Pathol 68:327, 1954.

68. Soscia JL, et al: Complete heart block due to a solitary gumma, Am J Cardiol 13:553, 1964.

69. Srivastava SC, Robson AO: Electrocardiographic abnormalities associated with subarachnoid hemorrhage, Lancet 2:431, 1964.

70. Stober T, Kunze K: Electrocardiographic alterations in subarachnoid hemorrhage: correlation between spasm of the arteries on the left side of the brain and T wave inversion and QT prolongation, J Neurol 227:99, 1982.

71. Surawicz B: Electrocardiographic pattern of cerebrovascular accident, JAMA 197:191, 1966.

72. Szilagyi N, Solomon SL: Variation in the form of the T wave in a case of partial heart block, Am Heart J 58:637, 1959.

73. Van Bruggen HW, et al: Convulsive syncope resulting from arrhythmia in a case of congenital deafness with ECG abnormalities, Am Heart J 78:81, 1969.

74. Wasserman F, et al: Electrocardiographic observations of patients with cerebrovascular accidents: report of 12 cases, Am J Med Sci 231:502, 1956.

75. Weintraub BM, McHenry LC Jr: Cardiac abnormalities in subarachnoid hemorrhage: a resumé, Stroke 5:384, 1974.

76. Yamour BJ, et al: Electrocardiographic changes in cerebrovascular hemorrhage, Am Heart J 99:294, 1980.

77. Yanowitz F, et al: Functional distribution of right and left stellate innervation to the ventricles: production of neurogenic electrocardiographic changes by unilateral alteration of sympathetic tone, Circ Res 18:416, 1966.

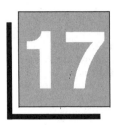

Deep T wave inversions: other noninfarctional causes

This chapter completes the discussion of major noninfarctional causes of deep T wave inversions begun in Chapter 15.

POSTTACHYCARDIA T WAVE PATTERN

Posttachycardia T wave pattern (Fig. 17-1) refers to the noninfarctional T wave inversions sometimes observed following bouts of supraventricular* or ventricular[21,46,53] tachycardia. It has the following characteristics:

1. *T wave morphology.* Usually symmetric, resembling the coronary T wave pattern; however, in most cases posttachycardia T waves have a somewhat broader base[46] (compare Figs. 14-2 and 17-1). Posttachycardia T wave inversions may be shallow or may in some cases reach striking dimensions suggestive of extensive ischemic damage. For example, inversions almost 20 mm deep[46] were noted in a 21-year-old man following a 24-hour episode of supraventricular tachycardia. The QT interval is also frequently prolonged with the posttachycardia T wave syndrome. However, abnormal Q waves and ST segment elevations are not seen.

2. *Topography of T wave changes.* May appear in any leads, though probably most common in the middle to lateral precordial and the inferior limb leads.[29,49] T wave inversions in the right precordial leads simulating anteroseptal ischemia have also been reported.[41]

3. *Temporal sequence.* In some cases resolving within hours, in others persisting for weeks or even months. Serial tracings over a period of days to weeks usually reveal a gradual diminution in T wave amplitude and an eventual return to baseline status.[13,29,49] No definite relationship has been established between the duration or rate of the preceding tachycardia and the amplitude or duration of the subsequent T wave inversions.[61]

4. *Incidence.* Not reported.

Etiology. The precise cause of the posttachycardia T wave pattern is unre-

---

*References 7, 13, 19, 29, 41, 49, 61.

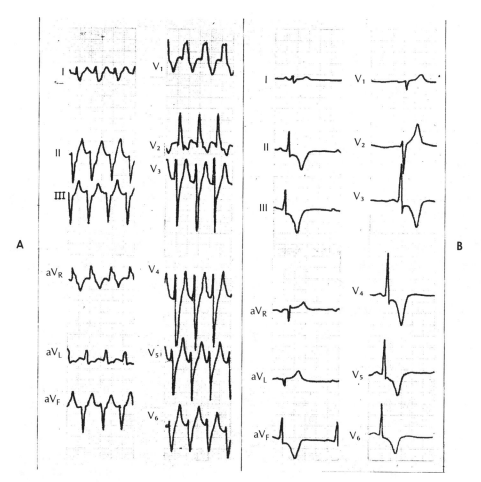

A

B

FIG. 17-1. This ECG is from a 21-year-old man with no evidence of organic heart disease, including normal cardiac catheterization and coronary arteriographic studies. **A,** Recorded during an episode of wide-complex (probably supraventricular) tachycardia. **B,** Recorded immediately after reversion to sinus rhythm 2 days later. (From Kernohan RJ: Br Heart J 31:803, 1969.)

solved. T wave inversions subsequent to ventricular tachycardia have been attributed to delayed repolarization in the region of increased automaticity.[30] However, this does not explain the mechanism of T wave inversions following supraventricular tachycardias, in which the focus of stimulation is in the atria or AV junction.

Nor is it clear whether these repolarization changes are functional or represent actual subclinical myocardial damage. No patients with the pattern have shown clinical signs of infarction or elevated enzyme levels in serial studies.[29,46,49] Furthermore, the young age of a number of patients with this pattern[13,29,46] and the absence of underlying heart disease or cardiac impairment following the episodes suggest a functional cause for the ECG changes.[46] On the other hand, the amplitude of the T waves and their persistence for extended periods in some cases raise the possibility of organic myocardial damage secondary to the tachycardia.[46]

T wave inversions may also occur in the beat following a single extrasystole (ventricular or supraventricular). Such *postextrasystolic T wave inversions* usually are found in patients with underlying cardiac disease.[16,31,36] Postextrasystolic T wave changes have been correlated with a shortening of phase 2 and a lengthening of phase 3 repolarization in the beat following the extrasystole.[16] Whether there is any relationship between the transient T wave changes that may occur following a single extrasystole (postextrasystolic T wave pattern) and the marked T wave inversions sometimes observed following prolonged bouts of ectopic tachycardia (posttachycardia pattern) remains to be determined.

The diagnosis of posttachycardia T wave inversions is one of exclusion that must be made with caution. Other causes of T wave inversions (p. 319), particularly ischemia or infarction, must be carefully excluded.

PACEMAKER T WAVE PATTERN

Several reports[8,9,20] have described a syndrome of massive T wave inversions occurring in nonpaced beats following the use of a ventricular pacemaker (Fig. 17-2). They have the following general characteristics:

1. *Morphology.* Usually more broadly based and blunter than the relatively narrow sharply inscribed T wave inversions of infarction (compare Figs. 14-2 and 17-2). Postpacemaker T wave inversions may exceed 15 mm in depth and be associated with pronounced QT prolongation.
2. *Topography.* Appear related to the site of pacemaker stimulation. Chatterjee et al.[8] observed T wave inversions in II, III, aV_F, and the lateral precordial leads when a pacemaker was implanted on the endocardium of the right ventricle or epicardium of the left ventricle. In two patients with pacemakers placed in the right ventricular outflow tract, the T wave inversions occurred primarily in V_1 and V_2.
3. *Amplitude and duration.* Directly related to the power of the pacing stimulus and the duration of pacing.[8] For example, Chatterjee et al.[8] found that the T wave inversions produced by just 10 minutes of endocardial pacing in one patient lasted only 15 minutes whereas those after 2 years of pacing in another persisted for more than a year.
4. *Incidence.* Not systematically studied. Chatterjee et al. found the pattern in 29 of 31 patients.
5. *Potassium salts.* No effect in two patients,[18] increased T wave negativity in a third.[8]

The significance of these T wave inversions is not clear. No evidence of myocardial infarction has been found in any of the cases. The results of cardiac enzyme studies were negative, and abnormal Q waves or ST elevations were never

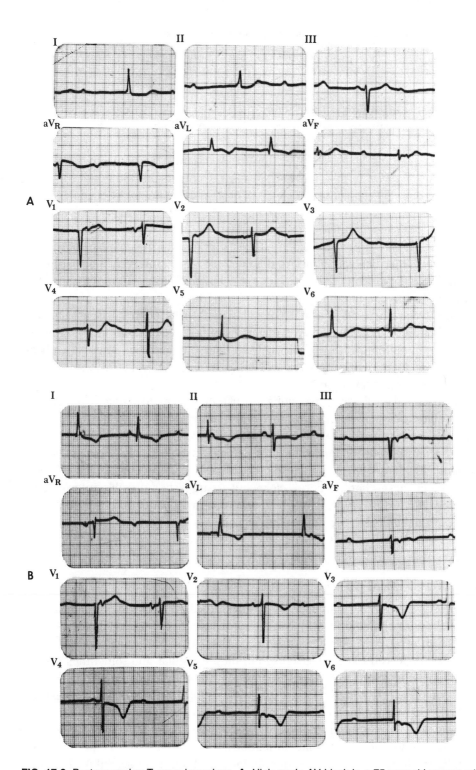

FIG. 17-2. Postpacemaker T wave inversions. **A,** High-grade AV block in a 75-year-old woman with dizzy spells. A temporary transvenous pacemaker was inserted into the right ventricle. **B,** Note on the routine ECG obtained 3 days later with the pacemaker turned off the deep diffuse T wave inversions, most prominent in the middle to lateral precordial leads. There was no clinical evidence of infarction, and serial cardiac enzyme studies were normal. (From Gould L, et al: Chest 63:829, 1973.)

seen in the postpacemaker beats. However, unlike purely functional T wave inversions, these postpacemaker changes did not normalize after potassium administration. Furthermore, their persistence for extended periods in some cases suggests the possibility of some type of slowly reversible, structural myocardial damage.[8]

Chatterjee et al.[8] suggested that the T wave changes were due to depolarization of the ventricles from an ectopic site. T wave inversions did not occur when the pacemaker spike was made to fall in the absolute refractory period or following atrial pacing.

The morphologic similarity of these postpacemaker T waves and the post-tachycardia T waves just described suggests a common mechanism (e.g., sustained ventricular depolarization from an ectopic site). However, the post-tachycardia T wave inversions may also be seen following supraventricular as well as ventricular tachycardias.

Deep T wave inversions also occur following Stokes-Adams attacks (Chapter 16). Although most of the reported instances of postpacemaker T wave changes have been in patients with underlying high-degree heart block, there have been no apparent intercurrent episodes of Stokes-Adams syndrome in any of these patients to account for them.[8]

Postpacemaker T wave inversions are usually not as irregular or as wide as the T waves that accompany cerebrovascular injury. However, Chatterjee et al.[8] presented an interesting example of wide irregular T wave inversions that appeared after the oral administration of potassium chloride in a patient whose baseline ECG had shown symmetric postpacemaker T wave inversions. The significance of these changes is not clear, but it suggests a possible interrelationship between the two types of deep T wave inversion patterns.

From the clinical viewpoint the postpacemaker T wave syndrome represents another important example of massive T wave inversions that may occur in the absence of myocardial infarction.

IDIOPATHIC LONG QT SYNDROMES

In 1957 Jervell and Lange-Nielsen[26] described a familial syndrome (autosomal recessive) characterized by congenital perceptive deafness, prolongation of the QT interval, and episodes of syncope and sometimes sudden death (surdocardiac or Jervell Lange-Nielsen syndrome). A similar and sometimes familial (autosomal dominant) syndrome (Romano-Ward) of QT prolongation associated with syncope and sudden death in the *absence* of deafness has since been described.[48] QT prolongation is a major substrate for high-grade ventricular tachyarrhythmias, in particular *torsade de pointes* ventricular tachycardia (which may degenerate into ventricular fibrillation).[47,50,62]

Bizarre alterations in T wave morphology, including occasional deep T wave inversions, have been reported in both variants of the idiopathic long QT syndrome.[18,32] The T waves may have a normal morphology (except for the prolonged QT interval), or they may be biphasic or deeply inverted.[4,58] Furthermore, they often show spontaneous lability and may vary in appearance under the influence of drugs, exercise, etc.[27] Abnormal Q waves or QRS prolongation are *not* seen in association with QT prolongation syndromes.

Prolongation of the QT interval in these patients is a reflection of delayed repolarization. The cause of this disturbance is not known. Necropsy study of one case[17] revealed degenerative changes in the sinus node; degenerative changes in the His bundle were seen in a second case.[43] However, focal lesions in the proximal conduction system cannot account for the generalized repolarization changes present in these patients.

Yanowitz, Preston, and Abildskov[60] have demonstrated that alterations in sympathetic tone in the dog can markedly affect the QT interval as well as the polarity of the T wave (p. 298). An imbalance in sympathetic innervation might also produce the patterns seen on the surface ECG in these unusual QT prolongation syndromes. This theory is supported by the clinical efficacy of left stellate ganglionectomy or beta blockade in preventing syncope or sudden death in some, though not all, subjects.[50] Altered sympathetic tone has also been cited as a possible cause of the marked repolarization abnormalities seen in some cases of cerebrovascular injury; it is tempting to suggest a possible common neurogenic mechanism to explain them. (This topic is discussed at greater length in Chapter 16.) Alternatively, patients with idiopathic long QT syndrome may have a primary myocardial defect selectively affecting repolarization.[62]

MITRAL VALVE PROLAPSE SYNDROME*

Mitral valve prolapse (sometime referred to as the "click-murmur" or "billowing mitral lealet" syndrome) is a disorder of unknown cause with distinctive auscultatory and electrocardiographic features.† Its auscultatory hallmark is a nonejection systolic click or clicks, often followed by a midsystolic to late systolic murmur. Angiographic or echocardiographic studies may reveal prolapse of one or both of the mitral valve leaflets into the left atrium, sometimes with mitral regurgitation ranging from mild to severe. Although varying degrees of left ventricular asynergy have been reported,[23] the coronary arteries are typically normal.[25] Echocardiographic studies have demonstrated the relatively common occurrence of this syndrome, particularly in women. In one prospective study[45] evidence of mitral valve prolapse appeared in about 6% of women. A number of families with several affected members have been reported.[14]

Clinically the patients may be entirely without symptoms. However, a num-

---

*This discussion focuses on the idiopathic or primary mitral valve prolapse syndrome. This syndrome can also occur as a secondary finding with other types of heart disease, including coronary disease and rheumatic valvulitis.[3]
†References 14,15,25,42,44.

ber will experience atypical or angina-like chest pain that, together with the ECG abnormalities described in the following paragraphs, often leads to a mistaken diagnosis of coronary artery disease.

Characteristics of the mitral valve prolapse syndrome that mimic coronary disease are outlined in the following list:

Inferolateral ST-T changes

Inferolateral Q waves (?)

Chest pain

High-grade ventricular or atrial arrhythmias

AV conduction disturbances

False-positive exercise stress test

Systolic murmur

Ventricular asynergy

Cerebral ischemic events[4]

The ECG abnormalities of this syndrome include ST-T changes and rarely noninfarctional Q waves.

1. *ST-T changes.* The most common abnormalities, seen in many but not all patients, are relatively nonspecific ST-T changes, including ST depressions, T wave flattening, and minimal T wave inversions (Fig. 17-3). These are characteristically notable in the inferior limb leads or lateral precordial leads. Occasionally T wave inversions will be more prominent and have a coronary or coved plane morphology that is strongly suggestive of ischemia.[25] However, even when marked, they rarely if ever exceed 5 mm in depth.

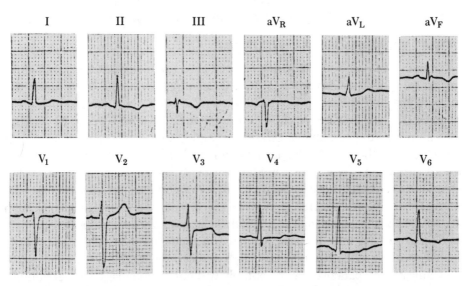

FIG. 17-3. ST-T changes associated with mitral valve prolapse. In this 34-year-old woman in whom mitral valve prolapse was documented angiographically, the coronary arteries were normal. Note the nonspecific ST-T abnormalities with slight T wave inversions in the lateral precordial and inferior leads. Failure to recognize this syndrome may lead to erroneous attribution of ST-T alterations to functional abnormalities, left ventricular strain, or coronary artery disease.

The ST-T complex may be quite labile. In one reported case[55] ST-T changes were elicited by sitting, hyperventilating, and performing a Valsalva maneuver. Amyl nitrite may also induce characteristic ST-T changes in patients whose baseline ECG is unremarkable.[25] False-positive stress tests have been reported in patients with mitral valve prolapse (Chapter 13). QT prolongation has been noted occasionally.

2. *Q waves.* Although the ST-T alterations just described are relatively common, noninfarctional Q waves have been reported in only a few instances. Barlow and Bosman[1] described one case of an 8-year-old girl whose ECG showed Q waves and T wave inversions in II, III, and aV_F and another of a 17-year-old boy with apparently noninfarctional Q waves and T wave inversions in the inferior limb leads and lateral precordial leads. Similarly, Lobstein et al.[34] reported a 20-year-old man with pseudoinfarctional Q waves in the inferolateral leads. In two other cases[57] QS waves were present in V_1 to V_3. Several patients have been reported with apparent infarct patterns but normal left ventriculograms and coronary arteriograms.[23,52]

The genesis of the ECG abnormalities in patients with this syndrome is still uncertain. Pocock and Barlow[44] suggested that the primary cause was the billowing mitral valve, which over time put traction on the papillary muscle apparatus, resulting in local ischemia with ST and T wave changes. Histologic examination of the mitral valve in patients with this syndrome[15] typically shows *redundancy* and *myxomatous degeneration* of the leaflets, without myocardial involvement. Early angiographic studies showing left ventricular asynergy in a number of these patients[22] suggested some type of underlying myocardial disease that was not histologically defined.

To date, however, there have been only tentative explanations for the repolarization abnormalities seen with this syndrome and no good explanation for the occasional appearance of pseudoinfarctional Q waves. The presence of pathologic Q waves in a patient with a systolic murmur should always suggest an alternative diagnosis, especially the likelihood of coronary artery disease with secondary papillary muscle dysfunction or hypertrophic cardiomyopathy (which is discussed in detail in Chapter 4). Mitral valve prolapse may be associated with pectus excavatum (p. 57), another cause of poor precordial R wave progression. Of related interest is that a number of young patients with mitral valve prolapse have been reported who had acute myocardial infarction with normal coronary arteriograms. The clinical picture in these cases was strongly suggestive of coronary vasospasm[10] (Chapter 8).

The clinical significance of the mitral valve prolapse syndrome is variable. In most of the patients who have had long-term follow-up, the syndrome appears to follow a benign course.[2] However, there are multiple reports of complications in these patients, including high-grade brady- or tachyarrhythmias, sudden death, bacterial endocarditis, and significant mitral regurgitation necessitating surgical treatment.[14,15,40,42] In addition, a number of patients may complain of bothersome chest pain that suggests angina pectoris or sometimes even myocardial infarction.[45] Mitral valve prolapse with ECG changes have been reported with Marfan's syndrome[6] and other connective tissue disorders.

The unexpected discovery of T wave inversions in the inferior or inferolateral leads of any patient should always prompt a careful search for a systolic click-murmur. However, patients with mitral valve prolapse evident at echocardiography or angiography do not always present the typical auscultatory findings (silent mitral valve prolapse).[25]

The nondiagnostic nature of the ECG findings in some patients with this syndrome underscores the need for caution in assessing apparently functional or nonspecifically abnormal ST-T patterns. A number of the many factors, normal as well as pathologic, that are associated with such nonspecific ST and T wave alterations are listed on pp. 8 and 9.

ARRHYTHMOGENIC RIGHT VENTRICULAR DYSPLASIA

Arrhythmogenic right ventricular dysplasia, a cause of prominent right precordial T wave inversion, is discussed in Chapter 4.

SELECTIVE CORONARY ARTERIOGRAPHY

Deep broad T wave inversions are characteristically observed during selective coronary arteriography (Fig. 17-4, A). As a rule the T wave vector shifts away from the perfused area*; thus injection of the right coronary artery with dye typically displaces the T wave vector superiorly and leftward (toward −60 degrees), producing deep T wave inversions in II, III, and aV_F, and left coronary artery injection usually displaces the T wave vector inferiorly and rightward (toward +120 degrees) in the frontal plane (Fig. 17-4, B), producing deep wave inversions in I and aV_L.

Injection of dye into the left coronary artery also produces a generally leftward shift in the frontal plane QRS axis, which has been attributed to transient left anterior hemiblock. Right coronary artery injection shifts the frontal plane QRS axis generally to the right, possibly secondary to transient left posterior hemiblock (Fig. 17-4).[38]

In summary: The left coronary response to selective arteriography is characterized by a rightward shift of the frontal plane T wave axis and a leftward shift of the QRS axis. The right coronary response is characterized by a leftward shift of the T wave axis and a rightward shift of the QRS axis.[11]

Marked T wave changes have also been reported in the precordial leads during selective coronary angiography. In one study[39] deep T wave inversions and ST depressions were observed in the right chest leads (V_1 and V_2) during right coronary artery injection and deep lateral T wave inversions were noted (V_5 and V_6) during left coronary angiography.

Slight ST segment deviations (usually less than 2 mm) may occur in the direction of the T wave changes (e.g., ST depression with T wave inversions).[22] Prominent U waves may also appear with prolongation of repolarization time (QU interval),[39] mimicking the appearance of the giant splayed T waves seen in some cases of cerebrovascular accident (Chapter 16).

---

*References 11, 22, 35, 37, 54.

Injection of right coronary artery with radiopaque dye

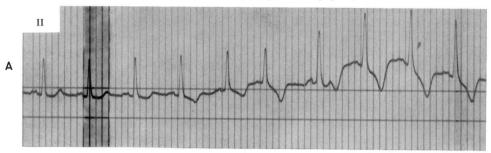

Injection of left coronary artery with radiopaque dye

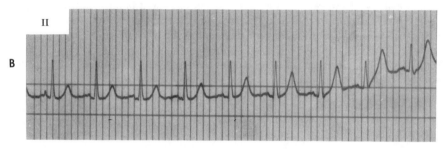

FIG. 17-4. QRS-T changes in lead II associated with selective coronary arteriography: **A,** injection into the right coronary artery produces deep T wave inversions; **B** injection into the left produces increased T wave positivity. (See text for details.)

The course of these ECG changes is rapid; they typically appear within 4 to 6 seconds of the injection of dye and resolve within 30 to 60 seconds.[22]

The typical left coronary and right coronary patterns may be modified by the type of coronary circulation or by the presence of significant coronary obstruction. For example, Maranhao et al.[37] observed these patterns only in patients with right coronary predominance. They found no (or only minimal) ECG alterations in the presence of left coronary predominance or a balanced coronary circulation. Similarly, no ECG changes were seen during selective coronary arteriography in a case of single coronary artery circulation.[22] In another series, McCans et al.[39] found no direct correlation between localization of ECG changes and the coronary circulation pattern.

Coronary artery disease can also modify the ECG response to coronary arteriography. Major coronary obstruction (left or right) may completely block the appearance of these changes.[22] In other cases of obstruction with collateralization a biphasic ECG response has been reported. For example, injection of a patent coronary artery may initially produce the expected ECG pattern, which is then followed by the pattern when the contralateral coronary is perfused. This biphasic response is probably due to late filling of the obstructed contralateral coronary artery through anastomotic collateral channels.

The deep T wave inversions associated with selective coronary arteriography are not caused by ischemia. Rather, they are probably related to local prolongation of repolarization produced by the relatively high sodium concentration of the radiopaque dye. Smith,

Harthorne, and Sanders[54] reproduced these T wave changes with both sodium-containing dyes and pure saline solutions. The higher the concentration of sodium, the more pronounced was the effect on repolarization. However, infusions of hypertonic mannitol, dextrose in water, hypoxic blood, or Ringer's solution did not produce comparable T wave inversions.

Increased extracellular sodium may act at the cell membrane level by prolonging the plateau phase of the action potential.[24] Perfusion of local areas of myocardium with high sodium concentrations therefore will lead to a regional prolongation in repolarization. Shabetai, Surawicz, and Hammill[51] observed that injection of the right coronary artery with dye or 3% saline caused local prolongation of right ventricular monophasic action potentials while left ventricular action potentials remained normal.

Ischemic T wave inversions seen during the chronic stage of infarction may be due to a localized prolongation of repolarization, resulting in displacement of the T wave vector away from the injured area. The local ionic changes underlying these inversions have not been elucidated. However, from a clinical point of view it is important to recognize that they can be elicited acutely during coronary arteriography. Equally important is the fact that they are evanescent and cannot explain any ST-T changes persisting after an angiographic study.

Nonspecific ST-T changes have been noted in some patients following intravenous pyelography.[33] More prominent ischemic appearing ST changes have also been reported,[5] particularly in elderly patients with underlying heart disease. It is not certain whether these are related to the hypertonic dye or to actual ischemia in the setting of organic heart disease. Ischemic changes were not seen in one survey of healthy subjects undergoing intravenous pyelography.[28]

OTHER CAUSES OF DEEP NONINFARCTIONAL T WAVE INVERSIONS

Other causes of deep T wave inversions are described in this text in the sections on left ventricular hypertrophy ("strain" pattern), apical hypertrophic cardiomyopathy, bundle branch blocks, dilated (congestive) cardiomyopathy, right ventricular overload ("strain" pattern), acute metabolic injury (e.g., transient ischemia), acute myocarditis, traumatic noncoronary injury (penetrating and nonpenetrating myocardial injury, lightning stroke), Friedreich's ataxia, chronic chagasic myocarditis, myocardial tumors, pericarditis, pheochromocytoma, and hypothermia. Isolated instances of T wave changes have also been reported in several unrelated conditions, including hypopituitarism,[56] acute iron intoxication,[59] and flecainide intoxication.[12]

REFERENCES

1. Barlow JB, Bosman CK: Aneurysmal protrusion of the posterior leaflet of the mitral valve, Am Heart J 71:166, 1966.
2. Barlow JB, Pocock WA: Mitral valve prolapse, the specific billowing mitral leaflet syndrome, or an insignificant nonejection systolic click. [Editorial], Am Heart J 97:277, 1979.
3. Barnett HJM, et al: Further evidence relating mitral valve prolapse to cerebral ischemic events, N Engl J Med 302:139, 1980.
4. Benhorin J, et al: Long QT syndromes. New electrocardiographic characteristics, Circulation 82:521, 1990.
5. Berg GR, et al: Electrocardiographic abnormalities associated with intravenous urography, N Engl J Med 289:87, 1973.
6. Bowers S: An electrocardiographic pattern associated with mitral valve deformity in Marfan's syndrome, Circulation 23:30, 1961.

7. Campbell M: Inversion of T waves after long paroxysm of tachycardia, Br Heart J 4:49, 1942.

8. Chatterjee K, et al: Electrocardiographic changes subsequent to artificial ventricular depolarization, Br Heart J 31:770, 1969.

9. Chatterjee K, et al: T-wave changes after artificial pacing, Lancet 1:759, 1969.

10. Chesler E, et al: Acute myocardial infarction with normal coronary arteries: a possible manifestation of billowing mitral leaflet syndrome, Circulation 54:203, 1976.

11. Coskey RL, Magidson O: Electrocardiographic response to selective coronary arteriography, Br Heart J 29:512, 1967.

12. Crijns HJGM, et al: Transient giant inverted T waves during flecainide intoxication, Am Heart J 113:314, 1987.

13. Currie GM: Transient inverted T waves after paroxysmal tachycardia, Br Heart J 4:149, 1942.

14. Devereux RB, et al: Mitral valve prolapse: causes, clinical manifestations, and management, Ann Intern Med 111:305, 1989.

15. Düren DR, et al: Long-term follow-up of idiopathic mitral valve prolapse in 300 patients: a prospective study, J Am Coll Cardiol 11:42:1988.

16. Edwards RE, Bailey JC: Postextrasystolic T wave, Am J Cardiol 28:536, 1971.

17. Fraser GR, et al: Congenital deafness associated with electrocardiographic abnormalities, fainting attacks, and sudden death: a recessive syndrome, Q J Med 33:361, 1964.

18. Garza LA, et al: Heritable QT prolongation without deafness, Circulation 41:39, 1970.

19. Geiger AJ: Electrocardiograms simulating those of coronary thrombosis after cessation of paroxysmal tachycardia, Am Heart J 26:555, 1943.

20. Gould L, et al: Pacemaker-induced electrocardiographic changes simulating myocardial infarction, Chest 63:829, 1973.

21. Graybiel A, White RD: Inversion of the T-wave in lead I or II in young individuals with neurocirculatory asthenia, with thyrotoxicosis, in relation to certain infections, and following paroxysmal ventricular tachycardia, Am Heart J 10:345, 1935.

22. Grendahl H, et al: Electrocardiographic changes during selective coronary arteriography, Acta Med Scand 191:493, 1972.

23. Gulotta SJ, et al: The syndrome of systolic click, murmer, and mitral valve prolapse: a cardiomyopathy? Circulation 49:717, 1974.

24. Hecht HH: Some observations and theories concerning the electrical behavior of heart muscle, Am J Med 30:720, 1961.

25. Jeresaty RM: Mitral valve prolapse-click syndrome, Prog Cardiovasc Dis 15:623, 1973.

26. Jervell A, Lange-Nielsen F: Congenital deaf-mutism; functional heart disease with prolongation of the Q-T interval and sudden death, Am Heart J 54:59, 1957.

27. Jervell A, et al: The surdo-cardiac syndrome: three new cases of congenital deafness with syncopal attacks and QT prolongation in the electrocardiogram, Am Heart J 72:582, 1966.

28. Kappelman N, et al: Electrocardiographic changes with intravenous pyelography in healthy individuals, Urology 9:88, 1977.

29. Kernohan RJ: Post-paroxysmal tachardia syndrome, Br Heart J 31:803, 1969.

30. Lepeschkin E: Modern electrocardiography, Baltimore, 1951, The Williams & Wilkins Co, vol 1.

31. Levine HD, et al: The clinical significance of postextrasystolic T-wave changes, Circulation 6:538, 1952.

32. Levine SA, Woodworth CR: Congenital deaf-mutism, prolonged QT interval, syncopal attacks, and sudden death, N Engl J Med 259:412, 1958.

33. Listchinsky M, et al: Electrocardiographic changes following intravenous pyelography, Israel J Med Sci 11:304, 1975.

34. Lobstein HP, et al: Electrocardiographic abnormalities and coronary arteriograms in the mitral click-murmur syndrome, N Engl J Med 289:127, 1973.

35. MacAlpin RN, et al: Electrocardiographic changes during selective coronary arteriography, Circulation 34:627, 1966.

36. Mann RH, Burchell HB: The significance of T wave inversion following ventricular extrasystoles, Am Heart J 47:504, 1954.

37. Maranhao V, et al: Temporary repolarization abnormalities during coronary artery visualization, Am Heart J 85:138, 1973.

38. Maytin O, et al: The genesis of the QRS changes produced by selective coronary arteriography, Circulation 41:247, 1970.

39. McCans JL, et al: Electrocardiographic changes in precordial leads during selective coronary angiography, J Electrocardiol 9:211, 1976.

40. Mills P, et al: Long-term prognosis of mitral-valve prolapse, N Engl J Med 297:13, 1977.

41. Myerson RM: Transient inversion of T waves after paroxysmal tachycardia, JAMA 148:193, 1952.

42. Nishimura RA, et al: Echocardiographically documented mitral-valve prolapse. Long-term follow-up of 237 patients, N Engl J Med 313:1305, 1985.

43. Phillips J, Ichinose H: Clinical and pathologic studies in the hereditary syndrome of a long QT interval, syncopal spells, and sudden death, Chest 58:236, 1970.

44. Pocock WA, Barlow JB: Etiology and electrocardiographic features of the billowing posterior leaflet syndrome: analysis of a further 130 patients with a late systolic murmur or nonejection systolic click, Am J Med 51:731, 1971.

45. Procacci PM, et al: Prevalence of clinical mitral-valve prolapse in 1169 women, N Engl J Med 294:1086, 1976.

46. Rakov HI: Prolonged benign T-wave inversion following paroxysmal ventricular tachycardia NY J Med 64:2100, 1964.

47. Ratshin RA, et al: Q-T interval prolongation, paroxysmal ventricular arrhythmia, and convulsive syncope, Ann Intern Med 75:919, 1971.

48. Romano C: Congenital cardiac arrhythmias, Lancet 1:658, 1965.

49. Sargin O, Demirkol C: Deeply inverted T-waves after supraventricular paroxysmal tachycardia, Dis Chest 48:321, 1965.

50. Schwartz PJ: Idiopathic long QT syndrome: progress and questions, Am Heart J 109:399, 1985.

51. Shabetai R, et al: Monophasic action potentials in man, Circulation 38:341, 1968.

52. Sloman G, et al: Arrhythmias on exercise in patients with abnormalities of the posterior leaflet of the mitral valve, Am Heart J 83:312, 1972.

53. Smith LB: Paroxysmal ventricular tachycardia followed by electrocardiographic syndrome with a report of a case, Am Heart J 32:257, 1946.

54. Smith RF, et al: Vectorcardiographic changes during intracoronary injections, Circulation 36:63, 1967.

55. Sreenivasan VV, et al: Posterior mitral regurgitation in girls due to posterior papillary muscle dysfunction, Pediatrics 42:276, 1968.

56. Surawicz B: The pathogenesis and clinical significance of primary T-wave abnormalities. In Schlant RD, Hurst JW (editors): Advances in electrocardiography, New York, 1972, Grune & Stratton Inc.

57. Tuqan SK, et al: Anterior myocardial infarction patterns in the mitral valve prolapse–systolic click syndrome, Am Heart J 58:719, 1975.

58. Van Bruggen HW, et al: Convulsive syncope resulting from arrhythmia in a case of congenital deafness with ECG abnormalities, Am Heart J 78:81, 1969.

59. Wallack MC, Winkelstein A: Acute iron intoxication in an adult, JAMA 229:1333, 1974.

60. Yanowitz F, et al: Functional distribution of right and left stellate innervation to the ventricles: production of neurogenic electrocardiographic changes by unilateral alteration of sympathetic tone, Circ Res 18:416, 1966.

61. Zimmerman SL: Transient T-wave inversion following paroxysmal tachycardia, J Lab Clin Med 29:598, 1944.

62. Zipes DP: Cardiac electrophysiology: promises and contributions, J Am Coll Cardiol 13:1329, 1989.

Review 4: Differential diagnosis of deep T wave inversions (Chapters 14 through 17)

The following outline reviews the major causes of prominent T wave inversions:

1. Primary T wave inversions
   a. Normal variant
      (1) Juvenile T wave pattern
      (2) "Early repolarization" variant
      (3) Hyperventilation
   b. Myocardial ischemia/infarction
   c. Left or right ventricular "strain"
   d. Neurocardiac syndromes
      (1) Cerebrovascular hemorrhage
      (2) Possibly related causes: radical neck dissection, bilateral carotid endarterectomy, QT prolongation—syncope syndromes, truncal vagotomy, Stokes-Adams syndrome
   e. Postpacemaker T wave pattern
   f. Posttachycardia T wave pattern
   g. Miscellaneous: mitral valve prolapse, dilated cardiomyopathy, hypertrophic cardiomyopathy (particularly apical variant), arrhythmogenic right ventricular dysplasia, pericarditis, Friedreich's ataxia, intermittent left bundle branch block, myocardial tumor
2. Secondary T wave inversions
   a. Left bundle branch block
   b. Right bundle branch block
   c. Wolff-Parkinson-White preexcitation syndrome
   d. Ventricular paced beats

Right precordial T wave inversions. Prominent T wave inversions in the right to middle precordial leads (V_1 to V_3) may have a number of causes. They are a normal variant in children and are not uncommon in young adults (especially women) as part of the juvenile pattern. The two most important pathologic causes of *primary* T wave inversions are anterior wall ischemia or infarction and right ventricular strain. The main cause of *secondary* T wave inversions, frequently seen in leads showing an rSR′ morphology, is right bundle branch block. Deep T wave inversions in the right to middle precordial leads have also been reported in normally conducted beats with intermittent left bundle branch block (Fig. 5-4).

T wave inversions in young adults. The unexpected finding of inverted T waves in otherwise healthy patients, especially young adults, raises a number of differential possibilities: the normal-variant juvenile pattern (p. 281) manifests itself as benign right precordial T wave inversions; ST segment elevations with sharply coved T wave inversions in the midprecordial to left precordial leads may occur as a normal variant, especially in young athletic men*; ST-T abnormalities in the inferior limb or lateral precordial leads suggest mitral valve prolapse (echocardiography may be needed to confirm, since the pathognomonic click-murmur is not present in every case; diffuse T wave inversions with a history of recent sustained palpitation suggest the posttachycardia T wave syndrome; T wave inversions in the right to middle precordial leads (V_1 to V_4) are seen with arrhythmogenic right ventricular dysplasia (p. 82); prominent T wave inversions may occur with pericarditis or myocarditis, cardiomyopathy, or intramyocardial tumors (p. 156); hyperventilation may induce transient T wave inversions, especially with the "early repolarization" pattern (p. 283); deep T wave inversions in the right to middle precordial leads are a characteristic finding with apical hypertrophic cardiomyopathy (p. 84).

Secondary T wave changes. Disturbances in repolarization secondary to depolarization abnormalities may be seen in the right precordial leads with right bundle branch block (in conjunction with an rSR' complex), in the left precordial leads (in conjunction with left bundle branch block), and also in association with the Wolff-Parkinson-White pattern, leading to discordance of the QRS and T wave vectors.

Miscellaneous and obscure causes of inverted T waves. A number of the less common factors sometimes associated with deep T wave inversions are listed on p. 316. Occasionally one encounters cases in which deep T wave inversions are present without any clearly identifiable cause. In older patients or in subjects at high risk for coronary disease such ECG abnormalities should be considered as indicative of ischemia until proved otherwise. In other cases deep T wave inversions may be attributable to a combination of factors that by themselves might produce only minor ST-T alterations but that when present together produce more marked repolarization abnormalities.

---

*Several other features of the athlete's resting ECG can simulate organic heart disease: (1) tall right precordial R waves, mimicking right ventricular hypertrophy or posterior infarction (Fig. 15-2); (2) tall left precordial voltage, suggesting left ventricular hypertrophy; (3) bradyarrhythmias (sinus bradycardia, sinus pauses, atrial and AV junctional escape beats) and ectopic atrial rhythms; and (4) first-degree and second-degree (Mobitz type 1, Wenckebach) AV block.[1,2]

REFERENCES

1. Huston TP, et al: The athletic heart syndrome, N Engl J Med 313:24, 1985.
2. Lichtman J, et al: Electrocardiogram of the athlete: alterations simulating those of organic heart disease, Arch Intern Med 132:763, 1973.

Tall positive T waves are sometimes as important a sign of myocardial ischemia as the deep T wave inversions discussed in Chapter 14. There are three major ischemic settings in which relatively tall positive T waves are encountered: (1) acute myocardial infarction, (2) acute transmural ischemia without infarction (Prinzmetal's angina), and (3) the chronic (evolving) phase of myocardial infarction (positive T waves *reciprocal* to deep T wave inversions). The term *hyperacute T wave* applies only to the T waves in the first two categories.

These patterns are discussed in this chapter. The nonischemic (normal and abnormal) conditions that also may be associated with prominent positive T waves are presented in Chapter 19.

HYPERACUTE T WAVES

Over 70 years ago Smith[15] called attention to the prominent T waves that appeared after coronary ligation in dogs. Clinicians since then have adopted the term *hyperacute*[14] to refer to the tall positive T waves sometimes seen with the earliest phase of acute myocardial infarction.[2,3,8,10,13,17] A more general definition has subsequently been proposed[5,6] that considers hyperacute T waves as a *primary repolarization abnormality characterized by a relative increase in T wave positivity caused by transmural myocardial ischemia.*

This new definition includes the well-recognized giant T waves seen in some patients with acute infarction (Figs. 18-1 to 18-5) or noninfarctional ischemia, as well as the more subtle but equally important repolarization changes seen with some cases of transmural ischemia. For example, in the latter situation T waves may be only relatively and not absolutely increased (Fig. 18-6). Occasionally with acute infarction the reciprocal ST depressions will actually exceed in amplitude these primary hyperacute changes[6] (Fig. 11-7). Perhaps the most subtle example of hyperacute pathophysiology is the so-called *paradoxical normalization (pseudonormalization) of T waves.*

Hyperacute T waves are of particular clinical importance because they may be the earliest ECG sign of infarction. Although ST elevations are often consid-

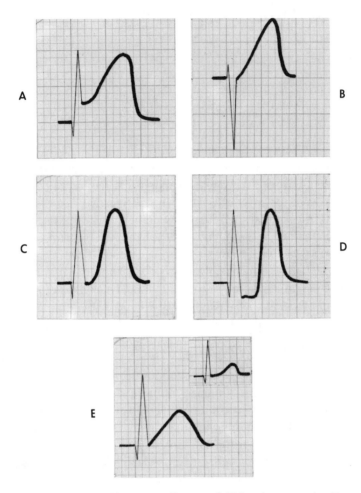

FIG. 18-1. Variable appearance of hyperacute T waves. **A,** Tall and asymmetric with an elevated ST takeoff (compare with Fig. 18-2, *A*). **B,** Tall and asymmetric with an isoelectric ST takeoff (Fig. 18-3, *A, V₂*). **C,** Tall and symmetric (parabolic) with an isoelectric ST takeoff (Fig. 18-4, *A*). **D,** Tall and symmetric (parabolic) with a slight ST depression (Fig. 18-5, *A*). **E,** Normal (or slightly increased) amplitude. This variant is characterized by an oblique rise of the ST segment at the J point. Normally (as shown in the *inset*) the ST is isoelectric and rises gradually into the T wave. During the hyperacute phase of infarction, however, it may have an abrupt takeoff from the baseline without actual elevation or prominence (Fig. 18-6, *A, aV_L*), giving it a dome shape. On any single ECG one or more of these T wave patterns may be present in the different leads.

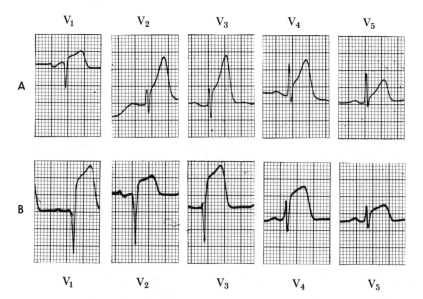

FIG. 18-2. Hyperacute phase of an anterior wall MI. **A,** Note the prominent asymmetric T waves with elevated ST segment takeoff. **B,** On the following day, notice now the evolution of a hyperacute pattern into the pattern of classic anterior infarction. Pathologic Q waves are now present in V_1 and V_2, with convex ST elevations in V_1 to V_5.

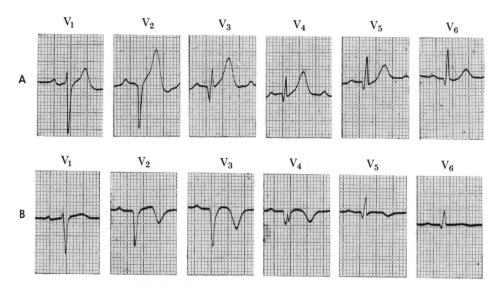

FIG. 18-3. Hyperacute T waves presaging an anterior wall infarction on serial strips from a patient with a previous history of infarction admitted with another episode of chest pain. **A,** Note the evidence of underlying anterior infarction with abnormal Q waves in V_2 to V_6. In addition, V_2 to V_4 show prominent (hyperacute) T waves. Note in V_2 that the T wave is broad and asymmetric, taking off directly from the J point. In V_3 and V_4 it has a more symmetric appearance, without significant ST elevation. **B,** On the next day, notice that the previous anterior wall infarct has extended, with QS waves now present in V_2 and V_3. The T waves have become inverted in the precordial leads and show the characteristic, relatively narrow, symmetric appearance of so-called "coronary" T waves.

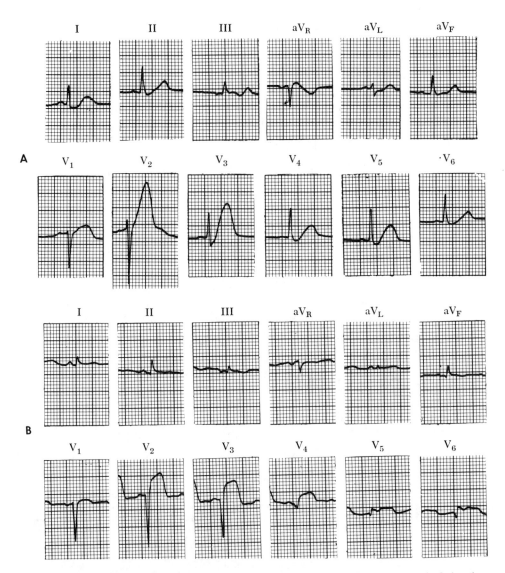

FIG. 18-4. Parabolic hyperacute T waves with an acute anterior wall infarction. Notice in **A** that they are unusually tall and symmetric. However, in **B** they are evolving into the classic anterior infarction pattern, with pronounced ST elevations and the presence of Q waves. (The QRS voltage also is significantly diminished.) Although usually such hyperacute T waves are tall and symmetric (Fig. 18-2, *A*), on occasion they will be symmetric like these in **A**.

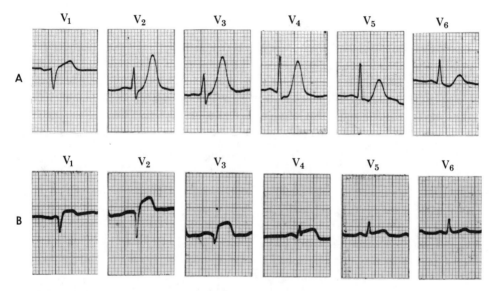

FIG. 18-5. Hyperacute phase of an anterior wall infarction. **A,** Tall symmetric T waves in the precordial leads are associated with slight ST depressions. These represent hyperacute changes presaging an anterior myocardial infarct. **B,** One day later, notice the classic pattern of an anterior wall infarction, with pathologic Q waves in V_1 to V_4 and convex ST elevations in V_1 to V_5.

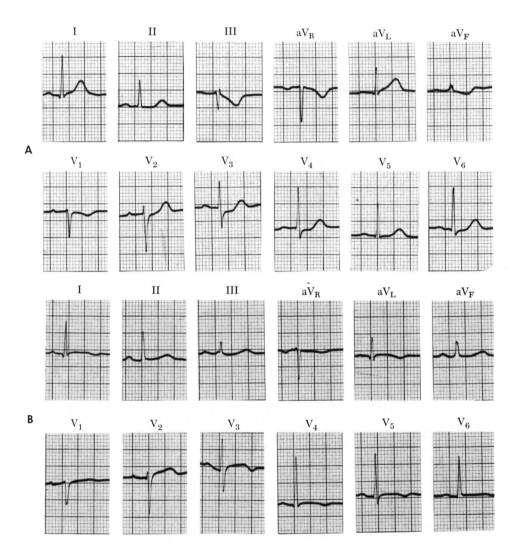

FIG. 18-6. Early subtle signs of an acute infarction. After several hours of chest pain, **A,** there is slight oblique straightening of the ST segment in aV_L with reciprocal ST depression in aV_F as well as some ST straightening in V_3 and V_4. On the following day, **B,** note the evolving T wave inversions in I, aV_L, and V_2 to V_5 along with decreased R wave amplitude in V_2. Cardiac enzymes were elevated.

ered the sine qua non of acute infarction, hyperacute T waves may precede them (as shown in Fig. 18-4).

Hyperacute T waves can have a variable morphology, depicted diagrammatically in Fig. 18-1. Additional examples are shown in Figs. 18-2 to 18-5. The hyperacute T wave may be asymmetric or symmetric (parabolic) and associated with elevated, isoelectric, or even slightly depressed ST segments. Furthermore, their amplitude need not be greatly increased. For example, in some cases the earliest sign of infarction is oblique straightening of the ST segment at the J point, producing a dome-shaped T wave of normal amplitude (Figs. 18-1, *E,* and 18-6, *A*).

Regardless of their morphology, hyperacute T waves caused by myocardial infarction are usually followed within 24 hours by pathologic Q waves and evolving ST-T changes. In rarer instances the hyperacute phase may persist for a longer time.

Pathogenesis of hyperacute T waves

The precise electrophysiologic basis for hyperacute T waves remains uncertain. The waveform presumably results from the same mechanisms that underlie ischemic ST deviations (current of injury) (discussed in Chapter 8). Acute subepicardial (and hence, transmural) ischemia shifts the repolarization (ST-T) vector toward the injured zone, reflecting systolic or diastolic injury currents. Acute ischemia may abbreviate the action potential duration. The earlier-repolarized acutely infarcted cells will carry a positive extracellular charge relative to the surrounding normal cells during electrical systole (QT interval). The ST-T vector consequently will be displaced toward the positive (ischemic) zone, causing increased T wave positivity. Relative positivity of the ST and T wave complex may also reflect a diastolic current of injury caused by lowering of the normal membrane resting potential (Fig. 8-9).

The ionic basis of early repolarization and diastolic depolarization is not resolved, although leakage of intracellular potassium secondary to ischemic membrane damage may be contributory. Increased extracellular potassium ion concentration lowers the membrane resting potential and shortens the action potential duration.[16] Systemic hyperkalemia also causes an increase in T wave positivity. However, morphologically, the broad-based hyperacute T waves differ from the more narrow-based "tented" T waves of hyperkalemia.

Early repolarization of acutely ischemic cells is a particularly attractive explanation for the occasional appearance of hyperacute T waves on the surface ECG in association with isoelectric ST segments. The isoelectric ST segment suggests that early in electrical systole the action potentials of ischemic and normal cells are relatively isopotential. However, early repolarization will tend to make the ischemic zone more electropositive late in electrical systole, when the T wave peak is being inscribed, which explains the selective increase in T wave amplitude without ST elevation. Concomitant early repolarization and diastolic depolarization would be predicted to cause both ST elevation and hyperacute T waves. Rarely ST depression will occur in conjunction with hyperacute T waves, probably reflecting a complex summation of epicardial and subendocardial injury currents.[5]

"Early repolarization" has also been cited as the mechanism underlying the ST elevations and tall positive T waves seen as a common normal variant (Chapter 9). The electrophysiologic basis of this functional repolarization variant remains undefined. However, the pattern probably reflects regional disparities in action potential duration, perhaps related to differences in autonomic tone. Support for the role of the sympathetic nervous system in the genesis of this pattern comes from the observation that isoproterenol and exercise usually diminish normal variant "early repolarization" ST elevations (pp. 205 and 207). The possible role of autonomic influences in the pathogenesis of ischemic early repolarization and hyperacute T waves is unknown.

An increase in T wave positivity has also been produced experimentally by warming the epicardium (which shortens subepicardial repolarization time) or by cooling the subendocardium (which lengthens subendocardial repolarization time).[9] The net effect in each case is to make the subepicardial layer repolarize more rapidly. The contribution of thermal differences to pathologic or physiologic early repolarization is unknown but probably insignificant.

As noted above, hyperacute T waves are not always indicative of acute infarction. They may also occur with acute reversible transmural ischemia and as such represent a variant of the Prinzmetal's angina pattern.[11] Such transient ST elevations or hyperacute T waves without evidence of actual infarction are generally due to coronary vasospasm (Chapter 8).

Paradoxical normalization (pseudonormalization) of T waves

The hyperacute phase of myocardial ischemia is classically associated with a notable increase in T wave amplitude in one or more leads. Occasionally the earliest hyperacute changes will appear only as subtle alterations in T wave contour or as a relative increase in T wave height without marked T wave positivity.

In cases in which the baseline ECG shows T wave flattening or inversion, the superimposition of hyperacute T waves can result in a paradoxical normalization (pseudonormalization) of the T waves.[7,12] This may occur with infarctional (Fig. 18-7) or noninfarctional (Fig. 18-8) ischemia. Paradoxical T wave normalization during episodes of noninfarctional ischemia represents a type of Prinzmetal's angina pattern (p. 180) and is usually associated with coronary artery spasm.[11]

The subtle manifestations of hyperacute T wave changes with paradoxical T wave normalization are illustrated in Fig. 18-7. This patient was admitted with a history of equivocal chest pain, and her ECG showed only nonspecific ST-T

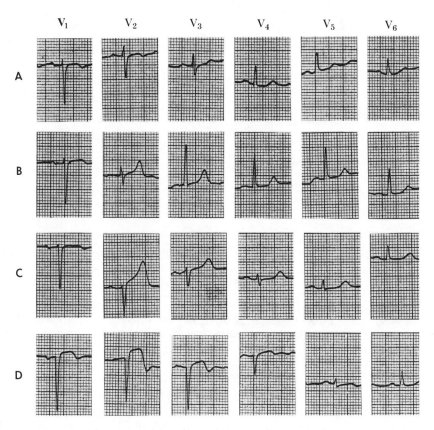

FIG. 18-7. Evolving anterior wall infarction. This patient, a 60-year-old woman, was admitted because of chest pain. **A,** Nonspecific ST-T changes are present: slight T wave inversions in V_1 and V_2, with minimal ST depression and T wave flattening in the other precordial leads. **B,** One day later, note the apparent normalization, with upright T waves now present across the entire precordium. Actually, increased T wave positivity (best seen in V_2) represents the earliest phase of hyperacute infarction. **C,** Two days later there is markedly increased T wave amplitude in V_2 (the classic hyperacute T wave), along with slow R wave progression in V_1 to V_4. **D,** On the following day, notice the typical pattern of an evolving anterior infarction: abnormal Q waves and coved plane T wave inversions in the right to middle precordial leads. This sequence of tracings illustrates the often subtle appearance of hyperacute T waves, which may be present with only a slight increase in their positivity or with only minimal rounding (see Fig. 18-6).

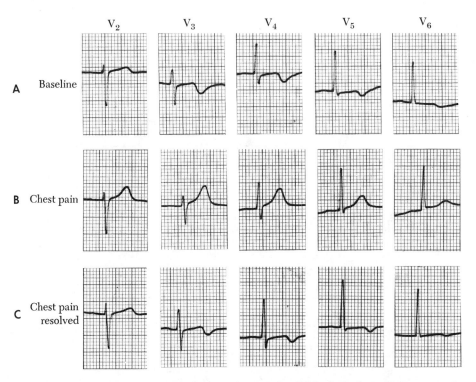

FIG. 18-8. Paradoxical T wave normalization. **A,** The baseline ECG of a patient with coronary artery disease shows ischemic T wave inversions. **B,** During an episode of chest pain, notice now the normalization of the T waves. **C,** Following resolution of the chest pain, the T waves have reverted to their baseline appearance.

changes. A subsequent ECG taken during an episode of chest pain in the hospital (Fig. 18-7, *B*) documented increased T wave positivity in the precordial leads. Follow-up ECGs revealed the typical changes of evolving anterior wall infarction. Without the advantage of a baseline ECG for comparison, the positive T waves in Fig. 18-7, *B*, could easily have been regarded as normal. However, taken in context the increase in T wave positivity in this case clearly represents the early hyperacute changes of myocardial infarction. Fig. 18-8 shows another example of paradoxical T wave normalization in a patient with acute ischemia but without evidence of acute infarction. As noted, paradoxical T wave normalization in the setting of noninfarctional ischemia appears to be equivalent to Prinzmetal's variant angina pattern and reflects transient transmural ischemia.[11] These examples illustrate the principle that a relative increase in T wave positivity can be as ominous as an increase in the amplitude of T wave inversions.

Paradoxical T wave normalization (discussed in Chapter 20) is a prime example of the limited sensitivity of the ECG in detecting acute ischemia.

Some patients with coronary artery disease may also have normalization of T waves during exercise stress testing. However, this sign is of limited diagnostic

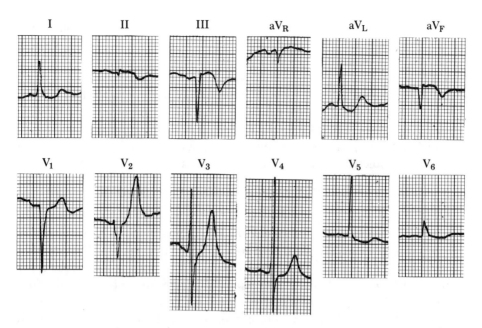

FIG. 18-9. Tall symmetrically positive T waves in a patient with the classic picture of an evolving inferior wall infarction. Abnormal Q waves in II, III, and aV_F are associated with slight ST elevations and deep terminal T wave inversions (coved plane T waves). Reciprocal ST depressions are apparent in I, aV_L, V_5, and V_6. Most striking are the reciprocally positive T waves in V_1 to V_4.

value because functional T wave inversions may normalize during exercise. In the study carried out by Aravindakshan et al.[1] complete normalization of inverted T waves occurred in 27% of patients with ischemic heart disease and 57% of subjects without evidence of coronary artery disease. Furthermore, even in patients with coronary artery disease, T wave normalization during exercise does not necessarily indicate acute ischemia.

Differential diagnosis. The hyperacute T waves of infarction may be mimicked by a number of common ECG patterns: tall positive T waves occur as a normal variant with the "early repolarization" pattern (Fig. 9-9); tall relatively narrow T waves are a hallmark of hyperkalemia (Fig. 6-2, A); prominent T waves, often with a high ST takeoff, are commonly observed in the right precordial leads with left ventricular hypertrophy (Fig. 4-1) and left bundle branch block (Fig. 5-1); tall positive T waves may also occur with cerebrovascular accidents (Fig. 19-1). (These patterns, as well as some less common simulators of hyperacute T waves, are discussed in Chapter 19.)

It is important to recognize that *not all tall positive T waves in patients with ischemia indicate the hyperacute phase of infarction.* Hyperacute T waves can occur with noninfarctional transmural ischemia (Prinzmetal's angina). Furthermore, as described in the following section, reciprocally tall positive T waves may be seen during the chronic phase of infarction (Fig. 18-9). The differential diagnosis of tall positive T waves is summarized on p. 345.

By way of summary: The term *hyperacute* describes the relative increase in T wave amplitude that can occur with acute transmural ischemia. Although such T waves are often notable for their greatly increased amplitude, the hyperacute phase of infarction or noninfarctional ischemia may also be associated with more subtle alterations in T wave morphology without much increase in T wave voltage or sometimes with paradoxical normalization of inverted T waves. Hyperacute T waves must be distinguished from reciprocally positive T waves seen during the evolving phase of myocardial infarction as well as from a number of nonischemic causes of tall positive T waves.

RECIPROCALLY POSITIVE T WAVES DURING THE CHRONIC PHASE OF INFARCTION

The evolving (subacute, chronic) phase of infarction is characterized by deep coved or coronary T wave inversions in leads that previously showed hyperacute T waves and ST elevations. During this chronic phase, reciprocally positive and symmetric T waves will typically be seen in leads facing the uninfarcted region[4] and may at times be mistaken for primary hyperacute changes.

T wave inversions during the chronic (evolving) phase of myocardial infarction reflect a regional delay in repolarization (Chapter 14). As a result the T wave vector shifts away from the infarcted zone (associated with T wave inversions in overlying leads) and toward the noninfarcted zone (associated with a reciprocal increase in T wave positivity).

For example, with inferoposterior wall infarction deep T wave inversions characteristically appear in II, III, and aV_F while reciprocally positive T waves may be seen in one or more of the precordial leads and sometimes in I and aV_L (Fig. 18-9); by contrast, with anterior wall infarction the T wave inversions in the precordial leads may be associated with reciprocally positive T waves in the inferior limb leads.

The pathogenesis of T wave changes seen during the chronic phase of myocardial infarction is discussed in Chapter 14.

REFERENCES

1. Aravindakshan V, et al: Electrocardiographic exercise test in patients with abnormal T waves at rest, Am Heart J 93:706, 1977.
2. Dressler W, Roesler H: High T waves in the earliest stage of myocardial infarction, Am Heart J 34:627, 1947.
3. Freundlich J: The diagnostic significance of tall upright T-waves in the chest leads, Am Heart J 52:749, 1956.
4. Glotzer S: Symmetrical T-waves in myocardial infarction, NY J Med 58:2667, 1958.
5. Goldberger AL: Hyperacute T waves revisited, Am Heart J 104:888, 1982.
6. Goldberger AL, Erickson R: Subtle ECG sign of acute infarction: prominent reciprocal ST depression with minimal primary ST elevation, PACE 4:709, 1981.
7. Haïat R, et al: L'inversion transitoire d'ondes T negatives chez les coronariens: un aspect électrocardiographique inhabituel de l'ischémie myocardique spontanée, Nouv Presse Med 5:3015, 1976.
8. Handjani AM: Significance of positive and peaked electrocardiographic T waves in

early diagnosis of ischemic heart disease, Chest 62:24, 1972.

9. Hellerstein HK, Liebow IM: Factors influencing the T-waves of the electrocardiogram. I. Effects of heating and cooling the endocardium and epicardium, Am Heart J 39:35, 1950.

10. Horwitz LD: Differential diagnosis of tall T waves in the resting electrocardiogram, South Med J 66:873, 1973.

11. Maseri A, et al: "Variant" angina: one aspect of a continuous spectrum of vasospastic myocardial ischemia, Am J Cardiol 42:1019, 1978.

12. Noble RJ, et al: Normalization of abnormal T waves in ischemia, Arch Intern Med 136:391, 1976.

13. Pinto IJ, et al: Tall upright T waves in the precordial leads, Circulation 36:708, 1967.

14. Schamroth L: The electrocardiology of coronary artery disease, Oxford, 1975, Blackwell Scientific Publications.

15. Smith FM: The ligation of coronary arteries with electrocardiographic study, Arch Intern Med 22:8, 1918.

16. Surawicz B: Relationship between electrocardiogram and electrolytes, Am Heart J 73:814, 1967.

17. Wasserburger RH, Corliss RJ: Prominent precordial T waves as an expression of coronary insufficiency, Am J Cardiol 16:195, 1965.

Tall positive T waves: nonischemic causes

NORMAL VARIANTS

The upper limits of normal for T wave magnitude have never been clearly established.[17] In previous studies T waves exceeding 8 mm (0.8 mV)[7] or 10 mm (1 mV)[10] were considered prominent. However, tall positive T waves greater than 10 mm are not uncommon in normal subjects, especially with the "early repolarization" pattern[16] (Fig. 9-9).

The early repolarization pattern (Chapter 9) consists of benign ST elevations in the midprecordial to left precordial leads. The elevated ST segments frequently terminate in a tall T wave, simulating the hyperacute phase of infarction (Fig. 9-9). These early repolarization T waves are stable over time, in contrast to the rapidly evolving hyperacute T waves. Hyperventilation, however, can induce marked terminal T wave inversions in leads showing benign early repolarization ST elevations[16] (Fig. 15-5).

The association of ST elevations with tall positive T waves in the benign "early repolarization" variant is of interest because of the observation that pathologic ST elevations and T wave prominences seen in acute infarction are also correlated with accelerated repolarization in the acutely ischemic zone (p. 190).

HYPERKALEMIA

Tall symmetric T waves constitute the earliest electrocardiographic sign of hyperkalemia. At a serum potassium concentration of approximately 5.5 mm Eq/L or higher they tend to become taller, peaked (tented), narrowed, and symmetric (Fig. 19-1). The QT interval may be shortened or normal[15] unless hypocalcemia is also present. These tall T waves are usually most prominent in the precordial leads (Figs. 6-2, *A*, and 19-1).

The narrowness and symmetry of hyperkalemic T waves help differentiate them from the prominent T waves seen during the hyperacute phase of infarction. The absence of reciprocal T wave inversions and QT prolongation distin-

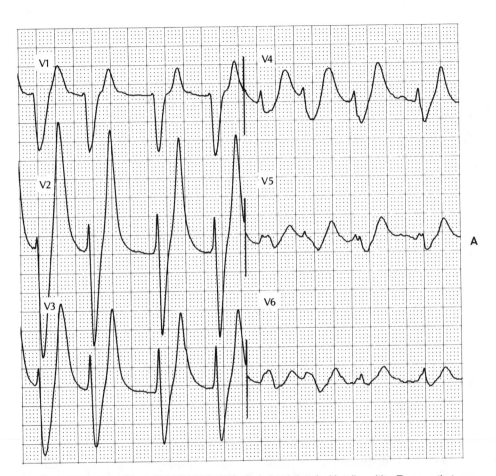

FIG. 19-1. Moderate to severe hyperkalemia typically is associated with tall positive T waves that may be mistaken for the hyperacute T waves of acute infarction. **A,** In this example from a 37-year-old man with renal failure, the initial serum potassium was markedly elevated (10.5 mEq/L). Note the absence of P waves and the wide QRS, typical of advanced hyperkalemia.   *Continued.*

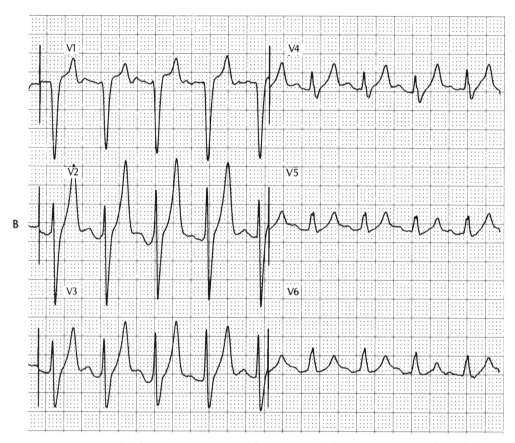

FIG. 19-1, cont'd. B, After therapy the serum potassium was still elevated ($\geq$7.4 mEq/L). Notice now the resumption of sinus rhythm with first-degree AV block and less prominent QRS prolongation. The T waves, however, remain tall and peaked, particularly in V_2 and V_3. They are usually narrower (more "tented") than the broad hyperacute T waves of acute ischemia or infarction. (Compare with Figs. 18-1 to 18-5.)

guishes the hyperkalemic T wave from the reciprocally positive T waves seen in the chronic phase of infarction.

Etiology. Surawicz[15] studied the effects of hyperkalemia on isolated rabbit myocardial fibers. The earliest effects of an increased serum potassium concentration on the action potentials of these individual fibers were (1) shortened duration of the action potential and (2) increased rate of phase-3 repolarization. These effects were noted at serum K^+ concentrations that produced only T wave peaking on the surface ECG.

Surawicz[15] suggested that the shortened action potential accounts for the abbreviated QT interval sometimes observed with hyperkalemia and that the change in slope of the repolarization curves of individual muscle fibers might be reflected on the conventional body surface ECG as the characteristic T wave peaking.

Tall positive T waves are also seen during the hyperacute phase of infarction. Like hyperkalemic T waves, they have been correlated with an acceleration in repolarization time (early repolarization phenomenon). Although hyperacute T waves may have a symmetric appearance (Fig. 18-4, *A*), they are generally more broad based than the typically narrow and symmetric T waves seen with hyperkalemia (Fig. 6-2, *A*).

Tall symmetrically positive T waves, as mentioned earlier, are also seen in leads facing uninjured areas of myocardium during the chronic phase of infarction (Fig. 18-9). The morphologic similarity between the symmetrically positive T waves of myocardial infarction and those of hyperkalemia is notable, especially since the former are associated with a regional prolongation in repolarization whereas the latter apparently reflect a generalized *increase* in the rate of myocardial repolarization.

Hypokalemia is not generally considered in the differential diagnosis of tall repolarization waves. The typical ECG findings of hypokalemia consist of ST segment depression and prominent U waves. There are, however, rare cases[12] of hypokalemia associated with giant upright U waves (approximately 10 mm tall) simulating the ECG pattern of *hyper*kalemia or hyperacute infarction. In these cases the serum potassium level was as low as 2.6 mEq/L, and the serum chloride level was approximately 50 mEq/L.

ACUTE HEMOPERICARDIUM

London and London[9] reported an ECG pattern associated with acute hemopericardium (caused by aortic or myocardial rupture) that consisted of tall positive T waves in the precordial leads. The ST segments were depressed, isoelectric, or elevated. In some cases the pattern was characterized by the sudden reversal of previously negative T waves. Bradyarrhythmias or tachyarrhythmias were also seen.

The T wave positivity of acute hemopericardium has been attributed to the hemolysis of red cells in the pericardium, producing a selective increase in epicardial potassium ion concentration. Experimentally Hellerstein and Katz[6] showed that local application of a potassium-rich solution to the epicardial surface increases T wave positivity in the overlying leads.

Electrocardiographic disturbances associated with cardiac rupture are also discussed in Chapter 21.

CEREBROVASCULAR ACCIDENT

In certain cases cerebrovascular accident causes massive T wave *inversions* (see Chapter 16). In others it produces tall *positive* T waves (Fig. 19-2). Byer, Ashman, and Toth[3] noted the association of tall upright T waves with cerebrovascular accident in 1947. Subsequent reports primarily describing cases of intracranial hemorrhage[1,8] have confirmed this observation.

The T waves seen in these patients are characteristically tall (exceeding 20 mm in one instance[11]), wide (with a prolonged QT interval), and symmetric. They are usually most prominent in the midprecordial to lateral precordial leads. Reciprocal T wave inversions are not seen. The duration of these neurogenic T waves is variable. In one reported case[11] they regressed within 5 days.

Their width and the associated QT prolongation usually distinguish these T waves from hyperkalemic T waves. The T waves associated with cerebrovascu-

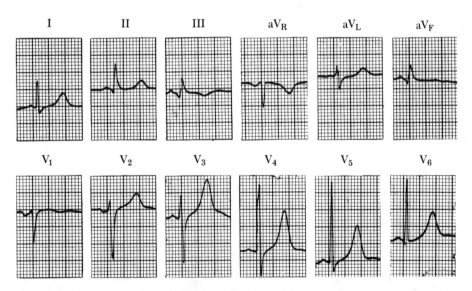

FIG. 19-2. Tall positive T waves with subarachnoid hemorrhage. Cerebrovascular accident (Figs. 16-1, 16-3, and 16-4) can produce deeply inverted T waves like those seen in the precordial leads of this tracing from a 58-year-old man. A follow-up ECG obtained 11 days later showed diminution of T wave voltage in the precordial leads. Note the borderline-wide Q waves in II, III, and aV_F consistent with an inferior wall infarction of indeterminate age. Tall positive T waves that occur with cerebrovascular accident at times will mimic the hyperacute T waves of infarction.

lar accident also do not undergo the characteristic evolution seen with the hyperacute T waves of infarction, and abnormal Q waves do not appear with them.

Etiology. The cause of both the tall positive and the deeply inverted T waves seen with cerebrovascular injury is still uncertain. Burch et al.[2] suggested that the unusual repolarization changes seen with cerebrovascular injury could be caused by a pronounced increase in sympathetic activity ("sympathetic storm") induced by hypothalamic stimulation. Yanowitz, Preston, and Abildskov[18] demonstrated that stimulation of the left stellate ganglion in dogs produced an increase in T wave positivity while stimulation of the right stellate ganglion produced increased T wave negativity in selected leads. QT prolongation occurred in both cases. These experimental findings may provide a model for the apparently paradoxical clinical observation that cerebrovascular accident is associated with tall positive T waves in some cases and deeply inverted T waves in others. (The possible role of the sympathetic nervous system in generating these repolarization changes is discussed in Chapter 16.)

LEFT VENTRICULAR HYPERTROPHY

Tall positive T waves may be seen in the right or left precordial leads with left ventricular hypertrophy.

1. *Right precordial T wave prominence.* Asymmetric T waves with a high ST takeoff are commonly seen in the right precordial leads with left ventricular hypertrophy. An identical pattern occurs with hypertrophic cardiomyopathy (Fig. 4-15) that may simulate the hyperacute phase of infarction (Chapter 4). Left bundle branch block may be associated with similar ST elevations and tall T waves in the right precordial leads (Fig. 19-4).

2. *Left precordial T wave prominence.* In the lateral precordial leads T waves with left ventricular hypertrophy usually are either flattened or inverted as part of the left ventricular "strain" pattern (p. 64). Occasionally, however, they will be tall and positive[2] (Figs. 19-5 and 19-6).

Cabrera[4] introduced a classification of left ventricular hypertrophy patterns that utilized the terms *systolic* and *diastolic* to distinguish overload variants depending on the polarity of the T waves in the lateral chest leads. The diastolic overload variant (Figs. 19-3 and 19-4), seen typically with chronic aortic regurgitation, mitral regurgitation, patent ductus arteriosus, and ventricular septal defect, consisted of tall positive T waves. The systolic overload variant, seen typically in patients with aortic stenosis or systemic hypertension, consisted of T wave inversions and corresponded to the classic "strain" pattern previously discussed (Fig. 4-1). The pathophysiologic basis for these differences is not certain. Considerable overlap has been noted between patients with diastolic and systolic overload conditions.[13] Furthermore, the reliability of this classification is questionable. T wave inversions are not uncommon in patients with chronic aortic regurgitation and generally indicate severe vol-

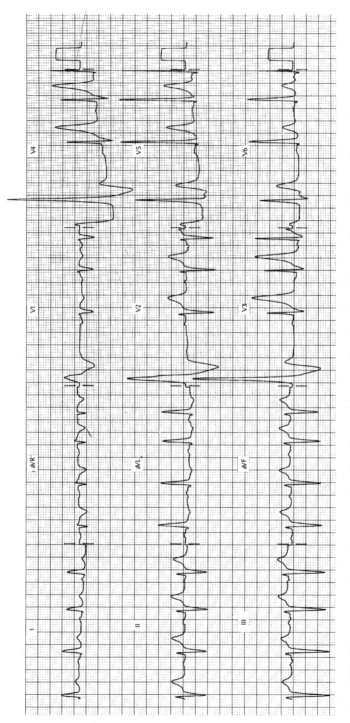

FIG. 19-3. Left ventricular "diastolic overload" pattern associated with tall positive T waves (V₃ to V₅) in a 76-year-old man who is without symptoms but has severe mitral regurgitation due to mitral valve prolapse. There is also evidence of the following: left ventricular hypertrophy, left atrial abnormality, left axis deviation, slight prolongation of the QRS, and atrial and ventricular ectopic beats.

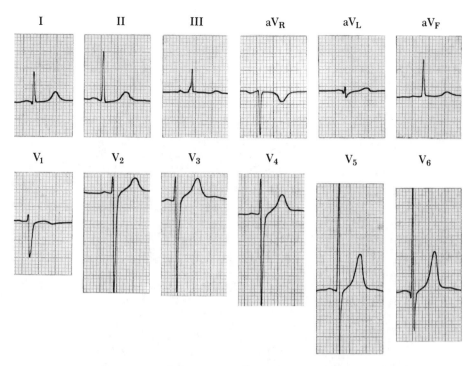

FIG. 19-4. Tall positive T waves with left ventricular diastolic overloading. Note the prominent precordial voltages compatible with left ventricular hypertrophy on this tracing from a 23-year-old man with ventricular septal defect. The positive T waves in V_5 and V_6 are associated with high-amplitude R waves. This pattern has been described in conditions that cause left ventricular diastolic overload. (Compare with Fig. 19-3 from a patient with mitral regurgitation.)

ume overload.[14] Finally, an abrupt conversion from diastolic to systolic overload patterns (upright T waves to T wave inversions) has been found in some patients with chronic aortic regurgitation following prosthetic valve replacement.[5]

LEFT BUNDLE BRANCH BLOCK

ST segment elevations with tall positive T waves in the right precordial leads are a common finding in uncomplicated cases of left bundle branch block (Figs. 4-17, C, 5-1, and 19-5), mimicking the hyperacute T waves of infarction. (The ST-T changes associated with left bundle branch block and their differential diagnosis are discussed in Chapter 5.)

ACUTE PERICARDITIS

The ST segment elevations seen with acute pericarditis are characterized by a diffuse distribution (Fig. 10-2); but, as noted in Chapter 10, they generally are of less magnitude than the changes seen with acute myocardial infarction.

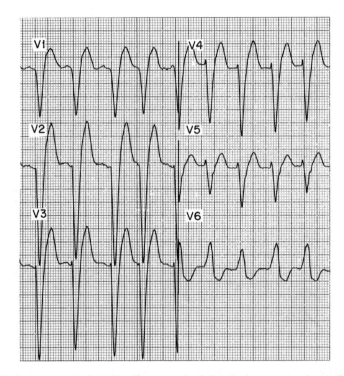

FIG. 19-5. ST elevations and tall positive T waves, simulating the hyperacute phase of infarction, are a common finding with left bundle branch block. Poor R wave progression, shown here, may also be seen without infarction in this conduction disturbance. The underlying rhythm is borderline sinus tachycardia with a single atrial premature depolarization (fourth beat). (Compare with Figs. 4-17, C, and 5-1.)

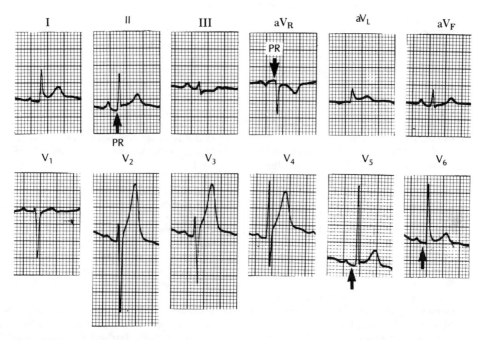

FIG. 19-6. Acute pericarditis simulating the hyperacute phase of myocardial infarction. Shortly after being admitted with substernal pressure, this 54-year-old white man complained of mild pleuritic chest discomfort. A loud three-component pericardial friction rub was detected. The tracing taken on the first hospital day shows slight ST elevations in I, II, aV$_L$, and V$_5$ and V$_6$, with reciprocal depressions in III and aV$_R$. Note the vaulting T waves in V$_2$ to V$_4$ associated with a high ST takeoff. These mimic the hyperacute changes of early infarction and are relatively rare with acute pericarditis. Subsequent tracings revealed diminishing amplitude of the precordial T waves. Serial cardiac enzymes were normal. Notice also the atrial current of injury patterns that have been described with acute pericarditis: elevation of the PR segment in aV$_R$, reciprocal PR depressions in II, aV$_F$, and V$_2$ to V$_6$ *(arrows)*. (See Figs. 10-1 and 10-2.)

Rarely the tall positive T waves of acute pericarditis will simulate the hyperacute ST-T alterations of infarction (Fig. 19-6).

REFERENCES

1. Burch GE, et al: A new electrocardiographic pattern observed in cerebrovascular accidents, Circulation 9:719, 1954.
2. Burch GE, et al: Acute myocardial lesions following experimentally induced intracranial hemorrhage in mice: a histological and histochemical study, Arch Pathol 84:517, 1967.
3. Byer E, et al: Electrocardiograms with large upright T waves and long Q-T intervals, Am Heart J 33:796, 1947.
4. Cabrera E: A clinical reevaluation of systolic and diastolic overloading patterns, Prog Cardiovasc Dis 2:219, 1959.
5. Goldberger AL: Deep T wave inversions following aortic valve replacement for chronic aortic regurgitation: possible conversion from diastolic to systolic overload pattern, J Electrocardiol 13:378, 1980.
6. Hellerstein HK, Katz LN: Electrical effects of injury at various myocardial locations, Am Heart J 36:184, 1948.
7. Horwitz LD: Differential diagnosis of tall T waves in the resting electrocardiogram, South Med J 66:873, 1973.
8. Kreus KE, et al: Electrocardiographic changes in cerebrovascular accidents, Acta Med Scand 185:327, 1969.
9. London RE, London SB: The electrocardiographic sign of acute hemopericardium, Circulation 25:780, 1962.
10. Pinto IJ, et al: Tall upright T waves in the precordial leads, Circulation 36:708, 1967.
11. Runge PJ, Bousvaros G: Giant peaked upright T waves in cerebrovascular accident, Br Heart J 32:717, 1970.
12. Sarma RN: Unusually tall and narrow U waves simulating hyperkalemic T waves: report of 2 cases of hypochloremic alkalosis with hypokalemia, Am Heart J 70:397, 1965.
13. Sedziwy L, Shillingford J: Cardiographic patterns in systolic and diastolic overload of the left ventricle, Br Heart J 23:533, 1961.
14. Spagnuolo M, et al: Natural history of rheumatic aortic regurgitation: criteria predictive of death, congestive heart failure, and angina in young patients, Circulation 44:368, 1971.
15. Surawicz B: Relationship between electrocardiogram and electrolytes, Am Heart J 73:814, 1961.
16. Wasserburger RH, Alt WJ: The normal RS-T segment elevation variant, Am J Cardiol 8:184, 1961.
17. Wasserburger RH, Corliss RJ: Prominent precordial T waves as an expression of coronary insufficiency, Am J Cardiol 16:195, 1965.
18. Yanowitz F, et al: Functional distribution of right and left stellate ganglion innervation to the ventricles: production of neurogenic electrocardiographic changes by unilateral alteration of sympathetic tone, Circ Res 18:416, 1966.

Review 5: Differential diagnosis of tall positive T waves (Chapters 18 and 19)

Unlike the long list of differential possibilities raised by Q waves or T wave inversions, tall positive T waves require consideration of only a limited number of conditions, outlined as follows:

1. Ischemic causes
   a. Hyperacute phase of myocardial infarction
   b. Acute transient transmural ischemia (Prinzmetal's angina)
   c. Chronic (evolving) phase of myocardial infarction (tall positive T waves reciprocal to primary deep T wave inversions)
2. Nonischemic causes
   a. Normal variants ("early repolarization" patterns)
   b. Hyperkalemia
   c. Acute hemopericardium
   d. Cerebrovascular hemorrhage
   e. Left ventricular hypertrophy
      (1) Right precordial leads usually in conjunction with left precordial ST depressions and T wave inversions
      (2) Left precordial leads sometimes in association with "diastolic" overload conditions
   f. Left bundle branch block (right precordial leads)
   g. Acute pericarditis

PART

III

Special Topics in the Electrocardiographic Diagnosis of Myocardial Infarction

This concluding section of the book focuses on a number of special problems related to the electrocardiographic diagnosis of myocardial ischemia and infarction: the limitations in sensitivity seen with coronary artery disease (Chapter 20), the patterns seen with some major complications of acute myocardial infarction (Chapter 21), and the wider context of other diagnostic tests also routinely used in the differential diagnosis of infarction, with emphasis on their inherent limitations and complementary uses (Chapter 22).

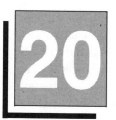

20 The electrocardiogram in coronary artery disease: limitations in sensitivity

This book has been devoted primarily to the specificity of the ECG in diagnosing ischemic heart disease. As such, its primary focus has been on conditions, both normal and pathologic, associated with patterns mimicking those of ischemia and infarction (false-positive diagnoses). False-negative diagnoses are also of obvious importance, and mention has been made throughout the text of the limitations in diagnostic sensitivity of the ECG. Sensitivity is defined as the probability that a test such as the ECG will show diagnostic abnormalities when a particular disease is present.[10,31] The purpose of this chapter is to review this topic, summarizing the settings in which electrocardiography may fail to yield a definite diagnosis of chronic or even acute ischemic heart disease.

NORMAL ECG WITH CHRONIC ISCHEMIC HEART DISEASE

A nondiagnostic or completely normal ECG does not exclude the presence of severe underlying coronary artery disease, including previous myocardial infarction. Normal ECGs are well-described in patients with coronary obstruction and even total occlusion of coronary vessels.[17,22] For example, Martinez-Rios et al.[22] reported 21 patients with entirely normal ECGs despite severe coronary disease, in some cases involving all three major arteries. Of note was their finding that in 19 of these 21 patients collateral circulation developed to the diseased vessels, suggesting one possible explanation for the preservation of a normal ECG despite total occlusion of a coronary artery. However, patients with ventricular wall motion abnormalities (asynergy) indicative of possible myocardial infarction also may have an entirely normal ECG at rest.[17]

Furthermore, a normal ECG is occasionally observed in patients with a well-documented infarct whose previous tracings showed pathologic Q waves.[15] In one series[5] complete normalization of the ECG was noted in 5.6% of cases with Q waves; in another study[16] Q waves disappeared in 6.7% of patients (see also p. 26).

As discussed on pp. 26 and 27, there are at least five possible mechanisms to account for the disappearance of Q waves following infarction: (1) recovery of electrical function by cells that are ischemic ("stunned") but not actually infarcted, (2) "scarring down" of the infarcted zone, (3) contrecoup effect, whereby a second, new, infarction may reciprocally increase QRS forces in the direction of the first infarct, neutralizing the loss of forces produced by the initial infarct,[6] (4) masking of Q waves by an intraventricular conduction disturbance, and (5) hypertrophy of myocardial fibers near the infarcted region.

NORMAL ECG WITH ACUTE ISCHEMIC HEART DISEASE

These observations underscore the limitations of the ECG in detecting chronic ischemic heart disease. Clinicians must also recognize that normal ECGs may be recorded even during episodes of acute ischemia. A normal ECG with angina pectoris is a well-documented finding. For example, in one study[29] 5 of 29 patients with significant coronary disease and an unstable pattern of angina pectoris failed to show ST-T changes during episodes of chest pain. Similarly, during exercise testing it is not uncommon for patients with documented coronary artery disease to complain of ischemic chest discomfort in the absence of ST abnormalities.[32]

In the next section, specific settings in which the sensitivity of the ECG for detecting acute ischemia may be limited are discussed—including stress electrocardiography, vasospastic angina, paradoxical T wave normalization, intraventricular conduction disturbances, and acute myocardial infarction.

Stress Electrocardiography

The limited sensitivity of stress electrocardiography in detecting coronary artery disease was introduced in Chapter 13. As a general rule the diagnostic sensitivity of exercise testing appears to be related to the extent of the coronary lesions. Thus in one review of the literature[18] the overall sensitivity of stress electrocardiography in patients with single-vessel disease was only 43% compared to 67% with two-vessel disease and 86% with three-vessel involvement.

The exercise test does appear highly sensitive,[3,9,19,26,33] though not specific,[7] in detecting left main coronary artery stenosis. For example, Weiner, McCabe, and Ryan,[34] reporting on 35 patients with 50% or greater luminal reduction of the left main coronary artery by angiography, found 97% of the patients to have a positive stress ECG (defined by ST depressions of 1 mm or more); furthermore, 91% had ST depressions of at least 2 mm. Comparable sensitivity has been reported in a number of other studies of left main disease.[3,22,26]

Thus the exercise ECG may be of limited sensitivity in detecting single- or double-vessel coronary artery disease. However, the fact that a patient is able to achieve 85% of the age-adjusted maximal predicted heart rate without anginal chest pain, hypotension, or significant ST depressions makes the presence of severe left main coronary stenosis highly unlikely.

The sensitivity of stress electrocardiography can be further reduced in a patient taking antiischemic medication (e.g., nitrate preparations, beta-adrenergic blocking agents, calcium antagonists) (p. 268).

The use of myocardial imaging with thallium-201 may enhance the sensitivity of stress electrocardiography in detecting reversible ischemia.[12] (Limitations in the diagnostic accuracy of thallium imaging are reviewed elsewhere.[7]) Because it may generate false-positive or false-negative results and because of its substantial added cost, the exercise thallium test generally is reserved for patients who have uninterpretable ST changes due to such factors as digitalis, bundle branch block, pacemaker patterns, or preexcitation (Chapter 13). Thallium scintigraphy also is helpful in assessing the *location* and *extent* of ischemia.

Vasospastic Angina

The electrocardiographic manifestations of vasospastic (variant or Prinzmetal's) angina are described in Chapter 8. Transient elevation of the ST segment appears to be a highly specific sign of reversible transmural ischemia caused by coronary vasospasm. However, the sensitivity of the ECG in detecting vasospasm is limited; during episodes of demonstrated vasospasm some patients will manifest ST depression or T wave inversions instead of ST elevations.[4,13,23,34] Furthermore, there are a number of well-documented cases[11,13,36] in which the ECG has remained entirely normal during episodes of coronary vasospasm. One report,[13] for example, showed that of 30 patients with vasospastic angina, 2 did not have ECG changes during the anginal attacks, and only 18 had ST elevation with all the episodes. *Failure to observe ST elevations with chest pain thus does not exclude the diagnosis of coronary vasospasm.*

Paradoxical T Wave Normalization

A special cause of a normal ECG with acute ischemia is the phenomenon of paradoxical normalization (pseudonormalization) of T waves (pp. 328 to 331). In patients with T wave inversions on their baseline recording the occurrence of acute transmural ischemia can increase T wave positivity sufficiently to "normalize" the T waves (Fig. 18-8). This may be seen during the earliest phase of acute infarction or with reversible coronary vasospasm (Prinzmetal's angina). Thus when a patient with "ischemic" chest pain has a normal ECG, it is important to repeat the tracing after resolution of the pain, to look for evidence of paradoxical T wave normalization. *Normalization of T wave inversions during exercise, however, is not necessarily diagnostic of ischemia* (p. 331). For example, this finding may occur with ventricular wall motion abnormalities without acute ischemia,[27] or with functional (benign) T wave inversions, or with abnormal but noncoronary T wave inversions.

Intraventricular Conduction Disturbances

Disturbances in the sequence of ventricular activation can mask both pathologic Q waves and ST-T changes of ischemia and infarction. The most important patterns that can hide the diagnosis of infarction are left bundle branch block, pacemaker patterns, and the Wolff-Parkinson-White syndrome (Chapter 5). Right bundle branch block, because it affects primarily the terminal phase of ventricular depolarization, does not generally mask pathologic Q waves. Furthermore, the secondary ST-T changes associated with right bundle branch block are seen exclusively in leads with an R' complex. By contrast, primary ischemic T wave inversions in the midprecordial to lateral precordial leads can usually also be detected in the presence of right bundle branch block (Fig. 5-9). (The diagnosis of ischemia and infarction in the presence of a bundle branch block is discussed in Chapter 5.)

With intermittent pacemaker patterns or intermittent left bundle branch block the diagnosis of ischemia or infarction may at times be made from the QRS complexes with normal intraventricular conduction. However, as previously described, ischemia can be overdiagnosed in such patients based on postpacemaker T wave inversions (Fig. 17-2) or T wave changes associated with intermittent left bundle branch block (Fig. 5-4).

Left anterior hemiblock, which is associated with orientation of early ventricular depolarization forces toward II, III, and aV_F, may mask the Q waves of inferior wall infarction (pp. 109 to 112).

Acute Myocardial Infarction

There are two major questions relating to the diagnostic sensitivity of the ECG in acute myocardial infarction. First, does a completely normal ECG in a patient with chest pain exclude infarction? Second, what percentage of patients with acute infarction will have diagnostic, as opposed to nonspecific, abnormalities?

Although the literature does not afford precise answers to these questions, the following general observations seem warranted. Normal ECGs with acute infarction have occasionally been reported.[28] However, a normal *series* of tracings over several days during the course of acute infarction is highly unusual. Indeed, in one retrospective autopsy study of 304 cases[35] ECG abnormalities were noted in all patients. Similarly, in another autopsy series[37] a normal ECG in association with acute infarction was observed in only 1 of 95 cases. Such reports based on postmortem data are probably biased to select more extensive infarcts, which are more likely to be associated with ECG changes. By contrast, normal or nearly normal ECGs are more likely to be seen with smaller infarcts, perhaps detectable only by minimal elevations in creatine kinase enzyme levels.

This speculation is supported by data from a large multicenter study in which the initial ECG was interpreted as normal in only 35 of 1024 patients (3.4%) with acute infarction at the time of emergency room presentation.[30] Patients with a normal ECG or with nonspecific ST-T changes had significantly smaller infarcts (based on peak creatine kinase values) and lower mortality rates than did patients with more diagnostic ECG findings.

Although an entirely normal ECG is extremely unusual with acute infarction, nondiagnostic (acute or chronic) abnormalities are relatively common. For example, in the retrospective autopsy series of Woods, Laurie, and Smith[37] only 82% of cases showed definite evidence of infarction based on Q wave criteria or an evolving injury pattern. Similarly, in a postmortem series reported by Weiss and Weiss[35] "specific" ECG abnormalities were seen in 85% of patients with acute infarction, excluding those with left bundle branch block. A more recent survey of 612 patients with clinical evidence of acute infarction based on chest pain and cardiac enzyme elevations[21] revealed "diagnostic" ECG changes in 531 cases (87% sensitivity). An additional 11 patients, although included in the group with nondiagnostic ST-T changes, had ST depressions of 2 mm or more, ST elevations without Q waves, or prominent T wave inversions. If these patients had been reclassified in the "diagnostic" category, the sensitivity of the ECG in acute infarction would have increased to 89%.

In addition to the intraventricular conduction delays just discussed, diagnostic difficulties can affect the electrocardiographic recognition of acute infarction in patients with prior infarcts. However, even in this subgroup the ECG appears relatively sensitive. For example, in one retrospective autopsy series[24] 17 of 21 patients with recurrent infarction showed diagnostic changes on their ECG. The authors suggested that diagnostic sensitivity might have been decreased in cases in which the acute infarct was superimposed on a zone of previous infarction.

Another important factor that can influence the sensitivity of the surface ECG in detecting acute ischemia or infarction is the location of the ischemic zone. ST segment monitoring of acute transmural ischemia induced by intracoronary balloon inflation during percutaneous transluminal angioplasty has indicated that complete occlusion of the left circumflex coronary artery is the *least* likely of all coronary artery occlusions to cause ST elevations on the surface 12-lead ECG. In particular, Berry et al.[2] reported such elevations in only 32% of patients with left circumflex occlusion, compared to 84% and 92% of patients with left anterior descending and right coronary artery occlusions respectively. On the other hand, the magnitude of *intracoronary* ST elevations was not significantly different among the groups.

Why is acute circumflex occlusion (usually leading to transmural posterolateral wall ischemia) less likely to be detected by ST elevations on a 12-lead ECG? The answer probably relates to a combination of geometric and anatomic factors.[2,25] A current of injury generated by the posterolateral wall may not project onto the conventional leads, which are aligned more to detect anterior or inferior ST elevations (seen typically with acute left anterior descending or right coronary occlusion). However, the *reciprocal* anterior lead ST depressions associated with acute posterolateral wall ischemia or infarction may lead to the mistaken diagnosis of anterior subendocardial ischemia (p. 238) in such cases.

Occasionally the diagnostic sensitivity of the ECG in detecting acute myocardial infarction can be enhanced by recording additional leads. For example, ST elevations in the right precordial leads (e.g., V_{3R} and V_{4R}) may support a diagnosis of acute right ventricular ischemia or infarction (Fig. 21-1). Left chest leads recorded an interspace or two above their usual positions have been advocated[20] for detecting so-called high lateral infarcts, but their use has not been systematically studied. (The enhancement of diagnostic sensitivity by using vectorcardiographic leads is taken up in Chapter 3.) Detailed discussions of this topic and of investigational techniques like body surface mapping (p. 31) and high-frequency electrocardiography[1,8] lie outside the scope of this book.

SENSITIVITY OF THE ECG: CONCLUSIONS

The sensitivity of the ECG in detecting myocardial ischemia and infarction is variable and the result of many factors. Nevertheless, several general conclusions can be made:

First, in the absence of left bundle branch block, pacemaker patterns, or a Wolff-Parkinson-White type of preexcitation, the ECG is highly sensitive in detecting *acute* myocardial infarction based on new Q waves or new repolarization abnormalities. Its sensitivity may be decreased by previous infarcts. However, an entirely normal series of ECGs recorded during acute infarction is extremely rare. Indeed, in patients with prolonged chest pain (e.g., lasting hours) but no ECG changes, alternative diagnoses should be considered. Normal or nondiagnostic ECGs can be recorded during other major cardiopulmonary disorders, including acute pericarditis, aortic dissection, or pulmonary embolism.

Second, the sensitivity of the ECG in detecting *chronic* myocardial infarction based on Q waves or major ST-T changes is considerably lower. Nondiagnostic repolarization abnormalities are commonly seen in this setting; and in a small percentage of cases, the ECG reverts entirely to normal in the weeks and months following an acute infarction.

Finally, the ECG is of only moderate sensitivity in detecting acute ischemia without actual infarction. Even stress electrocardiography has major limitations, particularly in the detection of single-vessel or double-vessel coronary disease.

Limitations in the sensitivity of other tests routinely used to diagnose myocardial infarction, including nuclear cardiology and cardiac enzyme analysis, are discussed in Chapter 22.

REFERENCES

1. Abhoud S, et al: High frequency electrocardiography of three orthogonal leads in dogs during a coronary artery occlusion, PACE 12:547, 1989.
2. Berry C, et al: Surface electrocardiogram in the detection of transmural myocardial ischemia during coronary occlusion, Am J Cardiol 63:21, 1989.
3. Blumenthal DS, et al: The predictive value of a strongly positive stress test in patients

with minimal symptoms, Am J Med 70:1005, 1981.

4. Cipriano PR, et al: Clinical courses of patients following the demonstration of coronary artery spasm by angiography, Am Heart J 101:127, 1981.

5. Cox CJ: Return to normal of the electrocardiogram after myocardial infarction, Lancet 1:1194, 1967.

6. Evans W: Cardiographic contrecoup in the course of cardiac infarction, Br Heart J 24:713, 1963.

7. Froelicher VF: Exercise and the heart: clinical concepts, ed 2, Chicago, 1990, Year Book Medical Publishers Inc.

8. Goldberger AL, et al: Effect of myocardial infarction on high-frequency QRS potentials, Circulation 64:34, 1981.

9. Goldschlager N, et al: Treadmill tests as indicators of presence and severity of coronary artery disease, Ann Intern Med 85:277, 1976.

10. Griner PF, et al: Selection and interpretation of diagnostic tests and procedures: principles and applications, Ann Intern Med 94:557, 1981.

11. Haïat R, et al: Angina pectoris without ST-T changes in patients with documented coronary heart disease, Am Heart J 105:883, 1983.

12. Hakki A-H, et al: Implications of normal exercise electrocardiographic results in patients with angiographically documented coronary artery disease: correlation with left ventricular function and myocardial perfusion, Am J Med 75:439, 1983.

13. Heupler F: Syndrome of symptomatic coronary arterial spasm with nearly normal coronary arteriograms, Am J Cardiol 45:873, 1980.

14. Iskandrian AS, et al: Role of exercise thallium-201 imaging in decision making, Arch Intern Med 146:1098, 1986.

15. Kalbfleisch JM, et al: Disappearance of the Q-deflection following myocardial infarction, Am Heart J 76:193, 1968.

16. Kaplan BM, Berkson DM: Serial electrocardiograms after myocardial infarction, Ann Intern Med 60:430, 1964.

17. Kedy K, et al: Severity and distribution of coronary artery disease in patients with normal resting electrocardiograms, J Electrocardiol 7:115, 1974.

18. Koppes G, et al: Treadmill exercise testing, Curr Probl Cardiol 7(8,9):1, 1977.

19. Lee TH, et al: Prospective evaluation: a clinical and exercise test model for the prediction of left main coronary artery disease, Med Decis Making 6:136, 1986.

20. Lepeschkin E: Modern electrocardiography, Baltimore, 1951, The Williams & Wilkins Co, vol 1.

21. Marriott P, et al: Discrepancies between electrocardiographic and enzyme evidence of myocardial infarction, Br Heart J 35:1240, 1973.

22. Martinez-Rios MA, et al: Normal electrocardiogram in the presence of severe coronary artery disease, Am J Cardiol 25:320, 1970.

23. Maseri A, et al: "Variant" angina: one aspect of a continuous spectrum of vasospastic myocardial ischemia, Am J Cardiol 42:1019, 1978.

24. Merrill S, Pearce ML: An autopsy study of the accuracy of the electrocardiogram in the diagnosis of recurrent myocardial infarction, Am Heart J 81:48, 1971.

25. Mizutani M, et al: ST monitoring for myocardial ischemia during and after coronary angioplasty, Am J Cardiol 66:389, 1990.

26. Nixon JV, et al: Exercise testing in men with significant left main coronary disease, Br Heart J 42:410, 1979.

27. Ogawa T, et al: Mechanisms of stress-induced ST elevation and negative T wave normalization studied by serial cardiokymogram in patients with a previous myocardial infarction, Am J Cardiol 65:962, 1990.

28. Prinzmetal M, et al: Clinical implications of errors in electrocardiographic interpretation: heart disease of electrocardiographic origin, JAMA 161:138, 1956.

29. Rahim A, et al: Electrocardiographic changes during chest pain in unstable angina, Br Heart J 39:1340, 1977.

30. Rouan GW, et al: Clinical characteristics and outcome of acute myocardial infarction in patients with initially normal or non-specific electrocardiograms (a report from the Multicenter Chest Pain Study), Am J Cardiol 64:1987, 1989.

31. Sox HC Jr: Probability theory and the interpretation of diagnostic tests. In Sox HC Jr (editor): Common diagnostic tests: uses and interpretation, ed 2, Philadelphia, 1990, American College of Physicians, p 16.

32. Weiner DA, et al: The predictive value of anginal chest pain as an indicator of coronary disease during exercise testing, Am Heart J 96:458, 1978.

33. Weiner DA, et al: Identification of patients with left main and three-vessel coronary disease with clinical and exercise test variables, Am J Cardiol 46:21, 1980.

34. Weiner L, et al: Spectrum of coronary arterial spasm: clinical, angiographic, and myocardial metabolic experience in 29 cases, Am J Cardiol 38:945, 1976.

35. Weiss MM, Weiss WH Jr: The electrocardiogram in myocardial infarction: diagnostic accuracy, Arch Intern Med 101:1126, 1958.

36. Whittle JL, et al: Variability of electrocardiographic responses to repeated ergonovine provocation in variant angina patients with coronary artery spasm, Am Heart J 103:161, 1982.

37. Woods JD, et al: The reliability of the electrocardiogram in myocardial infarction, Lancet 2:265, 1963.

The electrocardiogram in diagnosing the complications of acute myocardial infarction

The complications of acute myocardial infarction can be considered in two general categories, electrical and mechanical, reflecting the basic duality of cardiac function. Discussion of the recognition and management of arrhythmias and conduction disturbances lies outside the scope of this book. This chapter reviews the uses and limitations of the ECG in diagnosing the major mechanical complications of acute infarction—congestive heart failure and cardiogenic shock, right ventricular infarction, papillary muscle dysfunction or rupture, left ventricular free wall rupture, ventricular septal rupture, ventricular aneurysm, "pseudoaneurysm," pericarditis, and arterial and venous thromboembolic disease.

CONGESTIVE HEART FAILURE AND CARDIOGENIC SHOCK

"Pump failure" following acute myocardial infarction is a major complication, which will be manifested by the signs and symptoms of left-sided or right-sided heart failure and in the most severe cases by frank shock. Congestive heart failure and cardiogenic shock, though most common with extensive anterior Q wave infarction, may also be seen in the setting of inferoposterior infarction and with non–Q wave infarctions.[1] For example, in one large series,[34] congestive heart failure was noted in 55% of Q wave anterior infarcts, 37% of Q wave inferior infarcts, and 25% of non–Q wave infarcts.

Generally in patients with Q wave infarcts, the extent of the Q waves correlates with the extent of the underlying ventricular wall motion disorder. Thus patients with an acute anterior wall infarct with extensive loss of R waves across the precordial leads usually have marked impairment of ventricular function. Based on this principle, more detailed QRS criteria have been derived as indices of the pathologic size of an infarction[35] and of the left ventricular ejection fraction[54] in patients with a recent acute myocardial infarct. Although of investigational interest,[70] such indices are not as yet likely to have widespread clinical application because they exclude patients with left ventricular hypertrophy, intraventricular conduction delays, and multiple infarcts.

Furthermore, in unselected patients with chronic coronary disease, the ECG is likely to be of limited value in predicting ventricular function. Even patients with severe left ventricular failure caused by ischemic heart disease ("ischemic cardiomyopathy") may occasionally fail to show pathologic Q waves (p. 163).

Special causes of severe heart failure in the postinfarction setting, including right ventricular infarction, ventricular aneurysm, papillary muscle dysfunction, and ventricular septal defect, are discussed separately in the following sections.

RIGHT VENTRICULAR INFARCTION

The electrocardiographic features of acute right ventricular infarction (Chapter 2) were initially reported exclusively in the setting of inferoposterior infarcts,[36] though they have subsequently also been reported with anterior infarction.[12] The diagnosis of acute right ventricular infarction can usually be made by clinical findings in association with noninvasive and hemodynamic studies.

This diagnosis should be suspected in any patient with ECG evidence of inferoposterior infarction, particularly with elevated venous pressure.[15,19] Hypotension and even shock may be present. In addition to ST segment elevations in the inferior limb leads, the ECG often shows ST elevation in one or more of the right precordial leads (V_1 to V_3) or extra right precordial leads (V_{3R} to V_{6R}), reflecting a right ventricular or ventricular septal current of injury* (Fig. 21-1).

A number of studies[10,13,38,47] suggest that, of any single lead, V_{4R} may be the most useful since ST elevations (usually ≥ 1 mm) recorded by it have a relatively high sensitivity and specificity for acute right ventricular ischemia/infarction in the setting of inferior wall infarction. This pattern correlates strongly with that accompanying occlusion of a dominant right coronary proximal to the first right ventricular branch.[10] However, diagnostic confusion can arise for two reasons: first, acute anteroseptal infarction may cause ST elevations in the right precordial leads, and second, pure right ventricular infarction occasionally produces ST elevations as far left as V_4 or V_5.[27,37] Inspection of the *ST segment trend* from right to left chest leads therefore may be helpful in localizing the acute infarction: the magnitude of ST elevations from V_{4R} to V_2 typically will decrease with acute right ventricular infarction but increase with anterior wall infarction; furthermore, with acute right ventricular infarction, new Q waves will not evolve in V_1 to V_5.[27]

Echocardiography may show right ventricular dysfunction and dilation, and technetium-99m-pyrophosphate scans reveal "hot spot" uptake over the area of the right ventricle.[8,13]

Right-sided heart catheterization may be helpful in confirming right ventricular dysfunction with elevated end-diastolic pressures. Of particular importance

---

*References 13, 14, 17, 18, 57.

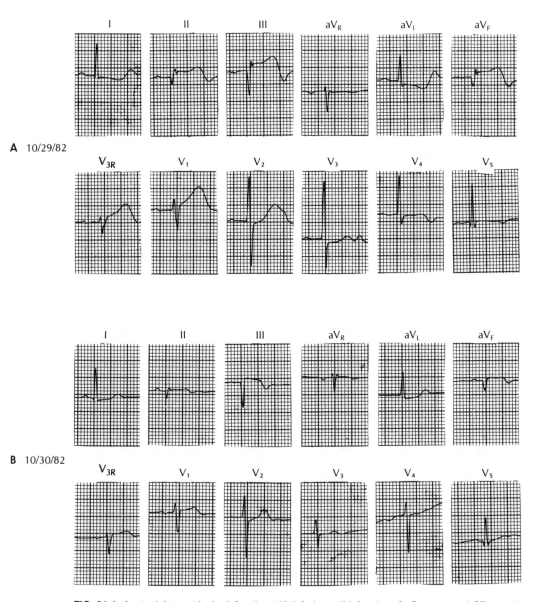

FIG. 21-1. Acute right ventricular infarction with inferior wall infarction. **A,** Q waves and ST elevations in II, III, and aV$_F$ are accompanied by ST elevations in the right precordial leads (V$_{3R}$ and V$_1$). ST-T changes in V$_5$ and V$_6$ are consistent with lateral wall ischemia. The ST depressions in I and aV$_L$ are probably reciprocal to an inferior wall current of injury. **B,** Note on the follow-up tracing the diminution of acute ST changes. The patient was hypotensive, and right-side heart catheterization showed elevated filling pressures but relatively low pulmonary capillary wedge pressure. He responded favorably to volume expansion therapy.

is the fact that the pulmonary capillary wedge pressure may be normal or low even in the presence of hypotension.[15] At other times it will be elevated as well. Acute right ventricular infarction may simulate the hemodynamic profile of constrictive pericarditis, with Kussmaul's sign (inspiratory rise in the mean right atrial pressure), equalization of left-sided and right-sided heart filling pressures, and a dip and plateau configuration to the right ventricular diastolic pressure curve.[48]

Recognition of right ventricular infarction is of major clinical importance. Volume expansion may be critical in patients who are hypotensive and have low or normal pulmonary capillary wedge pressure despite elevated systemic venous pressures. Patients with acute right ventricular infarction may also be at increased risk for the development of high-degree AV heart block[9] and for ventricular fibrillation during temporary pacing.[61]

PAPILLARY MUSCLE DYSFUNCTION OR RUPTURE

Papillary muscle dysfunction with mitral regurgitation can result from a variety of mechanisms in the setting of acute myocardial infarction. The syndrome may occur, for example, with ischemia or infarction of either the posteromedial or the anterolateral papillary muscles, with infarction of the myocardium subjacent to the papillary muscles, with marked left ventricular dilation, or with frank rupture of one of the papillary muscles.

No specific ECG pattern is associated with papillary muscle dysfunction. Burch, DePasquale, and Phillips[11] called attention to the association between ST-T changes consistent with subendocardial ischemia (Chapter 11) and clinical evidence of papillary muscle dysfunction (murmur of mitral regurgitation). However, similar ECG patterns (ST depressions and lateral T wave inversions) can occur in other settings, such as left ventricular hypertrophy or digitalis effect (p. 272). Patients with clinical evidence of papillary muscle dysfunction caused by myocardial infarction may have evidence of Q waves and ST elevations.[62]

Actual rupture of a papillary muscle is a major complication of infarction that usually leads to severe, life-threatening, acute mitral regurgitation. The ECG generally shows pathologic Q waves in either the anterior or the inferior leads, helping to localize the ruptured papillary muscle, although in some cases nonspecific ST-T changes may be the only ECG finding.[71] Rupture most commonly involves the posteromedial papillary muscle.[69,71]

Echocardiography will usually confirm evidence of a "flail" mitral valve, with severe mitral regurgitation documented during left ventriculography.

RUPTURE OF THE LEFT VENTRICULAR FREE WALL

Rupture of the left ventricular free wall, with ensuing pericardial tamponade, is an important cause of sudden death following acute myocardial infarction. It is most frequently noted during the first week or two following infarction.[7] Later rupture may also occur, particularly in the setting of ventricular "pseudoaneurysm" (discussed later).

Rupture of the left ventricle may occur with anterior or inferoposterior infarcts. Lateral wall involvement is relatively common. With occasional exceptions, the ECG shows pathologic Q waves.[7]

Clinically, acute rupture of the left ventricle causes cardiac arrest, usually with electromechanical dissociation.[7,26,53] Thus the ECG typically continues to show organized electrical activity for at least a brief time while the patient is pulseless and unconscious. Rupture of the heart is characteristically attended by abrupt slowing of the sinus rate and often the appearance of an AV junctional escape rhythm.[26,50,53] The mechanism of these bradyarrhythmias is not certain but may relate to vagal reflexes associated with pericardial tamponade.[26] Although electromechanical dissociation is a sensitive indicator of myocardial rupture, it is by no means specific and may be observed with extensive myocardial infarction without actual rupture.

Acute rupture of the heart also may be associated with new ST-T changes. In particular, London and London[44] described increased T wave positivity in patients with this complication (p. 337). However, this sign, which may be caused by local effects of potassium from hemolyzed erythrocytes, appeared in only one of six cases in another series.[26]

VENTRICULAR SEPTAL RUPTURE

Rupture of the interventricular septum has been estimated[55] to complicate as many as 1% to 3% of infarctions. In more than three quarters of the reported cases it has occurred during the first week after the infarct; and it seems to occur with about equal frequency in anterior and inferior wall infarcts. For example, in one literature review of 75 cases,[45] it complicated an anterior wall infarction in 38 patients and an inferior wall infarction in 37. Similarly, in a more recent series of 41 patients[55] the infarct was anterior in 22 cases and inferior in 19. This nearly equal representation of anterior and inferoposterior infarctions probably reflects the dual blood supply to the interventricular septum from both the anterior and the posterior circulation. However, the mortality rates are higher for patients with septal rupture and an inferoposterior wall infarction, possibly because of concomitant right ventricular dysfunction.[49,52] The ECG is highly useful in localizing the area of infarction. Pathologic Q waves were observed in 39 of the 41 patients studied by Radford et al.[55]

The diagnosis is usually made clinically on the basis of a new, usually loud, holosystolic murmur, with documentation of a significant step-up in oxygen content between the right atrium and right ventricle. Left ventriculography provides direct localization of the left-to-right shunt. Noninvasive documentation is usually possible with two-dimensional and Doppler echocardiography.

VENTRICULAR ANEURYSM

Left ventricular aneurysm, a major complication of acute myocardial infarction, may be associated with congestive heart failure, ventricular arrhythmias, and arterial thromboembolism. It is defined as a discrete, usually thinned, area of infarcted myocardium that bulges outward during systole and diastole.[3] Most such aneurysms are anterior (including anterolateral and anteroapical) in location, although inferoposterior aneurysms are occasionally seen.[33] The diagnosis may be suggested at physical examination by a rocking (dyskinetic) apical impulse. The chest radiograph occasionally shows an abnormal contour at the apex, with an actual bulge or squared-off configuration. Two-dimensional echocardiography, radionuclide radionuclide ventriculography, and left ventricular angiography may be used to diagnose a ventricular aneurysm.

The ECG may also be helpful in suggesting this complication, although the test is limited in both sensitivity and specificity. The classic ECG sign of ventricular aneurysm is persistent elevation of the ST segment (Fig. 8-5) for several weeks after an acute infarction[23,31,51,58] (p. 181). Mills et al.[51] reported that persistent ST elevation was a specific marker of "advanced ventricular asynergy," which included not just dyskinesis but severe hypokinesis and akinesis (assessed by left ventriculography). However, only 62% of the patients in their series with such wall motion abnormalities exhibited this ECG finding, comparable to the pooled sensitivities of ST elevations in detecting ventricular aneurysm based on their review of previous studies. In a subsequent two-dimensional echocardiographic study of 23 patients with persistent ST elevations after an anterior wall infarct, Arvan and Varat[3] observed dyskinetic wall motion in 22 but a frank aneurysm in only 10. Persistent elevation of the ST segments therefore does not necessarily indicate a discrete surgically resectable aneurysm.[3,42,49]

The mechanism for chronic ST elevations remains uncertain.[28,43] A persistent current of injury from viable but ischemic cells within the aneurysm has been suggested, as has mechanical stress caused by traction on the normal myocardium surrounding the aneurysm.

Latent ST elevations associated with a ventricular wall motion abnormality and sometimes a frank aneurysm may be unmasked during stress electrocardiography in patients with a prior Q wave infarct (p. 185).

Persistent ST elevations are generally seen in I, aV_L, and V_1 to V_6, reflecting the predominantly anterior location of ventricular aneurysms. Inferoposterior aneurysms are generally associated with changes in II, III, and aV_F and sometimes a tall R wave in V_1[46] (Fig. 3-11).

Another ECG sign of ventricular aneurysm has been described by El-Sherif[25]: the rSR' pattern in left surface leads. This sign consists of an rSR' or equivalent waveform with either a normal or a prolonged QRS duration in one or more of V_4 to V_7, I, aV_L, and vector lead X, or a lead recorded directly over the ventricular apex. A ventricular aneurysm was noted in 17 of 18 patients with this sign, although the sensitivity of the pattern was not studied. Presumably it

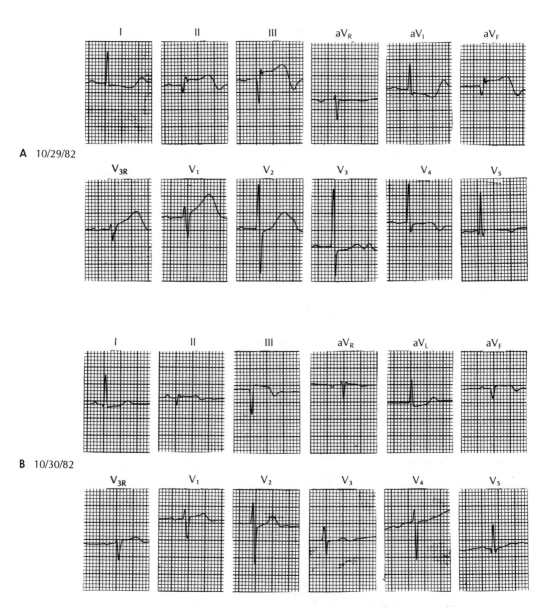

FIG. 21-2. Acute right ventricular infarction with inferior wall infarction. **A,** Q waves and ST elevations in II, III, and aV$_F$ are accompanied by ST elevations in the right precordial leads (V$_{3R}$ and V$_1$). ST-T changes in V$_5$ and V$_6$ are consistent with lateral wall ischemia. ST depressions in I and aV$_L$ are probably reciprocal to an inferior wall current of injury. **B,** Follow-up tracing. Note the diminution of acute ST changes. This patient was hypotensive, and right-side heart catheterization showed elevated filling pressures but a relatively low pulmonary capillary wedge pressure. The patient responded favorably to volume expansion.

is quite low. The mechanism of this rSR' pattern is not certain but may relate to a local conduction disturbance.

Other nonspecific ECG abnormalities can occur with ventricular aneurysm, including left axis deviation (caused by left anterior hemiblock) or right axis deviation[24] (caused by loss of apicolateral QRS forces). Marked left or right axis deviation may be associated with a prominent R wave in aV_R.[29] Ventricular tachyarrhythmias, which may be refractory to conventional therapy, also may occur.

After left ventricular aneurysmectomy the ECG sometimes shows regression of ST segment elevations and loss of pathologic Q waves.[16,30,56,68] No consistent correlation has been noted between the postoperative ECG and changes in clinical status. For example, ST elevations may persist in patients who are clinically improved, and lessening of ST elevations may be seen in patients who are either unimproved[34] or actually worse[68] after surgery.

A pattern of persistent ST elevations simulating those of ventricular aneurysm rarely arises in noncoronary settings, including cardiac sarcoidosis (p. 154), cardiac echinococcosis (p. 157), myocarditis (Fig. 6-1), and metastatic ventricular tumors (p. 155).

Ventricular aneurysm may be associated also with a persistently positive technetium-99m-pyrophosphate myocardial scintigram (Chapter 22).

In summary: Persistent ST elevations are a highly specific though only moderately sensitive sign of usually severe ventricular asynergy, but not necessarily frank aneurysm formation. A left precordial rSR' or equivalent complex may also be highly specific in detecting wall motion disorders, but it lacks sensitivity.

VENTRICULAR PSEUDOANEURYSM

A relatively rare but important complication of acute myocardial infarction is a so-called pseudoaneurysm.[33,67] Unlike a true aneurysm, in which the ventricle is scarred but intact, a pseudoaneurysm is associated with actual rupture of the wall. Although acute rupture of the free wall generally leads to pericardial tamponade and cardiac arrest (p. 361), in some cases the tear is at least temporarily sealed off by pericardium and hematoma. A "false" aneurysmal sac may then be formed.

Pseudoaneurysms are of particular importance because of their high incidence of late rupture. They may occur following either inferoposterior or anterior wall infarcts. However, about 60% involve the diaphragmatic or posterolateral aspect of the left ventricle, in contrast to true aneurysms, which generally involve the apical or anterolateral walls.[33]

The ECG generally localizes the region of the infarct. Persistent ST segment elevations, the pattern associated with true aneurysm, are sometimes but not invariably present.[67]

Clinically patients with pseudoaneurysms may have persistent pericarditis or congestive failure. A holosystolic murmur, mimicking mitral regurgitation or a ventricular septal defect, may be associated with ejection of blood through the ventricular tear.

The posteroanterior chest radiograph will often show a double density behind the cardiac silhouette, and the lateral film may show an abnormal retrocardiac density in cases of posterolateral aneurysm.[33] Ventricular angiography provides the definitive diagnosis, although noninvasive imaging with two-dimensional echocardiography and gated blood pool scans may be possible in selected cases.[2]

In summary: Pseudoaneurysm of the left ventricle is suggested by the clinical findings already mentioned, particularly in the presence of an inferoposterior infarction. Surgical therapy is generally indicated because of the high incidence of late rupture.

PERICARDITIS

Pericarditis is a common complication of acute myocardial infarction, reported in 7% to 25% of cases, with even higher estimates based on postmortem examination.[22,60,65,66] Clinically the diagnosis is most securely made in the presence of a pericardial friction rub, usually detected between 18 and 98 hours after infarction. Pericarditis that occurs within only a few hours of infarction may carry a particularly bad prognosis.[60] Pleuritic chest pain is commonly but not invariably present. Some patients will have pleuritic pain without an audible rub. Delayed postinfarction pericarditis (Dressler's syndrome) also occurs.

Postinfarction pericarditis has been reported primarily in patients with Q wave infarct patterns,[41,60] reflecting some degree of transmural infarction, but it may occur with non–Q wave infarcts as well. The occurrence of pericarditis with only ST-T changes in acute infarction probably also reflects a certain degree of transmural necrosis despite the absence of Q waves[64] (Chapter 2). In one large multicenter study[65] pericarditis (defined by a pericardial rub) was noted in 25% of patients with Q wave infarction as compared to only 9% of patients with a non–Q wave infarct ($p < 0.0001$). Pericarditis is more common with anterior than with inferoposterior infarcts.[41,60] Tofler et al.[65] reported that patients with pericarditis had significantly larger infarcts, a higher incidence of congestive heart failure and atrial tachyarrhythmias, and significantly greater mortality rates at 12-month follow-up than did patients without this complication.

The classic electrocardiographic changes of pericarditis are described in Chapter 10. Acute pericarditis is characteristically associated with diffuse ST elevations resulting from a generalized ventricular current of injury, sometimes followed by the appearance of T wave inversions. The differential diagnosis of pericarditis and acute myocardial infarction is described on p. 216.

When pericarditis complicates acute myocardial infarction, typical ECG changes of the former do not usually occur. For example, one study[60] reported diffuse ST elevations in only 6 of 38 patients with pericarditis complicating

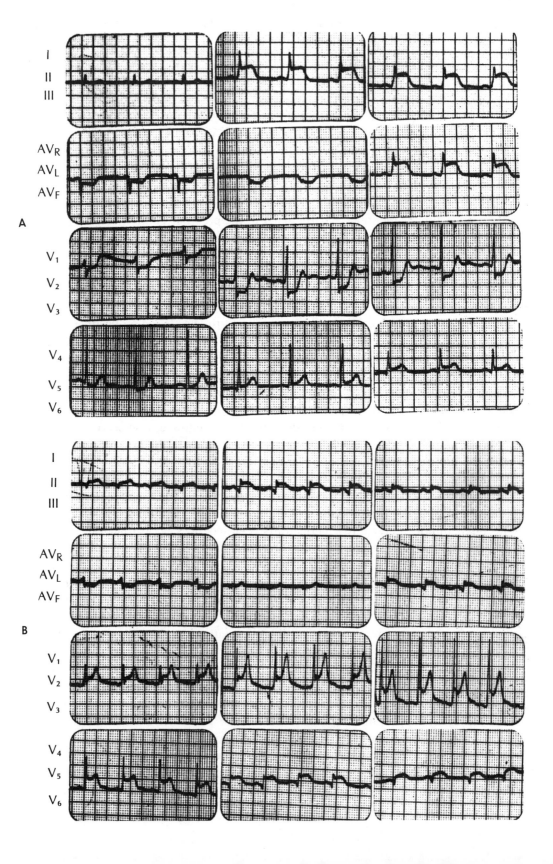

FIG. 21-3. **A,** Acute inferolateral wall infarction with ST elevations in II, III, aV_F, and V_6 and reciprocal ST depressions in V_1 to V_3. **B,** Note 72 hours later the diffuse ST elevations, consistent with a clinical diagnosis of pericarditis. Q waves in II, III, aV_F, and V_5 and V_6 and tall R waves in V_1 indicate an evolving posteroinferolateral infarct. (From Sawaya JI, et al: Am Heart J 100:144, 1980.)

acute infarction. In most cases the ECGs showed only the pattern of the evolving infarct. Less commonly diffuse ST elevations may be seen,[6] simulating the appearance of a new or extending infarct (Fig. 21-3).

Generally the ECG is an insensitive marker of the pericarditis of acute infarction.[40] This may be related to two major factors: First, pericarditis associated with infarction is often localized to the area overlying the infarct; more global inflammation occurs less commonly. Second, the repolarization changes of pericarditis may be masked by changes of greater magnitude associated with infarction.

ECG changes consistent with pericarditis also have been described in Dressler's syndrome,[21] the apparently delayed type of inflammatory reaction sometimes seen weeks to months following an acute infarction. Dressler's syndrome may represent a continuation of the pericarditis associated with acute infarction rather than a separate syndrome with a delayed onset.[39]

ARTERIAL AND VENOUS THROMBOEMBOLIC DISEASE

Mural thrombus formation at the site of myocardial infarction is an important complication because of the risk of arterial embolization. Mural thrombi are most common after acute anterior wall infarcts,[4,32] although they have been reported with inferoposterior infarcts as well.[5] In one series of patients studied with two-dimensional echocardiography,[4] mural thrombi were noted in 12 of 35 patients with an anterior wall infarct but in none of 35 patients with an inferior infarct. Among the patients with anterior wall infarction, mural thrombi are most often seen in association with more severe wall motion abnormalities (akinesis or dyskinesis) and larger infarcts.[4,63] However, Asinger et al.[4] reported that neither the extent or location of Q waves nor the degree of persistent ST elevations 3 days after an anterior infarction were predictive of mural thrombus formation.

Myocardial infarction is also a risk factor for pulmonary thromboembolism secondary to venous stasis or (occasionally) right ventricular mural thrombi. (The ECG patterns associated with pulmonary embolism are discussed in Chapter 4.) The ECG, as noted, lacks both sensitivity and specificity in this condition. Acute right ventricular strain may produce new right precordial T wave inversions or Q waves in III and aV_F that are misinterpreted as signs of a new or extending myocardial infarct (Fig. 4-3).

REFERENCES

1. Abbott JA, Scheinman MM: Nondiagnostic electrocardiogram in patients with acute myocardial infarction: clinical and angiographic correlations, Am J Med 55:608, 1973.
2. Alter BR, et al: Noninvasive diagnosis of left ventricular pseudoaneurysm by radioangiography and echography, Am Heart J 101:236, 1981.
3. Arvan S, Varat M: Persistent ST-segment elevation and left ventricular wall motion abnormalities: a two-dimensional echocardiographic study, Am J Cardiol 53:1542, 1984.
4. Asinger RW, et al: Incidence of left ventricular thrombosis after acute transmural myocardial infarction: serial evaluation by two-dimensional echocardiography, N Engl J Med 305:298, 1981.
5. Asinger RW, et al: Observations on detecting left ventricular thrombus with two-dimensional echocardiography: emphasis on avoidance of false positive diagnoses, Am J Cardiol 47:145, 1981.
6. Barnes A: Electrocardiographic pattern observed following acute coronary occlusion complicated by pericarditis, Am Heart J 9:734, 1934.
7. Bates RJ, et al: Cardiac rupture—challenge in diagnosis and management, Am J Cardiol 40:429, 1977.
8. Bellamy GR, et al: Value of two-dimensional echocardiographic, electrocardiographic, and clinical signs in detecting right ventricular infarction, Am Heart J 112:304, 1986.
9. Braat SH, et al: Right ventricular involvement with acute inferior wall myocardial infarction identifies high risk of developing atrioventricular conduction disturbances, Am Heart J 107:1183, 1984.
10. Braat SH, et al: Value of lead V4R for recognition of the infarct coronary artery in acute inferior myocardial infarction, Am J Cardiol 53:1538, 1984.
11. Burch GE, et al: The syndrome of papillary muscle dysfunction, Am Heart J 75:399, 1968.
12. Cabin HS, et al: Right ventricular myocardial infarction with anterior wall left ventricular infarction: an autopsy study, Am Heart J 113:16, 1987.
13. Candell-Riera J, et al: Right ventricular infarction: relationships between ST segment elevation in V_{4R} and hemodynamic, scintigraphic, and echocardiographic findings in patients with acute inferior myocardial infarction, Am Heart J 101:281, 1981.
14. Chou TC, et al: Electrocardiographic diagnosis of right ventricular infarction, Am J Med 70:1175, 1981.
15. Cohn JN, et al: Right ventricular infarction: clinical and hemodynamic features, Am J Cardiol 33:209, 1974.
16. Cokkinos DV, et al: Left ventricular aneurysm: analyses of electrocardiographic features and post resection changes, Am Heart J 82:149, 1971.
17. Coma-Canella I, et al: Electrocardiographic alterations in leads V1 to V3 in the diagnosis of right and left ventricular infarction, Am Heart J 112:940, 1986.
18. Croft CH, et al: Detection of acute right ventricular infarction by right precordial electrocardiography, Am J Cardiol 50:421, 1982.
19. Dell'Italia LJ, et al: Physical examination for exclusion of hemodynamically important right ventricular infarction, Ann Intern Med 99:608, 1983.
20. deMarchena EJ, et al: Angiographically demonstrated isolated acute right ventricular infarction presenting as ST elevation in leads V1-V3, Am Heart J 113:391, 1987.
21. Dressler W: The post-myocardial infarction syndrome, Arch Intern Med 102:28, 1959.
22. Dubois C, et al: Frequency and significance of pericardial friction rubs in the acute phase of myocardial infarction, Eur J Cardiol 6:766, 1986.
23. Dubnow MH, et al: Postinfarction ventricular aneurysm: a clinico-morphologic and electrocardiographic study of 80 cases, Am Heart J 70:753, 1965.
24. Eliaser M Jr, Konigsberg J: Electrocardiographic findings in cases of ventricular aneurysm, Arch Intern Med 64:493, 1939.
25. El-Sherif N: The rsR' pattern in left surface leads in ventricular aneurysm, Br Heart J 32:440, 1970.
26. Friedman HS, et al: Clinical and electrocardiographic features of cardiac rupture following acute myocardial infarction, Am J Med 50:709, 1971.
27. Geft IL, et al: ST elevations in leads V1-V5 may be caused by right coronary artery occlusion and acute right ventricular infarction, Am J Cardiol 53:991, 1984.
28. Gewirtz H, et al: Mechanism of persistent ST segment elevation after anterior myocar-

dial infarction, Am J Cardiol 44:1269, 1979.

29. Goldberger E, Schwartz SP: Electrocardiographic patterns of ventricular aneurysm, Am J Med 4:243, 1948.

30. Gooch AS, et al: Persistent ST segment elevation in left ventricular aneurysm before and after surgery, Am Heart J 98:11, 1979.

31. Gorlin R, et al: Prospective correlative study of ventricular aneurysm: mechanistic concept and clinical recognition, Am J Med 42:512, 1967.

32. Gueret P et al: Effects of full-dose heparin anticoagulation on the development of left ventricular thrombosis in acute transmural myocardial infarction, J Am Coll Cardiol 8:419, 1986.

33. Higgins CB, et al: False aneurysms of the left ventricle, Radiology 127:21, 1978.

34. Hutter AM Jr, et al: Nontransmural myocardial infarction: comparison of hospital and late clinical course of patients with that of matched patients with transmural anterior and transmural inferior myocardial infarction, Am J Cardiol 48:595, 1981.

35. Ideker RE, et al: Evaluation of a QRS scoring system for estimating myocardial infarct size. II. Correlation with quantitative anatomic findings for anterior infarcts, Am J Cardiol 49:1605, 1982.

36. Isner JM, Roberts WC: Right ventricular infarction complicating left ventricular infarction secondary to coronary artery disease, Am J Cardiol 42:885, 1978.

37. Kataoka H, et al: Massive ST-segment elevation in precordial and inferior leads in right ventricular myocardial infarction, J Electrocardiol 21:115, 1988.

38. Klein HO, et al: The early recognition of right ventricular infarction: diagnostic accuracy of the electrocardiographic V_{4R} lead, Circulation 67:558, 1983.

39. Kossowsky WA, et al: Reappraisal of the post myocardial Dressler's syndrome, Am Heart J 102:954, 1981.

40. Langendorf R: The effect of diffuse pericarditis on the electrocardiographic pattern of recent myocardial infarction, Am Heart J 22:86, 1941.

41. Lichstein E, et al: Pericarditis complicating acute myocardial infarction: incidence of complications and significance of electrocardiogram on admission, Am Heart J 87:246, Am Heart J 87:246, 1974.

42. Lindsay J Jr, et al: Relation of ST-segment elevation after healing of acute myocardial

infarction to the presence of left ventricular aneurysm, Am J Cardiol 54:84, 1984.

43. Lindsay J Jr, et al: Significance of persistent ST-elevation after healing of anterior wall acute myocardial infarction, Am J Cardiol 63:1404, 1989.

44. London RE, London SB: The electrocardiographic sign of acute hemopericardium, Circulation 25:780, 1962.

45. Longo EA, Cohen LS: Rupture of interventricular septum in acute myocardial infarction, Am Heart J 92:81, 1976.

46. Loop FD, et al: Posterior ventricular aneurysms: etiologic factors and results of surgical treatment, N Engl J Med 288:237, 1973.

47. Lopez-Sendon J, et al: Electrocardiographic findings in acute right ventricular infarction: sensitivity and specificity of alterations in right precordial leads V4R, V3R, V1, V2, and V3, J Am Coll Cardiol 6:1273, 1985.

48. Lorell B, et al: Right ventricular infarction: clinical diagnosis and differentiation from cardiac tamponade and pericardial constriction, Am J Cardiol 43:465, 1979.

49. Mann JM, Roberts WC: Acquired ventricular septal defect during acute myocardial infarction: analysis of 38 unoperated necropsy patients and comparison with 50 unoperated necropsy patients without rupture, Am J Cardiol 62:8, 1988.

50. Meurs AAH, et al: Electrocardiogram during cardiac rupture by myocardial infarction, Br Heart J 32:232, 1970.

51. Mills RM, et al: Natural history of S-T segment elevation after acute myocardial infarction, Am J Cardiol 35:609, 1975.

52. Moore CA, et al: Postinfarction ventricular septal rupture: the importance of location of infarction and right ventricular function in determining survival, Circulation 74:45, 1986.

53. Morgensen L, et al: Studies of myocardial rupture with tamponade in acute myocardial infarction. II. Electrocardiographic changes, Chest 61:6, 1972.

54. Palmeri ST, et al: A QRS scoring system for assessing left ventricular function after myocardial infarction, N Engl J Med 306:4, 1982.

55. Radford MJ, et al: Ventricular septal rupture: a review of clinical and physiologic features and an analysis of survival, Circulation 64:545, 1981.

56. Richter S, et al: Functional significance of electrocardiographic changes after left ven-

tricular aneurysmectomy, J Electrocardiol 11:247, 1978.

57. Robalino BD, et al: Electrocardiographic manifestations of right ventricular infarction, Am Heart J 118:138, 1989.

58. Rosenberg B, Messinger WJ: The electrocardiogram in ventricular aneurysm, Am Heart J 37:267, 1949.

59. Sadaniantz A, et al: Relationship of persistent S-T segment elevation and left ventricular wall motion abnormalities, Am J Noninvas Cardiol 3:105, 1989.

60. Sawaya JI, et al: Early diagnosis of pericarditis in acute myocardial infarction, Am Heart J 100:144, 1980.

61. Sclarovsky S, et al: Ventricular fibrillation complicating temporary pacing in acute myocardial infarction: significance of right ventricular infarction, Am J Cardiol 48:1160, 1981.

62. Shelburne JC, et al: A reappraisal of papillary muscle dysfunction: correlative clinical and angiographic study, Am J Med 46:862, 1969.

63. Spirito P, et al: Prognostic significance and natural history of left ventricular thrombosis in patients with acute anterior myocardial infarction: a two-dimensional echocardiographic study, Circulation 72:774, 1985.

64. Spodick DH: Q-wave infarction versus S-T infarction: nonspecificity of electrocardiographic criteria for differentiating transmural and nontransmural lesions, Am J Cardiol 51:913, 1983.

65. Tofler GH, et al: Pericarditis in acute myocardial infarction: characterization and clinical significance, Am Heart J 117:86, 1989.

66. Toole JC, Silverman ME: Pericarditis of acute myocardial infarction, Chest 67:647, 1975.

67. Van Tassel RA, Edwards JE: Rupture of the heart complicating myocardial infarction: analysis of 40 cases including nine examples of left ventricular false aneurysm, Chest 61:104, 1972.

68. Vasilomanolakis EC, et al: The effect of left ventricular aneurysmectomy on the electrocardiogram: a study of 77 patients and review of the literature, J Electrocardiol 15:173, 1982.

69. Vlodaver Z, Edwards JE: Rupture of ventricular septum or papillary muscle complicating myocardial infarction, Circulation 55:815, 1977.

70. Wagner GS: Clinical usefulness of quantitative ECG methods for evaluating ischemic and infarcted myocardium, Cardiol Clin 5:447, 1987.

71. Wei JY, et al: Papillary muscle rupture in fatal acute myocardial infarction: a potentially treatable form of cardiogenic shock, Ann Intern Med 90:149, 1979.

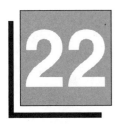

Epilogue: electrocardiography in the differential diagnosis of myocardial infarction, an integrated approach

This book has been devoted to the electrocardiographic differential diagnosis of myocardial infarction. Yet the ECG is only one of several noninvasive aids used in the assessment of ischemic heart disease. In evaluating patients with possible acute myocardial infarction the clinician must rely most on the history and serum cardiac enzymes in addition to the ECG. Echocardiography and radionuclide imaging may be particularly useful in selected cases.

PATIENT HISTORY

The diagnostic uses and limitations of the ECG in the setting of myocardial infarction have been described in detail. It is also important to recognize that the same problems of limited sensitivity and specificity apply to other tests routinely used in diagnosing acute infarction. For example, reliance on patient history may lead to underdiagnosis or overdiagnosis. At one extreme the history may be completely insensitive, as in the case of "silent" myocardial infarction.[6] It is not uncommon to encounter a patient with electrocardiographic or angiographic evidence of prior infarction who does not give any diagnostic history. In other cases the patient may complain of dyspnea caused by pulmonary edema, without actual chest pain. The history may also lack specificity. Severe chest pain always raises the specter of myocardial infarction, but identical symptoms can occur in a variety of other cardiac and noncardiac problems (e.g., pulmonary embolism, aortic dissection, and acute cholecystitis).[9]

The patient history may be particularly useful in timing the onset and duration of ischemia. The ECG by itself is not a precise temporal marker of infarction. Q waves can appear within mintues, hours, or days. Although suggestive of acute infarction, ST segment elevations may occur with noninfarctional ischemia (Prinzmetal's angina) and persist for weeks or longer after an actual infarction in the presence of underlying left ventricular asynergy. Similarly T wave inversions, although associated with the subacute or chronic phase of infarction, may appear within minutes or days and persist indefinitely. The only ECG pattern virtually specific for acute infarction is the combination of Q waves with a "monophasic" current of injury (ST elevations so marked that the end of the QRS and beginning of the ST segment are not separable), as seen in Figs. 2-1, 8-1, and 18-2.

CARDIAC ENZYMES

The other test of particular help in dating the onset of infarction is analysis of serum "cardiac" enzymes.[8,13,14] The most useful enzymes are creatine kinase (CK) and lactate dehydrogenase (LDH). Cardiac enzyme analysis and electrocardiography are the two most important laboratory tests for diagnosing acute infarction; they should be employed in a complementary way, with careful regard for their diagnostic limitations and uses.

The sensitivity of cardiac enzymes is a function of two key variables: the size and timing of the infarct. The peak enzyme levels correlate in a general way with the amount of myocardium infarcted.[6] The timing of infarction is also of critical importance.

For example, CK levels may not begin to rise for several hours after the onset of acute infarction despite acute ECG changes and chest pain. They then peak and return to normal, usually within 96 hours. Stated another way, the diagnostic sensitivity of creatine kinase is low very early and also several days after an acute infarction. Thus a normal CK level as measured by conventional electrophoretic techniques cannot be used to exclude infarction in the acute emergency evaluation of chest pain.

The LDH has an even longer course following infarction; it may not begin to rise for 6 to 10 hours but may stay elevated 1 to 2 weeks. Thus LDH can provide increased sensitivity in detecting a relatively recent infarction when the ECG no longer shows acute changes and the CK level has returned to normal.

The specificity of cardiac enzyme analyses is relatively high when isoenzyme determinations are performed. Although CK is found in many different tissues, the MB (myocardial band or fraction) is highly specific for heart muscle.[15] Elevation of the MB (whose exact value depends on the assay and the laboratory) is therefore strongly suggestive of myocardial infarction. However, an elevated MB in the absence of acute myocardial infarction occasionally has been reported in a number of other conditions (summarized in Table 22-1). Some of these (myocarditis [p. 216], myocardial trauma [p. 135], muscular dystrophy [p. 143], hypothermia [p. 230], and subarachnoid hemorrhage [p. 300], as well as certain athletics) may also be associated with pseudoinfarct ECG patterns. Elevation of the CK-MB is not characteristic of pulmonary embolus or pericarditis,[13*] two important conditions whose electrocardiographic patterns can simulate those of acute infarction.

It is important to recognize that the time course of the MB may differ from that of the total CK level following acute infarction: the MB tends to return to normal more rapidly. Thus a negative CK-MB in a patient with an elevated total creatine kinase also does not exclude the possibility of recent infarction.

Isoenzyme analysis may enhance the diagnostic specificity of LDH, a relatively ubiquitous enzyme. There are five LDH isoenzymes. Normally LDH_2 exceeds LDH_1.[14] Acute

---

*An elevated CK-MB in a patient with apparent pericarditis strongly suggests concurrent myocarditis (p. 216) or myocardial infarction.

TABLE 22-1. Causes of an elevated CK-MB

Specific factors	Comments
False elevations	
Spillover of CK-MM	Prevented by diluting sample
Isoenzyme variants	Detected by electrophoresis
Nonspecific fluorescence	Uncommon problem of qualitative electrophoresis assay
Myocardial damage	
Myocardial infarction	Total CK may be normal
*Myocarditis (or myopericarditis)	Occasional finding
*Myocardial puncture or trauma	Including intracardiac injections, cardiac surgery
Systemic disease with cardiac involvement	
*Muscular dystrophy	Peripheral CK-MB also found
*Hypothermia	Probably reflects myocardial damage
Hyperthermia	Associated with anesthesia
Reye's syndrome	Rare reports
Peripheral source of CK-MB	
Myositis	May have cardiac involvement
Rhabdomyolysis	Reflects abnormal regeneration
*Certain athletics	Examples: marathon runners, football players
Prostate surgery	Prostatic source
Cesarean section	Uterine source
Gastrointestinal surgery	Gastrointestinal source
Miscellaneous	
Renal failure	Source unknown
*Subarachnoid hemorrhage	May reflect myocardial damage
Hypothyroidism	Decreased clearance

*May also be associated with electrocardiographic pseudoinfarct patterns.
Modified from Lee TH, Goldman L: In Sox HC Jr (editor): Common diagnostic tests: uses and interpretation, ed 2, Philadelphia, 1990, American College of Physicians.

myocardial infarction causes a reversal of this ratio ("LDH flip"). Although helpful, the same type of LDH isoenzyme profile has been reported with hemolysis and certain types of renal injury (e.g., renal infarction).[16]

RADIONUCLIDE IMAGING

Radionuclide imaging of the heart may be valuable in diagnosing an equivocal infarction and estimating its size. Two radiopharmaceutical agents have been employed primarily for this purpose: technetium-99m-pyrophosphate (which accumulates in the infarcted myocardium) and thallium-201 (which is excluded from zones of ischemia or infarction).[5] However, the sensitivity and specificity of imaging acute infarcts with these agents are limited.

For example, the *sensitivity* of technetium-99m-pyrophosphate scans is reduced when they are performed within a few hours of an infarction: they are negative at first and become negative again after 7 to 10 days. Thus, as with cardiac enzymes, scans performed outside a relatively narrow time frame may be misleadingly normal. This false negativity is common with small and non–Q wave infarcts,[11] precisely the settings in which other tests also may yield equivocal results.

The *specificity* of technetium-99m-pyrophosphate scans is limited; among the causes of positive scintigrams are several noncoronary conditions (dilated cardiomyopathy, myocardial contusion, myocardial tumor, DC cardioversion, cardiac amyloidosis) that are associated with pseudoinfarct patterns. The major conditions with positive[99mTc] myocardial scans that have been reported include

Acute myocardial infarction
Unstable angina pectoris[1]*
Chronic myocardial infarction[12]
Left ventricular aneurysm[12]
Dilated (congestive) cardiomyopathy[1]
Myocardial contusion (p. 135)
Myocardial tumor (p. 155)
Calcified heart valves[10]
DC cardioversion[1]
Cardiac amyloidosis[17] (see also p. 141)

Because of these limitations in sensitivity and specificity, the current clinical use of technetium-99m-pyrophosphate scanning is very restricted. The test may be helpful for confirming the presence of acute infarction with borderline enzyme changes or an equivocal ECG. These scans may also be helpful in localizing the site and relative extent of acute infarction in patients whose ECGs show left bundle branch block, pacemaker patterns, or the Wolff-Parkinson-White type of preexcitation, all of which generally mask acute ischemic changes (Chapter 5).

Radionuclide imaging of infarcts also may be performed with thallium-201, a potassium analogue. In contrast to technetium-99m-pyrophosphate, which accumulates in the infarcted myocardium, thallium distribution is dependent on blood flow and therefore will be diminished or absent in ischemic or infarcted zones.[5] Myocardial infarction thus results in an area of decreased radionuclide uptake with thallium (a "cold spot"), as opposed to the "hot spot" seen with technetium-99m-pyrophosphate scintigraphy.

However, the *sensitivity* of thallium-201 scanning for diagnosing myocardial infarction has important limitations. In one series,[16] the sensitivity of the test in detecting acute infarction, confirmed by diagnostic ECG and enzyme changes, was only 82%. The sensitivity appears highest within the first 6 hours of infarction (in contrast to [99mTc] imaging and CK analysis) and decreases after 24 to 48 hours. The specificity of thallium-201 scanning for acute infarction is limited because decreased uptake occurs transiently with reversible ischemia, or may persist after the acute phase of the infarct.

The uses and limitations of thallium-201 scintigraphy with *exercise testing* are discussed in Chapters 13 and 20.

---

*Some of these cases likely include recent or prior infarcts.

ECHOCARDIOGRAPHY

Echocardiography may play an important role in the differential diagnosis of infarction.[3] Demonstration of regional ventricular wall motion disorders is consistent with but not diagnostic of ischemic damage. Cross-sectional (two-dimensional) studies may be particularly helpful in confirming the complications of myocardial infarction discussed in Chapter 21, including left ventricular thrombi, true and false aneurysms, flail mitral valve caused by papillary muscle infarction, and sometimes ventricular septal defect. In addition, dilation of the right ventricle may be seen with right ventricular infarction, and in some cases pericardial effusion may accompany the pericarditis of infarction.

Echocardiography also may be very useful in recognizing many of the multiple simulators of infarction that have been discussed. The major causes of pseudoinfarct patterns that can be diagnosed with or suggested by echocardiography are as follows:

Complete corrected transposition of the great vessels (Chapter 3)
Right ventricular hypertrophy (Chapter 4)
Acute cor pulmonale due to pulmonary embolism (Chapter 4)
Arrhythmogenic right ventricular dysplasia (Chapter 4)
Left ventricular hypertrophy (Chapter 4)
Hypertrophic cardiomyopathy (Chapter 4)
Cardiac amyloidosis (Chapter 7)
Acute myocarditis (Chapter 6)
Cardiac echinococcosis (Chapter 7)
Chronic constrictive pericarditis[15] (Chapter 7)
Dilated (congestive) cardiomyopathy (Chapter 7)
Intramyocardial tumors (Chapter 7)
Mitral valve prolapse (Chapter 17)

Use of the echocardiogram in differentiating some of the common causes of a tall R wave in V_1,[7] including normal variants, posterior infarction, right ventricular hypertrophy, and hypertrophic cardiomyopathy, is discussed on pp. 53, 72, and 83.

INTEGRATED APPROACH TO THE DIAGNOSIS OF INFARCTION: CONCLUSIONS

The purpose of this brief concluding chapter has been to outline the ways that other key tests complement the electrocardiographic diagnosis of infarction. In some cases additional tests will help secure the diagnosis. In others a noninvasive test such as the echocardiogram will be needed to confirm the suspicion of a condition associated with a pseudoinfarct pattern (e.g., hypertrophic cardiomyopathy). Careful recognition of both the limitations and the applications of these tests is essential. The electrocardiogram, like all other diagnostic tests, should be viewed therefore not simply as an isolated end point in clinical diagnosis but as an integral and dynamic aid in patient care.

REFERENCES

1. Ahmad M, et al: Limited clinical diagnostic specificity of technetium-99m stannous pyrophosphate myocardial imaging in acute myocardial infarction, Am J Cardiol 39:50, 1977.
2. Dunn RF, et al: Comparison of thallium-201 scanning in idiopathic dilated cardiomyopathy and severe coronary artery disease, Circulation 68:804, 1982.
3. Feigenbaum H: Echocardiography, ed 4, Philadelphia, 1986, Lea & Febiger.
4. Goldberger AL, O'Konski MS: Utility of the routine electrocardiogram before surgery and on general hospital admission. Critical review and new guidelines. In Sox HC Jr (editor): Common diagnostic tests: uses and interpretation, ed 2, Philadelphia, 1990, American College of Physicians, p 67.
5. Holman LB: Nuclear cardiology. In Braunwald EB (editor): Heart disease: a textbook of cardiovascular medicine, ed 3, Philadelphia, 1988, WB Saunders Co, p 311.
6. Kannel WB, Abbott RD: Incidence and prognosis of unrecognized infarction: an update on the Framingham study, N Engl J Med 311:1144, 1984.
7. Kramer NE, et al: Differentiation of posterior myocardial infarction from right ventricular hypertrophy and normal anterior loop by echocardiography, Circulation 58:1057, 1978.
8. Lee TH, Goldman L: Serum enzyme assays in the diagnosis of acute myocardial infarction: recommendations based on a quantitative analysis. In Sox HC Jr (editor): Common diagnostic tests: uses and interpreta-tion, ed 2, Philadelphia, 1990, American College of Physicians, p 35.
9. Levine HJ: Difficult problems in the diagnosis of chest pain, Am Heart J 100:108, 1980.
10. Marcus ML, Kerber RE: Present status of the 99m technetium pyrophosphate infarct scintigram, Circulation 56:335, 1977.
11. Massie B, et al: Myocardial scintigraphy with technetium-99m stannous pyrophosphate: an insensitive test for nontransmural myocardial infarction, Am J Cardiol 43:186, 1979.
12. Olson HG, et al: Prognostic value of a persistently positive technetium-99m stannous pyrophosphate myocardial scintigram after myocardial infarction, Am J Cardiol 43:889, 1979.
13. Roberts R, Sobel BE: Creatine kinase isoenzymes in the assessment of heart disease, Am Heart J 95:521, 1978.
14. Vasudevan G, et al: Lactic dehydrogenase isoenzyme determination in the diagnosis of acute myocardial infarction, Circulation 57:1055, 1978.
15. Voelkel AG, et al: Echocardiographic features of constrictive pericarditis, Circulation 58:871, 1978.
16. Wackers FJ, et al: Value and limitations of thallium-201 scintigraphy in the acute phase of myocardial infarction, N Engl J Med 295:1, 1976.
17. Wizenberg TA, et al: Value of positive myocardial technetium-99m pyrophosphate scintigraphy in the noninvasive diagnosis of cardiac amyloidosis, Am Heart J 103:468, 1982.

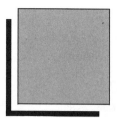

Index